OXFORD MEDICAL PUBLICATIONS

End of Life Care in the ICU

Oxford Specialist handbooks published and forthcoming

General Oxford Specialist Handbooks
A Resuscitation Room Guide
Addiction Medicine
Perioperative Medicine, Second Edition
Post-Operative Complications, second edition

Oxford Specialist Handbooks in Anaesthesia
Cardiac Anaesthesia
General Thoracic Anaesthesia
Neuroanaesthesia
Obstetric Anaesthesia
Paediatric Anaesthesia
Regional Anaesthesia, Stimulation and Ultrasound Techniques

Oxford Specialist Handbooks in Cardiology
Adult Congenital Heart Disease
Cardiac Catheterization and Coronary Intervention
Echocardiography
Fetal Cardiology
Heart Failure
Hypertension
Nuclear Cardiology
Pacemakers and ICDs

Oxford Specialist Handbooks in Critical Care
Advanced Respiratory Critical Care

Oxford Specialist Handbooks in End of Life Care
End of Life Care in Cardiology
End of Life Care in Dementia
End of Life Care in Nephrology
End of Life Care in Respiratory Disease
End of Life Care in the Intensive Care Unit

Oxford Specialist Handbooks in Neurology
Epilepsy
Parkinson's Disease and Other Movement Disorders
Stroke Medicine

Oxford Specialist Handbooks in Paediatrics
Paediatric Endocrinology and Diabetes
Paediatric Dermatology
Paediatric Gastroenterology, Hepatology, and Nutrition
Paediatric Haematology and Oncology
Paediatric Nephrology
Paediatric Neurology
Paediatric Radiology
Paediatric Respiratory Medicine

Oxford Specialist Handbooks in Psychiatry
Child and Adolescent Psychiatry
Old Age Psychiatry

Oxford Specialist Handbooks in Radiology
Interventional Radiology
Musculoskeletal Imaging

Oxford Specialist Handbooks in Surgery
Cardiothoracic Surgery
Hand Surgery
Hepato-pancreatobiliary Surgery
Oral Maxillo Facial Surgery
Neurosurgery
Operative Surgery, Second Edition
Otolaryngology and Head and Neck Surgery
Plastic and Reconstructive Surgery
Surgical Oncology
Urological Surgery
Vascular Surgery

End of Life Care in the ICU
From advanced disease to bereavement

Edited by

Graeme Rocker

Department of Medicine (Division of Respirology)
Dalhousie University, Halifax
Canada

Kathleen A Puntillo

Department of Physiological Nursing
University of California, San Francisco
USA

Élie Azoulay

Director Assistant of the Medical-ICU
Saint Louis Hospital, Paris
France

Judith E Nelson

Division of Pulmonary, Critical Care, and Sleep Medicine,
Hertzberg Palliative Care Institute,
Mount Sinai School of Medicine, New York
USA

Series editor

Max Watson

Consultant in Palliative Medicine
Northern Ireland Hospice, Belfast
UK, and
Honorary Consultant
The Princess Alice Hospice, Esher
UK

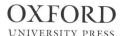

OXFORD
UNIVERSITY PRESS

OXFORD
UNIVERSITY PRESS

Great Clarendon Street, Oxford OX2 6DP

Oxford University Press is a department of the University of Oxford.
It furthers the University's objective of excellence in research, scholarship,
and education by publishing worldwide in

Oxford New York

Auckland Cape Town Dar es Salaam Hong Kong Karachi
Kuala Lumpur Madrid Melbourne Mexico City Nairobi
New Delhi Shanghai Taipei Toronto

With offices in

Argentina Austria Brazil Chile Czech Republic France Greece
Guatemala Hungary Italy Japan Poland Portugal Singapore
South Korea Switzerland Thailand Turkey Ukraine Vietnam

Oxford is a registered trade mark of Oxford University Press
in the UK and in certain other countries

Published in the United States
by Oxford University Press Inc., New York

© Oxford University Press, 2010

British Library Cataloguing in Publication Data
Data available

Library of Congress Cataloging-in-Publication Data
Data available 1006039716

Typeset by Cepha Imaging Private Ltd., Bangalore, India
Printed in China
on acid-free paper through
Asia Pacific Offset Ltd

ISBN 978–0–19–923924–5

10 9 8 7 6 5 4 3 2 1

Oxford University Press makes no representation, express or implied, that the drug dosages in
this book are correct. Readers must therefore always check the product information and clinical
procedures with the most up to date published product information and data sheets provided by
the manufacturers and the most recent codes of conduct and safety regulations. The authors and
publishers do not accept responsibility or legal liability for any errors in the text or for the misuse
or misapplication of material in this work.

Some of the medication discussed in this book may not be available through normal channels
and only available by special arrangements. Other examples used in research studies and recommended in international guidelines are unlicensed or may be subject to being used outside of their
licensed dosage ranges within the UK. We suggest consulting the BNF and local prescribing guide-
lines/protocols before using unfamiliar medication.

Foreword

The rates of Intensive Care Unit (ICU) utilisation at the end of life increase significantly with age and with the number of co-existing chronic illnesses, at least in developed societies. Indeed, despite concern over the appropriateness and quality of care provided in ICU's at the end of life, analyses suggest that nearly 40% of deaths in the USA occur in hospital and some 22% following ICU admission. The age-specific rates of ICU usage at the end of life is highest for infants (43%) and falls to around 14% for patients aged over 85 years.

The implications of such figures are several. Firstly, knowledge of the extent of critical care resources, at least in developed countries, would seem to be vital to guide policy decisions. Secondly, the way in which these resources are employed should be the subject of informed debate, particularly with regard to their allocation in response to the many demands placed upon them.

This book concerning end-of-life care as applied in the critical care setting, edited by Graeme Rocker and colleagues with contributions from leaders in the medical, nursing and allied health professions, provides an international perspective which is therefore both timely and likely to prove of significant value to a wide audience. The chapters employ a variety of styles, ranging from the (necessarily) factual and informative (e.g. concerning legal issues and conflict resolution), to that based upon personal experience. Whilst the latter may not attract the attention of the scientific community focussed upon evidence-based research, in the circumstances within which intensive care professionals practise end-of-life care, recollection and experience are all-important. Secondly, the contributions are inclusive, and range from pharmacological reviews (relating to the application of symptomatic relief) to the spiritual and ethical. Thirdly, the need for effective research and the means by which this can be accomplished in what is by definition a disparate group of patients managed (one hopes) in an individualistic and patient-centred manner, is particularly welcome. Fourthly, a disease-specific approach accommodates the clinical relevance of underlying conditions (e.g. malignancy); and the use of other patient groupings (e.g. by age) recognises the complexity of practice in this arena. Finally, sections dealing with conflict resolution, the development of clinical ethics committees and the significance of euthanasia, are particularly valuable.

As one practising in a healthcare environment where intensive care resources are, as a percentage of overall healthcare expenditure, significantly constrained compared to other developed societies, my hope is that this book will be widely available not only within the critical care community, but also for consultation by those practising in lower dependency areas. The wealth of knowledge that it contains is a reflection of advances not only in technical knowledge but also of the importance of the clinician experience in an environment that should be focussed on patient care. This clinician wishes this volume had been available to him when he started in critical care practice twenty years ago.

Timothy W. Evans

Preface

The ideas that culminated in the publication of this handbook began with Becky, a woman who lived and died at the age of 21 with cystic fibrosis. Becky's experience in the intensive care unit (ICU) during her last year of life had profound and lasting effects on many and in the end, her death was a release for her, for those who loved her, and also a release, in a different way, for the ICU team.

Becky's long and final illness illustrated many of the special and important issues that underpin the provision of quality palliative care in the ICU for patients and their families. Death is a frequent event in ICUs around the world though we cannot predict with sufficient accuracy for whom or when death will occur. Palliative care should be part of the comprehensive treatment plan for all patients in critical care units and their families, and we need to educate ourselves in this essential body of knowledge and skill. We recognize that the terms 'palliative care' and 'end-of-life care' may be interpreted in different ways in different settings and while we wish to promote the concept of quality palliation at any stage of an ICU illness, we accept the variable use of these terms throughout this book.

In the past decade, the science of ICU palliative care has advanced rapidly on many fronts. This handbook is intended to provide a convenient reference source for busy ICU practitioners. Our contributors include experts from four continents, who bring differing, yet complementary, perspectives on palliative care in the ICU. Sometimes, they write on the same or on a similar topic, but we feel that their unique perspectives promote a greater understanding of world views on palliative and end-of-life care.

We hope that these diverse contributions and reflections will resonate with ICU clinicians, and stimulate and support efforts to ensure the provision of quality palliative care in all ICUs

Graeme Rocker

Contents

Detailed contents ix
Contributors xv
Symbols and abbreviations xxiii

1	Introduction	1
2	Improving palliative and end-of-life care	41
3	Symptom control	51
4	Caring for families in the ICU	83
5	Cultural issues, spirituality, and hope	127
6	Teamwork, relationships, and moral distress	155
7	Legal issues and conflict resolution	189
8	Cardiopulmonary resuscitation	221
9	Withholding and withdrawal of life support	241
10	Lessons learnt	281
11	Personal reflections	293
12	Special situations	305
13	Organ and tissue donation	341
14	Research issues	347
15	Web-based resources	355

Appendix 359
Index 363

Detailed contents

Contributors *xv*

Symbols and abbreviations *xxiii*

1 Introduction   1

Diagnosing dying *2*
Anna Towers

The ICU: a place for palliative care *4*
Graeme Rocker, Deborah Cook

Care of the dying patient in the ICU, part 1:
  a global overview *12*
Malcolm Fisher

Care of the dying patient in the ICU, part 2:
  some current challenges *18*
Malcolm Fisher

Triage in the ICU *22*
Maité Garrouste-Orgeas, Jean Carlet

Older patients in the ICU *28*
Maité Garrouste-Orgeas, Jean Carlet

Complications of cancer and ICU admission decisions *34*
Frédéric Pène, Adeline Max, Jean-Paul Mira

2 Improving palliative and end-of-life care   41

Barriers to high-quality ICU palliative care *42*
Judith E Nelson

Evaluation of palliative care quality *46*
Judith E Nelson

3 Symptom control   51

Common symptoms in ICU patients at high risk of dying: an
  introduction *52*
Jennifer McAdam, Shoshana Arai, Kathleen Puntillo

Symptom relief for the imminently dying patient *54*
Kathleen Puntillo, Cathy Schuster

Pain *60*
Kathleen Puntillo, Shoshana Arai, Jennifer McAdam

Dyspnoea *66*
Shoshana Arai , Jennifer McAdam, Kathleen Puntillo

Anxiety 68
Jennifer McAdam, Shoshana Arai, Kathleen Puntillo

Delirium in the critically ill patient at the end of life: issues and
   management 74
Yoanna Skrobik

Sleep disturbances 78
Shoshana Arai, Jennifer McAdam, Kathleen Puntillo

Thirst/dry mouth 80
Shoshana Arai, Jennifer McAdam, Kathleen Puntillo

4   Caring for families in the ICU   **83**

Families of dying patients: an introduction to meeting their needs 84
Alexandre Lautrette, Élie Azoulay

From admission to bereavement: the patient- and family-centred
   care approach 88
Heather MacDonald

Relationships and iatrogenic suffering: part 1 94
David Kuhl

Conducting an ICU family conference: a VALUES approach 104
J Randall Curtis

Decision-making for patients who lack capacity to decide: the
   surrogate in the ICU 112
Alexandre Lautrette, Élie Azoulay, Jeffrey Watts, Bertrand Souweine

Observational studies of families of patients who died in the
   ICU 118
Élie Azoulay, Graeme Rocker

5   Cultural issues, spirituality, and hope   **127**

Cultural issues and palliative care in the ICU 128
Kerry Bowman

Influence of ICU culture on end-of-life care 134
Peter Dodek

Spiritual care in the ICU 140
Michele Shields, Denah Joseph

Considering hope in the context of palliative care in the ICU 146
Christy Simpson

The social and financial impact on the families of ICU patients: a view
   from the US 150
Sandy Swoboda

6 Teamwork, relationships, and moral distress 155

The role of teams in palliative ICU care *156*
Vicki Spuhler

Collaboration as an essential element of palliative
ICU care *160*
Vicki Spuhler

Relationships and iatrogenic suffering: part 2 *162*
David Kuhl

Educating trainees in the ICU: the value of death rounds *168*
Martha E Billings, Catherine L Hough, J Randall Curtis

Moral distress in critical care health care workers *174*
Freda DeKeyser Ganz

Burnout syndrome in ICU nurses and physicians *180*
Bara Ricou, Paolo Merlani

The rapid response system: a role in risk reduction *186*
F Rubulotta, P Calzavacca, M DeVita

7 Legal issues and conflict resolution 189

Palliative care in the ICU through a legal lens *190*
Jocelyn Downie

The Mental Capacity Act (UK) *196*
Graeme Rocker

Difficult cases *200*
Malcolm Fisher

Conflicts, negotiations, and resolution: a primer *202*
Thomas J Prendergast

The ethics consultant and clinical ethics committees *208*
Jean-Claude Chevrolet, Philippe Jolliet

Euthanasia: the Belgian experience *214*
*Ruth Piers, Nele Van Den Noortgate, Wim Schrauwen,
Dominique Benoit*

8 Cardiopulmonary resuscitation 221

Discussing cardiopulmonary resuscitation: a personal
(semi-structured) approach *222*
Stephen Workman

Cardiopulmonary resuscitation: an overview of outcomes *230*
Peter G Brindley, Gurmeet Singh

A decision aid for communication with hospitalized patients about cardiopulmonary resuscitation preference *234*
Christopher Frank, Jeannette Suurdt, Daren Heyland

Cardiopulmonary resuscitation: a decision aid for patients in hospital and their families *236*

9 Withholding and withdrawal of life support   241

Discussions about withdrawal of life support in the ICU: a perspective from the UK *242*
Simon L Cohen

Decisions to forgo life support: a perspective from Europe *246*
Thomas Fassier, Élie Azoulay

Limitation of life support in an Australian ICU *250*
Malcolm Fisher

ICU care during withdrawal of life support: a personal perspective from Canada *252*
Graeme Rocker

Withdrawal of ventricular assist device support *258*
Jane MacIver, Heather J Ross

Life support after cardiac arrest *262*
Virginie Lemiale, Nancy Kentish-Barnes, Alain Cariou

Withholding and withdrawing life support: Muslim perspectives *268*
Fekri Abroug, Lamia Ouanes Besbes

Withdrawal and withholding of life-sustaining therapies: protocolized approaches *274*
Judith E Nelson

The Liverpool Care Pathway for patients dying in intensive care in the UK *276*
Jane Harper, Laura Chapman

10 Lessons learnt   281

Hope and caring amidst prognostic uncertainty: a physician's perspective *282*
John E Heffner

Don't rush to a bad decision *286*
Duncan Young

'I am sorry, but I have no idea who you are.' *290*
John Myburgh

11 Personal reflections 293

A sister's tale 294
Vicki Guy

A Vietnam veteran's story 298
Harold MacAloney

Hope—a wife's perspective 300
Alison McCallum

Organ and tissue donation: a mother's plea for 'a gentle ask' 302
Denice Klavano

12 Special situations 305

Chronic critical illness 306
Judith E Nelson

Ventilatory support and palliative care in amyotrophic
   lateral sclerosis 312
Jesus Gonzalez Bermejo, Amélie Hurbault, Christophe Coupé,
Vincent Meininger, Thomas Similowski

Cystic fibrosis 318
Walter Robinson

Integrating paediatric palliative care into the paediatric
   intensive care unit 322
Stephen Liben

Palliative care in the trauma intensive care unit 328
Anne C Mosenthal

Non-invasive positive pressure ventilation for acute respiratory
   failure near the end of life: overview and outcomes 334
Tasnim Sinuff

Use of non-invasive positive pressure ventilation for
   patients who have declined intubation: controversy
   and justification 338
Tasnim Sinuff

13 Organ and tissue donation 341

Organ and tissue donation in the ICU 342
Sam D Shemie

14 Research issues 347

Conducting research at the end of life 348
Damon Scales, Niall Ferguson

Randomized controlled trials and ethical principles at the end of life:
a personal view 352
Didier Dreyfuss

15 Web-based resources   355

Web-based resources 356
Judith E Nelson

Appendix 359
Index 363

Contributors

Fekri Abroug
Intensive Care Unit
CHU F.Bourguiba
Tunisia
Withholding and withdrawing life support: Muslim perspectives

Shoshana Arai
Assistant Adjunct Professor
Department of Physiological Nursing
University of California
San Fransisco, USA
Common symptoms in ICU patients at high risk of dying: an introduction
Pain
Dyspnoea
Anxiety
Sleep disturbances
Thirst/dry mouth

Élie Azoulay
Professor of Medicine
Pulmonary Medicine and Critical Care;
Director Assistant of the Medical-ICU
Saint Louis Hospital
Paris, France
Families of dying patients: an introduction to meeting their needs
Decision-making for patients who lack capacity to decide: the surrogate in the ICU
Observational studies of families of patients who died in the ICU
Decisions to forgo life support: a perspective from Europe

Dominique Benoit
Intensive Care Department, Medical Unit
Ghent University Hospital
Gent, Belgium
Euthanasia: the Belgian experience

Martha E Billings
Senior Fellow
Division of Pulmonary and Critical Care Medicine
University of Washington
Seattle, USA
Educating trainees in the ICU: the value of death rounds

Kerry Bowman
University of Toronto
Mount Sinai Hospital
Cultural issues and palliative care in the ICU

Peter G Brindley
Associate Professor
Critical Care Medicine
University of Alberta Hospital
Edmonton, Canada
Cardiopulmonary resuscitation: an overview of outcomes

P Calzavacca
Institute of Anaesthesia and Intensive Care Medicine
Policlinico di Catania University Hospital
Italy
The Rapid Response System: a role in risk reduction

Alain Cariou
Réanimation Médicale
Chochin Hospital
Paris, France
Life support after cardiac arrest

Jean Carlet
French National Authority for Health (HAS)
Saint Denis, France
Triage in the ICU
Older patients in the ICU

Laura Chapman

Consultant in Palliative Medicine
Royal Liverpool and Broadgreen
University Hospitals
Liverpool
*The Liverpool Care Pathway for
patients dying in intensive care in
the UK*

Jean-Claude Chevrolet

Intensive Care Service
University Hospital
Geneva, Switzerland
*The ethics consultant and clinical
ethics committees*

Simon L Cohen

Consultant Physician
Intensive Care Unit
University College Hospital
London, UK
*Discussions about withdrawal
of life support in the ICU:
a perspective from the UK*

Deborah Cook

McMaster University, Ontario
Canada
The ICU: a place for palliative care

Christophe Coupé

Clinical Psychologist
ALS Centre
University Hospital Pitié
Salpêtrière
Paris, France
*Ventilatory support and pallia-
tive care in amyotrophic lateral
sclerosis*

J Randall Curtis

Professor of Medicine
Division of Pulmonary and
Critical Care Medicine
Harborview Medical Center
University of Washington
Seattle, USA
*Conducting an ICU family
conference: a VALUES approach
Educating trainees in the ICU: the
value of death rounds*

Freda DeKeyser Ganz

Head, Masters Program
Hadassah-Hebrew University
School of Nursing
Jerusalem, Israel
*Moral distress in critical care
health care workers*

M DeVita

Institute of Anaesthesia and
Intensive Care Medicine
Policlinico di Catania University
Hospital
Italy
*The Rapid Response System: a
role in risk reduction*

Peter Dodek

Center for Health Evaluation and
Outcome Sciences and Program in
Critical Care Medicine
St. Paul's Hospital & University of
British Columbia
Vancouver, Canada
*Influence of ICU culture on
end-of-life care*

Jocelyn Downie

Canada Research Chair and
Professor
Faculties of Law and Medicine
Dalhousie University
Halifax, Canada
*Palliative care in the ICU through
a legal lens*

Didier Dreyfuss

Professor of Medicine
Director of Medical-Surgical ICU
Hôpital Louis Mourier,
Colombes;
Assistance Publique,
Hôpitaux de Paris
Université Paris-Diderot
Paris, France
*Randomized controlled trials
and ethical principles at the end
of life: a personal view*

Thomas Fassier

Service de Réanimation Médicale
et d'Assistance Respiratoire
Hôpital de la Croix Rousse –
Hospices Civils de Lyon
Lyon, France
*Decisions to forgo life support: a
perspective from Europe*

Niall D Ferguson

Interdepartmental Division
of Critical Care Medicine
University of Toronto
Toronto, Canada
*Conducting research at the
end of life*

Malcolm Fisher

Professor
Departments of Medicine and
Anaesthesia
University of Sydney;
Senior Staff Specialist
Intensive Care Unit
Royal North Shore Hospital;
Senior Clinical Executive
Northern Sydney Central Coast
Area Health;
Visiting Intensivist
North Shore Private Hospital
Sydney, Australia
*Care of the dying patient in the
ICU, part 1: a global overview
Care of the dying patient in the
ICU, part 2: some current
challenges
Difficult cases
Limitation of life support in an
Australian ICU*

Christopher Frank

Associate Professor
Department of Medicine
Division of Geriatric Medicine
Queen's University
Kingston, Canada
*A decision aid for communication
with hospitalized patients about
cardiopulmonary resuscitation
preference*

Maité Garrouste-Orgeas

Medical ICU
Saint Joseph Hospital
Paris, France
*Triage in the ICU
Older patients in the ICU*

Jesus Gonzalez Bermejo

Pneumologist
Intensive Care Unit and ALS Centre
University Hospital Pitié Salpêtrière
Paris, France
*Ventilatory support and palliative
care in amyotrophic lateral sclerosis*

Vicki Guy

Department of Nursing
QEII Health Sciences Centre
Halifax, Canada
A sister's tale

Jane Harper

Consultant in Intensive Care and
Anaesthesia
Royal Liverpool University Hospital
Liverpool
*The Liverpool Care Pathway for
patients dying in intensive care in
the UK*

John E Heffner

Adjunct Professor of Medicine
Garnjobst Chair of Medical
Education
Providence Portland Medical Center
Oregon Health and Science
University
Portland, USA
*Hope and caring amidst
prognostic uncertainty:
a physician's perspective*

Daren Heyland

Professor
Department of Medicine
Queen's University;
Clinical Evaluation Research Unit
Kingston General Hospital
Kingston, Canada
*A decision aid for communication
with hospitalized patients
about cardiopulmonary
resuscitation preference*

Catherine L Hough
Assistant Professor
Division of Pulmonary and
Critical Care Medicine
University of Washington
Seattle, USA
*Educating trainees in the ICU:
the value of death rounds*

Amélie Hurbault
Clinical Psychologist
Intensive Care Service
University Hospital Pitié
Salpêtrière
Paris, France
*Ventilatory support and
palliative care in amyotrophic
lateral sclerosis*

Philippe Jolliet
Intensive Care Service
University Hospital
Geneva, Switzerland
*The ethics consultant and clinical
ethics committees*

Denah Joseph
Spiritual Care Services
University of California
San Fransisco Medical Centre
San Fransisco, USA
Spiritual care in the ICU

Nancy Kentish-Barnes
FAMIREA Study Group
Service de Réanimation Médicale
Hôpital Saint Louis
Paris, France
Life support after cardiac arrest

Denice Klavano
Certified Tissue Bank Specialist
Regional Tissue Bank
Capital District Health Authority
Halifax, Canada
*Organ and tissue donation: a
mother's plea for 'a gentle ask'*

David Kuhl
Director
Centre for Practitioner Renewal
Providence Heath Care/University
of British Columbia;
Associate Professor
Department of Family Practice,
Faculty of Medicine
University of British Columbia
Vancouver, Canada
*Relationships and
iatrogenic suffering:
part 1
Relationships and
iatrogenic
suffering: part 2*

Alexandre Lautrette
Assistant Director of the
Medical-ICU
University Hospital
Université d'Auvergne
Clermont-Ferrand, France
*Families of dying patients:
an introduction to meeting
their needs
Decision-making for
patients who lack capacity
to decide: the surrogate in the ICU*

Virginie Lemiale
Service de Réanimation Médicale
Hôpital Cochin – Saint Vincent de
Paul – La Roche Guyon
Paris, France
Life support after cardiac arrest

Stephen Liben
The Montreal Children's Hospital
Montreal, Canada
*Integrating paediatric palliative
care into the paediatric intensive
care unit*

Harold MacAloney
Former Registered Nurse
Nova Scotia, Canada
A Vietnam veteran's story

Heather MacDonald
Clinical Nurse Specialist
(Critical Care)
Halifax Infirmary
Halifax, Canada
*From admission to bereavement:
the patient- and family-centred
care approach*

Jane MacIver
Divisions of Cardiology and
Transplantation
Toronto General Hospital
Toronto, Canada
*Withdrawal of ventricular assist
device support*

Adeline Max
Medical Intensive Care Unit
Cochin Hospital, AP-HP
Paris, France
*Complications of cancer and ICU
admission decisions*

Jennifer McAdam
Assistant Professor of Nursing
Dominican University
San Rafael, USA
*Common symptoms in ICU
patients at high risk of dying: an
introduction
Pain
Dyspnoea
Anxiety
Sleep disturbances
Thirst/dry mouth*

Alison McCallum
Family Physician,
Halifax, Canada
Hope: a wife's perspective

Vincent Meininger
Professor of Neurology
ALS Centre
University Hospital Pitié
Salpêtrière
Paris, France
*Ventilatory support and palliative
care in amyotrophic lateral sclerosis*

Paolo Merlani
Intensive Care Service
University Hospitals
University of Geneva
Geneva, Switzerland
*Burnout syndrome in ICU nurses
and physicians*

Jean-Paul Mira
Medical Intensive Care Unit
Cochin Hospital, AP-HP
Université Paris Descartes
Paris, France
*Complications of cancer and ICU
admission decisions*

Anne C Mosenthal
Associate Professor Surgery
Chief, Division Surgical Critical Care
New Jersey Medical School
University of Medicine and
Dentistry of New Jersey
Newark, USA
*Palliative care in the trauma
intensive care unit*

John Myburgh
Professor of Critical Care
Medicine
University of New South Wales;
Department of Intensive Care
Medicine
St George Hospital;
The George Institute for
International Health
Sydney, Australia
*'I am sorry, but I have no idea who
you are.'*

Judith E Nelson
Professor of Medicine
Division of Pulmonary, Critical
Care, and Sleep Medicine
Hertzberg Palliative Care Institute
Mount Sinai School of Medicine
New York, USA
*Barriers to high-quality
ICU palliative care
Evaluation of palliative care
quality
Withholding and withdrawal of
life-sustaining therapies: protocol-
ized approaches
Chronic critical illness
Web-based*

Lamia Ouanes Besbes
Intensive Care Unit
CHU F.Bourguiba
Monastir, Tunisia
*Withholding and withdrawing
life support: Muslim
perspectives*

Frédéric Pène
Medical Intensive Care Unit
Cochin Hospital, AP-HP
Université Paris Descartes
Paris, France
*Complications of cancer
and ICU admission decisions*

Ruth Piers
Department of Geriatric Medicine
Ghent University Hospital
Ghent, Belgium
*Euthanasia: the Belgian
experience*

Thomas J Prendergast
Associate Professor of Medicine
and Anesthesiology;
Program Director
Pulmonary and
Critical Care Medicine
Dartmouth Hitchcock Medical
Center,
Lebanon, USA
*Conflicts, negotiations, and
resolution: a primer*

Kathleen Puntillo
FAAN Professor of Nursing
Department of Physiological
Nursing
University of California
San Francisco, USA
*Common symptoms in ICU patients
at high risk of dying: an introduction
Symptom relief for the imminently
dying patient
Pain
Dyspnoea
Anxiety
Sleep disturbances
Thirst/dry mouth*

Bara Ricou
Intensive Care Service
University Hospitals
University of Geneva
Geneva, Switzerland
*Burnout syndrome in ICU nurses
and physicians*

Walter Robinson
Pulmonary Division
Vanderbilt Children's Hospital;
Centre for Biomedical Ethics
and Society
Vanderbilt University
Nashville, USA
Cystic fibrosis

Graeme Rocker
Professor of Medicine
Department of Medicine
(Division of Respirology)
Dalhousie University
Halifax, Canada
*The ICU: a place for palliative care
Observational studies of families
of patients who died in the ICU
ICU care during withdrawal of life
support: a personal perspective
from Canada
The Mental Capacity Act (UK)*

Heather J Ross
Divisions of Cardiology and
Transplantation
Toronto General Hospital
Toronto, Canada
*Withdrawal of ventricular assist
device support*

F Rubulotta
Institute of Anaesthesia and
Intensive Care Medicine
Policlinico di Catania University
Hospital
Italy
*The Rapid Response System: a
role in risk reduction*

Damon C Scales
Interdepartmental Division of
Critical Care Medicine
University of Toronto
Toronto, Canada
*Conducting research at the end
of life*

Wim Schrauwen
Clinical Psychologist
Department of Medical Oncology
and Palliative Care
Ghent University Hospital
Gent, Belgium
*Euthanasia: the Belgian
experience*

Cathy Schuster
Clinical Nurse IV
Medical-Surgical ICU
University of California,
San Francisco Medical Centre
San Francisco, USA
*Symptom relief for the imminently
dying patient*

Sam D Shemie
Division of Critical Care
Montreal Children's Hospital;
Professor of Paediatrics
McGill University
Montreal, Canada;
Loeb Chair in Organ and Tissue
Donation
University of Ottawa;
Canadian Blood Services
Ottawa, Canada
*Organ and tissue donation
in the ICU*

Michele R Shields
Director
Spiritual Care Services
University of California
San Francisco Medical Centre
San Francisco, USA
Spiritual care in the ICU

Thomas Similowski
Professor of Pneumology
Intensive Care
University Hospital Pitié
Salpêtrière
Paris, France
*Ventilatory support and pallia-
tive care in amyotrophic lateral
sclerosis*

Christy Simpson
Associate Professor
Ethics Collaborations Coordinator
Department of Bioethics
Dalhousie University
Halifax, Canada
*Considering hope in the context of
palliative care in the ICU*

Gurmeet Singh
Assistant Clinical Professor
Critical Care Medicine and Cardiac
Surgery
University of Alberta Hospital
Edmonton, Canada
*Cardiopulmonary resuscitation: an
overview of outcomes*

Tasnim Sinuff
Department of Critical Care
Medicine
Sunnybrook Health Sciences
Center
Toronto, Canada
*Non-invasive positive pressure
ventilation for acute respiratory
failure near the end of life*

Yoanna Skrobik
Critical Care Medicine
Université de Montréal and
McGill University;
Intensive Care Unit
Maisonneuve-Rosemount Hospital
Montreal, Canada
*Delirium in the critically ill patient
at the end of life: issues and
management*

Bertrand Souweine
Director of the Medical-ICU
University Hospital
Université d'Auvergne
Clermont-Ferrand, France
*Decision-making for patients who
lack capacity to decide: the
surrogate in the ICU*

Vicki Spuhler
Nurse Manager RICU
Intermountain Medical Center
Murray, USA
*The role of teams in palliative
ICU care
Collaboration as an essential
element of palliative ICU care*

Jeannette Suurdt
Research Associate
Clinical Evaluation Research Unit
Kingston General Hospital
Canada
*A decision aid for communication
with hospitalized patients about
cardiopulmonary resuscitation
preference*

Sandy Swoboda
Johns Hopkins University Schools
of Medicine and Nursing
Baltimore, USA
*The social and financial impact
on the families of ICU patients: a
view from the US*

Anna Towers
Associate Professor
Palliative Care Division
McGill University
Montreal, Canada

Nele Van Den Noortgate
Department of Geriatric Medicine
Ghent University Hospital
Gent, Belgium
*Euthanasia: the Belgian
experience*

Jeffrey Watts
Professor
Université d'Auvergne
Clermont-Ferrand, France
*Decision-making for patients who
lack capacity to decide: the sur-
rogate in the ICU*

Stephen Workman
The Queen Elizabeth Health
Sciences Center
Halifax, Canada
*Discussing cardiopulmonary
resuscitation: a personal (semi-
structured) approach*

Duncan Young
Clinical Director
Adult Intensive Care Unit
John Radcliffe Hospital
Oxford, UK
Don't rush to a bad decision

Symbols and abbreviations

°C	degree centigrade
~	approximately
>	greater than
<	less than
≥	equal to or greater than
≤	equal to or less than
®	registered
™	trademark
AACN	American Association of Critical Care Nurses
ABG	arterial blood gases
ACLS	advanced cardiac life support
AIDS	acquired immunodeficiency syndrome
ALS	amyotrophic lateral sclerosis
a.m.	*ante meridiem* (before noon)
AML	acute myelogenous leukaemia
ARDS	acute respiratory distress syndrome
ARF	acute respiratory failure
ASY	asystole
BiPAP	bi-level positive airway pressure
BiVAD	Bi-ventricular assist device
BOOP	bronchiolitis obliterans with organizing pneumonia
BOS	burnout syndrome
CA	cardiac arrest
CAM-ICU	ICU-adjusted confusion assessment method
CCU	coronary care unit
CF	cystic fibrosis
CFRD	cystic fibrosis-related diabetes
CHF	congestive heart failure
CJD	Creutzfeldt–Jakob disease
CMV	cytomegalovirus
CNS	central nervous system
CO_2	carbon dioxide
COPD	chronic obstructive pulmonary disease
CPR	cardiopulmonary resuscitation

CT	computed tomography
DCD	donation after cardiac death
DFLST	decisions to forego life-sustaining therapies
DIOS	distal intestinal obstruction syndrome
dL	decilitre
DNI	do not intubate
DNR	do not resuscitate
DRS	delirium rating scale
DSM	diagnostic and statistical manual of mental disorders
ECG	electrocardiogram
ECMO	extracorporeal membrane oxygenation
EEG	electroencephalogram
e.g.	*exempli gratia* (for example)
ELISA	enzyme-linked immunosorbent assay
ER	emergency room
FEV1	forced expiratory volume in 1 minute
FIO_2	fraction of inspired oxygen
g	gram
GCS	Glasgow coma score
G-CSF	granulocyte colony-stimulating factor
GP	general practitioner
GVHD	graft-versus-host disease
h	hour
HDU	high dependency unit
HIV	human immunodeficiency virus
HSCT	haematopoietic stem cell transplantation
ICD	implantable cardio-defibrillators
ICDSC	intensive care delirium screening checklist
ICU	intensive care unit
i.e.	*id est* (that is)
IM	intramuscular
IMCA	independent mental capacity advocate
IV	intravenous
kPa	kilopascal
LCP	Liverpool Care Pathway
LOD	logistic organ dysfunction
LPA	lasting power of attorney
LVAD	Left ventricular assist device
MBI	Maslack burnout inventory
MBI–HSS	Maslach burnout inventory–human services survey
MCA	Mental Capacity Act

MDT	multidisciplinary team
MET	medical emergency team
mg	milligram
mL	millilitre
mmHg	millimetre mercury
MRI	magnetic resonance imaging
NaCl	sodium chloride
NH	nursing home
NIV	non-invasive ventilation
NPPV	non-invasive positive pressure ventilation
NREM	non-rapid eye movement
NRS	numerical rating scale
NSAID	non-steroidal anti-inflammatory drug
OHCA	out-of-hospital cardiac arrest
OPALS	Ontario Pre-hospital Advanced Life Support
p	probability
p.m.	*post meridiem* (after noon)
PaCO$_2$	partial pressure of carbon dioxide in arterial blood
PEA	pulseless electrical activity
PEEP	positive end expiratory pressure
PFCC	patient- and family-centred care
PICU	paediatric intensive care unit
PO	*per os* (by mouth)
PRN	*pro re nata* (when necessary)
PS	performance status
PTSD	post-traumatic stress disorder
QoL	quality of life
RA	respiratory arrest
RASS	Richmond agitation sedation scale
RCT	randomized controlled trial
REM	rapid eye movement
ROSC	return of spontaneous circulation
RN	respiratory nurse
RRS	rapid response system
RRT	rapid response team
RT	respiratory therapist
RVAD	Right ventricular assist device
SAPS	simplified acute physiology score
SAS	sedation-agitation scale
SC	subcutaneously
SCCM	Society of Critical Care Medicine

SOFA	sequential organ failure assessment
SpO$_2$	saturation of peripheral oxygen
SSEP	somatosensory evoked potential
SSRI	specific serotonin reuptake inhibitor
UK	United Kingdom
US	United States
VAD	ventricular assist device
VADS	vertical analog dyspnoea scale
VAS	visual analogue scale
VF	ventricular fibrillation
vs	versus
VT	ventricular tachycardia
WLST	withdraw (withdrawal of) life-sustaining therapy

Introduction

Diagnosing dying *2*
Anna Towers

The ICU: a place for palliative care *4*
Graeme Rocker, Deborah Cook

Care of the dying patient in the ICU,
   part 1: a global overview *12*
Malcolm Fisher

Care of the dying patient in the ICU,
   part 2: some current challenges *18*
Malcolm Fisher

Triage in the ICU *22*
Maité Garrouste-Orgeas, Jean Carlet

Older patients in the ICU *28*
Maité Garrouste-Orgeas, Jean Carlet

Complications of cancer and ICU admission decisions *34*
Frédéric Pène, Adeline Max, Jean-Paul Mira

Diagnosing dying

How do we know that a patient is dying?

Setting and respecting goals of care and the provision of quality palliative care should be the overriding concerns that inform and guide decisions about whether, when and when not to admit a dying patient to an intensive care unit (ICU).

Some standard teaching[1-3] provides some guidance as follows:

Assuming that there is agreement between referring clinical teams and the ICU, a patient is likely to be dying and unlikely to benefit from ICU admission if several of the following conditions and signs are present within the phases described below:

- Irreversible failure of a vital organ (heart, lungs, kidneys, liver, brain).
- Advanced cachexia.
- Irreversible delirium.

Phases of dying (irrespective of diagnosis)

Early signs (usual time prognosis: days to weeks)

Patients:

- Are very weak/irreversibly bedbound.
- Show little or no interest in food and fluid intake.
- Unable to take oral medications.
- Spend increasing time sleeping and/or show increasing signs of delirium.

Mid-stage

- Increasing obtundation.
- Pooling of secretions (failure of swallowing reflex).

Late signs (usual time prognosis: hours to days)

- Coma.
- Changes in respiratory pattern: apnoeas, irregular breathing, presence of pulmonary congestion with secretions that the patient cannot expectorate.
- Fever (likely from aspiration).
- Skin mottling.

The presence and time course of these signs varies, but in general they signal that goals may need to be redefined. Information should be imparted sensitively to families and to the patient if appropriate. Families are often unaware that death is imminent and they will likely be distressed if they are not prepared. Be clear that the patient is dying, but also that it is difficult to be certain when, so a relatively wide time range should be mentioned as part of these discussions.

It is essential to address and relieve suffering whatever the timing of dying. Poorly relieved suffering before a person dies is remembered by families and can cause intense distress in the months and years to come.

References

1. Furst CJ, Doyle D (2005). The terminal phase. In: Doyle D, Hanks G, Cherny N, Calman K (eds), *Oxford textbook of palliative medicine*, 3rd edn, pp 1117–33. Oxford University Press, New York.
2. Twycross R, Lichter I. The terminal phase. In: Doyle D, Hanks GWC, MacDonald N, eds. *Oxford Textbook of Palliative Medicine*. 2nd ed. Oxford, England: Oxford University Press; 1998: 977–992.
3. Weissman DE (2005). *Syndrome of imminent death. Fast fact and concept #3*, 2nd edn, End-of-life palliative education resource centre. Available from: http://www.eperc.mcw.edu.

The ICU: a place for palliative care

Introduction

A century ago, Sir William Osler gave us this guidance … 'It is much more important to know what sort of a patient has a disease than what sort of disease a patient has.'

If we remember this, plus the more modern advice that 'the care of the patient begins with the caring for the patient', and if we treat patients under our care during the end of their life as we would someone we love in our family, we should not go far wrong.

Many publications have documented the suboptimal care of dying patients, particularly in the ICU. In most of the developed countries in the world, we have been largely a 'death denying society', and many patients die institutionalized and technologically supported, some as victims of the 'medicalization of the dying process'. In contrast, over the last decade, the 'humanization of the dying process' has been the focus of numerous clinical, policy, and research efforts to improve end-of-life care for critically ill patients. In the following sections, we re-emphasize some key strategies occurring socially and appearing in the literature, drawing on some of our own personal experiences as well.

Promoting social change through professional initiatives

Professional societies, hospitals, clinicians, investigators, ethicists, patients, families, and the media have all called for social change to improve end-of-life-care. Professional societies continue to underpin efforts in this direction. Several years ago, in a landmark publication, Danis and colleagues called for earlier and more frequent integration of palliative care into critical care. More recently, the Robert Wood Johnson Foundation's Promoting Excellence in End-of-Life Care Project in the US supported an ICU Working Group. The mandate of this group was to galvanize clinical, educational, and research activities promoting excellence in end-of-life care for critically ill patients.

Reflecting this renewed interest, most national and international ICU conferences now hold symposia on end-of-life care. For example, the European Society of Intensive Care Medicine, the International Symposium of Intensive Care and Emergency Medicine, the American Thoracic Society, the Society of Critical Care Medicine, the American Association of Critical Care Nurses, and the American College of Chest Physicians routinely have sessions on this topic. Notably, the 2004 International Consensus Conference addressed this issue, reflecting recognition of the need to globalize these initiatives for social change, yet adapting them to different norms, religions, and cultures around the world.

Documents intended to guide decisions about the administration, withholding, or withdrawal of life support in the ICU have been summarized in a recent review of 49 publications representing professional society statements, consensus statements, and interest groups. Sources were independent academics, professional organizations, and health care organizations. Almost half were produced collectively by committees or consensus conference methods. These tools differed in format and focus, characterized as 'decision schemas' (involving clinical practice algorithms), 'decision guides' (reviewing legal or professional positions), and 'decision counsels' (more discursive and focusing typically on ethical issues). Tools addressed common life support issues such as advance directives, ICU admission and discharge criteria, whether nutrition and hydration decisions are different from decisions about other types of life support, and the 'double effect'. In summary, published tools for guiding life support decisions differ widely in their genesis, authorship, format, focus, practicality, and in their attention to, and positions on, key life support dilemmas. Future research is needed on how users interpret and apply the messages in these tools, and what their impacts are on practice, quality of care, participant experiences, and patient outcomes.

Further reading

1. Danis M, Federman D, Fins JJ, et al. (1999). Incorporating palliative care into critical care education: principles, challenges, and opportunities. Crit Care Med **27**, 2005–13.
2. Carlet J, Thijs LG, Antonelli M, et al. (2004). Challenges in end-of-life care in the ICU. Statement of the 5th International Consensus Conference in Critical Care, Brussels, Belgium, April 2003. Intensive Care Med **30**, 770–84.
3. Cook DJ, Rocker G, Giacomini M, Sinuff T, Heyland DK (2006). Understanding and changing attitudes toward withdrawal and withholding of life support in the ICU. Crit Care Med **24**(Suppl), S317–23.
4. Giacomini M, Cook DJ, DeJean D, Shaw R, Gedge E (2006). Decision tools for life support: a review and policy analysis. Crit Care Med **34**, 864–70.
5. American Thoracic Society (2008). Palliative care for patients with respiratory diseases and critical ilnesses: an official American Thoracic Society clinical policy statement. Am J Respir Crit Care Med **177**, 912–27.

Legitimizing research in end-of-life care

Over a decade ago, end-of-life research was deemed less rigorous than other clinical or basic science research, and received much less peer review funding. This situation has changed today. For example, the Canadian Institutes for Health Research (equivalent to the Medical Research Council in the UK) recently committed to actively support investigations in palliative and end-of-life care (see http://www.cihr-irsc.gc.ca/services/funding/opportunities/institutes/2003/rfa_8_palliative_care_e.shtml).

Benefits of this change in focus is evidenced by the training of career scientists in this field and the formation of collaborative research networks that advance our understanding of this aspect of care. Recently, a multidisciplinary group in the US described an end-of-life research agenda to help advance the field (see 'Further reading'). Long-standing collaborations in Canada and newer collaborations in Europe (*FAMIREA) have also been particularly successful.

Today, more ICU journal clubs discuss publications in end-of-life care, offering an opportunity to educate trainees, the ICU team, and others about end-of-life research initiatives in critical care.

Further reading

1. Rubenfeld GD, JR Curtis (2001). End-of-life care in the intensive care unit: a research agenda. Crit Care Med **29**, 1–11.
2. Azoulay E, Pochard F, Chevret S, et al. (2002). Impact of a family information leaflet on effectiveness of information provided to family members of intensive care unit patients: a multicentre, prospective, randomized, controlled trial. Am J Respir Crit Care Med **165**, 438–42.
3. Cook D, Rocker G, Marshall J, et al., for the Level of Care Study Investigators and the Canadian Critical Care Trials Group (2003). Withdrawal of mechanical ventilation in anticipation of death in the intensive care unit. N Engl J Med **349**, 1123–32.

* FAMIREA is the contraction between **FAMI**ly and ICU (**REA**nimation in French). The group includes 97 ICUs from all over France.

Determining what dying patients need

It is a reasonable assumption that patients dying in the ICU want good symptom control, to have their wishes respected, and to be surrounded by their loved ones. We should directly approach critically ill patients or their loved ones to determine what they need and want or expect from the ICU team. We should not assume that what we think or value will be the same for all our patients and families; many errors of judgement begin with a false assumption. A better understanding of our patients as human beings is likely to prevent much of the conflict that arises when there are clashes of hopes or expectations expressed by patients, families, and the ICU teams caring for them.

Differing populations have identified factors that are uniquely important to them regarding end-of-life care. Maintaining hope was a unique theme of cancer patients; pain control was of paramount importance to acquired immunodeficiency syndrome (AIDS) patients. Patients who had chronic obstructive pulmonary disease (COPD) wanted education about the diagnosis, prognosis, and treatment; they also wanted to know what dying might be like and to do some advance care planning. A more recent Canadian multicentre study identified factors most important to patients' concepts of quality end-of-life care. For 440 patients, elements of end-of-life care rated as 'extremely important' most frequently were:

- 'To have trust and confidence in the doctors looking after you' (56% of respondents).
- 'Not to be kept alive on life supports when there is little hope for a meaningful recovery' (56%).
- 'That information about your disease be communicated to you by your doctor in an honest manner' (44%).
- 'To complete things and prepare for life's end (life review, resolving conflicts, saying goodbye)' (44%).

Further reading

1. Curtis JR, Wenrich MD, Carline JD, et al. (2002). Patients' perspectives on physician skill in end-of-life care: differences between patients with COPD, cancer, and AIDS. *Chest* **122**, 356–62.
2. Heyland DK, Dodek P, Rocker G, et al. (2006). What matters most in end-of-life care: perceptions of seriously ill patients and their family members. *CMAJ* **174**, 627–33.

Determining what families of dying patients need

Caring for dying critically ill patients should go hand in hand with caring for their families. Anxiety and depression are common in family members visiting the ICU. While we cannot eliminate these symptoms, strategies such as compassionate communication, providing information brochures, and grief counselling can help (see 📖 in 'Families of dying patients: an introduction to meeting their needs' p84 and 📖 'Conducting an ICU family conference: a VALUES approach' p104).

Asking family members about the quality of care they received provides insights into areas ripe for quality improvement. A recent study of family satisfaction from the US has demonstrated that satisfaction with care was greater among the bereaved than among family members of ICU survivors. While at first blush counterintuitive, this finding highlights the power of frequent effective communication that likely occurs when prognosis, values, preferences, and hopes are addressed for dying patients in the ICU.

Studies in French ICUs have indicated a major reluctance of more than half of families to participate in end-of-life decision-making. A recent report from the US underscores the frequency of psychiatric symptoms that can develop or progress in bereaved family members who participate in end-of-life decision-making. These studies underscore the need to try to understand family members with respect to both their information needs and their wishes for involvement in decision-making.

Bereavement

Reducing the burdens of bereavement has not been a traditional focus for clinicians within the ICU. Nevertheless, it is likely to be an area where some of our most valuable contributions can be made. A randomized trial from France demonstrated the impact that a simple information brochure can have. Other groups arrange formal follow-up with families after a death (see 📖 in 'From admission to bereavement: the patient- and family-centred care approach' p88). Being available as an attending physician or a senior nurse offering meetings if there are any unresolved questions that families have, conducting memorial services, sending sympathy cards to grieving family members, and celebrating lives lived, these are all example of activities that families find helpful when dealing with loss. Our care for families should not end when the doors close behind them after a death in the ICU. Families need to know they are not alone.

Further reading

1. Nelson JE, Angus DC, Weissfeld LA, et al. (2006). End-of-life care for the critically ill: a national intensive care unit survey. *Crit Care Med* **34**, 2547–53.
2. Siegel MD, Hayes E, Vanderwerker LC, Loseth DB, Prigerson HG (2008). Psychiatric illness in the next of kin of patients who die in the intensive care unit. *Crit Care Med* **36**, 1722–8.
3. Wall RJ, Curtis JR, Cooke CR, Engelberg RA (2007). Family satisfaction in the ICU: differences between families of survivors and non-survivors. *Chest* **132**, 1425–33.
4. Lautrette A, Darmon M, Megarbane B, et al. (2007). A communication strategy and brochure for relatives of patients dying in the ICU. *N Engl J Med* **356**, 469–78.

Talking less and listening more

A recent study in the US demonstrated the need for clinicians to listen more than they talk during family conferences. From 51 audio-taped family conferences, physicians monopolized the available time (71% of the time) with families speaking infrequently (only 29% of the time). Family satisfaction ratings with the conferences clearly demonstrated that physicians should talk less and listen more. Increased proportion of family speech was also associated with decreased family ratings of conflict with the physician.

Some simple approaches can lessen the jargon and improve the clarity of any conversation in the ICU. For example, instead of saying 'cardiac arrest', we should say 'his heart stopped'. Instead of saying 'vent', we should say 'breathing machine'. Instead of saying she is 'stable', underscore that 'she is critically ill and might die'. These are examples of language that can serve as the foundation for direct communication, augmented by explanatory passages and compassionate listening.

Ensuring input from all members of the health care team

End-of-life care can be improved by understanding the perspectives of all members of the ICU team. Nurses and physicians often have different perspectives on end-of-life care. Most feedback described in the literature is from family members, which may be based only on a single experience. However, registered nurses (RN) and respiratory therapists (RT) perspectives incorporate the experience of many ICU deaths. One study of RNs and RTs who reflected on 98 withdrawals of life-sustaining therapy in the ICU led to the following suggestions.

In Canada and USA RTs are members of the multidisciplinary ICU team with responsibility for initiating and maintaining mechanical ventilators and oxygen therapy.

On preparing for death
- 'There should be more RN involvement in the process. Doctors should regard RN and RT concerns and information more seriously. I sometimes feel the bedside nurse's opinion is not taken seriously.' [RN]

On standardizing life support withdrawal procedures
- 'Try to develop standardized way of doing things, not each intensivist doing his/her own thing.' [RT]
- 'Although individual cases will require different plans of action, it would be nice to have a protocol or policy written up that could be reviewed by the doctor, nurse, and RT prior to initiating the procedures.' [RT]

On the ICU environment
- 'We should have been quieter when having rounds outside the room for another patient [when] a lot of family was gathered. Family appeared bothered by closing doors tighter.' [RN]

Further reading
1. Rocker GM, Cook DJ, O'Callaghan CJ, et al. (2005). Canadian nurses' and respiratory therapists' perspectives on withdrawal of life support in the intensive care unit. *J Crit Care* **20**, 59.

Initiating quality improvement

Quality improvement initiatives in end-of-life care in the ICU can be driven by sentinel events or can develop as part of a planned local or national programme.

Several years ago in Halifax, Nova Scotia, a first-degree murder charge was laid against an ICU physician regarding treatment of a dying patient (later dismissed). A retrospective review of all deaths in two university-affiliated ICUs in Halifax was conducted with institutional support. Accordingly, policies were developed to address key issues such as:
- More comprehensive recording of symptoms (dyspnoea, pain, agitation), and their management.
- Open-ended orders with no fixed upper limit (for opioids or benzodiazepines).
- A DNR order protocol to help clarify resuscitation preferences.
- A 'withdrawal of life support' checklist to prompt clinicians to:
  - Consult with referring physicians.
  - Obtain a second physician's opinion about life support withdrawal.
  - Discontinue technologic interventions incongruent with palliation.
  - Document patient and family discussions with the entire ICU team.
  - Offer spiritual care to the family.

Other interdisciplinary approaches to end-of-life quality improvement include the concept of implementing 'death rounds' into ICU practice as described by Dr Billings and colleagues (see 📖 in 'Educating trainees in the ICU: the value of death rounds' p168). More recent interventions and their successes or failings in an ICU setting have been described by Curtis and Engelberg in a 2006 supplement to Critical Care Medicine. For a more general approach to quality assurance initiatives, see 📖 Evaluation of palliative care quality, p46.

Further reading

1. Rocker GM (2003). End-of-life care in Canada after a murder charge in an ICU. *Intensive Care Med* **29**, 2336–7.
2. Hough CL, Hudson LD, Salud A, Lahey T, Curtis JR (2005). Death rounds: end-of-life discussions among medical residents in the intensive care unit. *J Crit Care* **20**, 20–5.
3. Curtis JR, Cook DJ, Wall RJ, *et al.* (2006). Intensive care unit quality improvement: a 'how-to' guide for the interdisciplinary team. *Crit Care Med* **34**, 211–8.
4. Curtis JR, Engelberg RA (2006). Measuring success of interventions to improve the quality of end-of-life care in the intensive care unit. *Crit Care Med* **34**(11 Suppl), S341–7.
5. Mularski RA, Curtis JR, Billings JA, *et al.* (2006). Proposed quality measures for palliative care in the critically ill: a consensus from the Robert Wood Johnson Foundation Critical Care Workgroup. *Crit Care Med* **34**(11 Suppl), S404–11.

Educating future clinicians: what do they need?

Residency programmes provide a great opportunity to influence end-of-life care in the present and in the future. Whether or not residents are adequately prepared for the task, they play a key role in some end-of-life decisions in the ICU: 50% of the CPR directives established in the first 24 hours of ICU admission in one international Level of Care Study were established by residents and affirmed by attending physicians.

Excellent skills are necessary for current and future nurses and physicians to participate effectively in the administration, withholding, and withdrawal of life support. Some key findings from a self-administered multicentre survey of ICU residents before and after their ICU rotation were as follows:

- Confidence in the withdrawal of life support discussions was primarily associated with resident involvement in family meetings.
- Residents recommended experiential, case-based, patient-centred curricula.

They need:

- Hands-on learning of the practical and ethical aspects of life support withdrawal, in preference to learning from lectures and textbooks.
- To observe expert role models and to proceed gradually toward individually supervised responsibility.

Future studies to improve the end-of-life education for clinicians would ideally test interactive educational approaches that have been shown to most effectively change a clinician's behaviour in other settings. These initiatives must incorporate cultural diversity and sensitivity training in today's world. These initiatives would ideally be designed to improve end-of-life care in any hospital setting, not just in the ICU.

Further reading

1. Cook DJ, Guyatt GH, Rocker G, *et al.*, for the Canadian Critical Care Trials Group (2001). Cardiopulmonary resuscitation directives on admission to the intensive care unit: an international observational study. *Lancet* **358**, 1941–5.
2. Stevens L, Cook DJ, Guyatt G, Griffith L, Walter S, McMullin JP (2002). Education, ethics, and end-of-life decisions in the intensive care unit. *Crit Care Med* **30**, 290–6.
3. Gorman TE, Ahern SP, Wiseman J, Skrobik Y (2005). Residents' end-of-life decision-making with adult hospitalized patients: a review of the literature. *Acad Med* **80**, 622–33.

Seeking and using patient and personal feedback

Simple questions can increase the confidence of patients and families in their interactions with ICU teams. For example, why would we not ask on a consistent basis 'how can we best help you at this difficult time?' If we do this, we open doors to help and share some intimacy, which can lead to compelling ideas about ways to improve end-of-life care.

We should ask grieving family members for feedback on their experience; this may be particularly important in teaching institutions, where families interact with many clinicians in training. A single comment can have huge potential for practice improvement. For example, here is a direct quotation from a son of an ICU patient in a plea to a medical resident after his mother died:

'Please don't rush. Make me feel like I am the most important person in the world to you right now. Listen twice as much as you talk. Don't just use your mouth; show me how you feel with your eyes.'

Some clinicians keep a personal diary of their own end-of-life clinical experiences and some ICUs hold formal multidisciplinary rounds to debrief each death in the ICU. Informal interchanges help us to understand different perspectives on the nature of the dying process and help health care teams deal with their own bereavement issues.

Encouraging the bereaved persons (whether families or staff) to talk or write about their experiences can be very powerful. The experiences of an oncology nurse whose sister died after a long ICU illness is described later in this book (see 📖 Ch. 11). The submission of her manuscript to a critical care journal initiated an innovative section dedicated to the bedside experience in the Journal of Critical Care.

While we are addressing family bereavement in the ICU and learning to initiate interventions to reduce depression following bereavement and post-traumatic stress disorder symptoms, we have been slow to recognize that the ICU staff also deal with challenging emotional reactions. We also need to find ways to reduce the effects of vicarious suffering (for sections on moral distress see 📖 p174 and iatrogenic suffering p162).

If we become more familiar with our own emotions through being in touch with ourselves and with our colleagues, and by taking part in regular discussions about death and dying in the ICU, we will be able to reach out more effectively and empathetically to the patients and families for whom we care.

Conclusions

It is our responsibility to provide high quality end-of-life care in the ICU, and to implement and evaluate numerous emerging interventions that may ease the dying process for patients, their families, and the ICU team. While many of our institutions have 'closed' ICUs in which patient care is intensivist-led, all our ICUs should be open to innovative strategies to improve and optimize the care of the dying. To accompany a thematic edition of the Journal of Palliative Care dedicated to ICU patients, editor Dr David Roy wrote:

'The time for decisions about life-prolonging treatment is a time marked by great uncertainty, stress and distress, anguish, and by the threats of impending loss. Preparing for these decisions, making them, and compassionate caring for the sick and for their families involved in these decisions and in the aftermath of these decisions are all integral elements of palliative care. If the ICU is so often the place where such decisions have to be made and lived through, then the ICU is a place for palliative care.'

Further reading

1. Roy D (2000). The times and places of palliative care. *J Palliat Care* **16**(Suppl), S3–4.
2. Cook DJ, Rocker GM, Heyland DK (2004). Dying in the ICU: interventions to improve end-of-life care. *Can J Anesthes* **51**, 266–72.

Care of the dying patient in the ICU, part 1: a global overview

Introduction

Recently, Angus and colleagues reported that in the US, 1 in 5 Americans die in an intensive care setting. That equates to 500,000 deaths in an ICU annually.[1] UK data indicates 12,258 ICU deaths (18.6% of ICU admissions) in England, Wales, and Northern Ireland).[2] Worldwide the doubling of persons over the age of 65 by 2030 will impose huge challenges to our heath care systems and we will require a system-wide expansion in ICU care for dying patients unless there is rationing or more effective advanced care planning, and a huge increase in capacity to care for dying patients in other settings.

Historical perspective

- In the early days of modern medicine, the lack of effective therapies was accompanied by well-developed medical skills in the management of death and dying.
- After World War II, improved support of ventilation and circulation ushered in a more technological approach to medicine.
- This seduced the medical profession to the point where death became a failure and the skills to deal well with death and dying were largely lost.
- This era was followed by a period of changes in society's expectations and a relative disenchantment with technology (e.g. more rational use of Swan Ganz catheters, extracorporeal membrane oxygenation (ECMO), etc.).
- The new era was one of a more humane approach to care.
- The goal of survival at any cost has been supplanted by a need to avoid prolonged dying in the absence of a reasonable expectation of return to function acceptable to the patient.
- More recently, various workers have begun to apply scientific methodology to the study of end-of-life issues. The results are of considerable interest although it is still unknown how well the results from one country apply to another.
- This increasingly humane approach is best encapsulated in the words of GR Dunstan, the Emeritus Professor of Moral and Social Philosophy at the University of London who stated in 1985:

'The success of intensive care is not to be measured only by the statistics of survival, as though each death were a medical failure. It is to be measured by the quality of lives preserved or restored, the quality of the dying of those in whose interest it is to die, and by the quality of relationships involved in each death.'

- More informed and demanding consumers mean that we should be moving away from what appeared to be an unacceptable incidence of unwelcome and suboptimal treatment that seemed to be a feature of critical care reported in SUPPORT.

- How patients die in ICUs is similar in many parts of the world (for an example from Australia, see Table 1.1).
- Worldwide, the incidence of withdrawal or withholding of treatment prior to death is common in ICUs in developed countries and ranges between 40 to 80% of patients.
- Decisions that result in withholding or withdrawal of life support are reached every week in most modern day medical/surgical ICUs.

Table 1.1 Mechanism of death in 480 consecutive patients in Royal North Shore Hospital, Sydney, Australia

Full treatment	9.0%
Brain death	10.5%
CPR only withheld	11.5%
Life support withheld	22.0%
Life support withdrawn	47.0%

How end-of-life decisions are made

Consideration should be given to initiating end-of-life discussions when:
- The patient makes such a request.
- A relative or significant other, in relation to an incompetent patient, makes such a request.
- A member of the patient's health care team raises this matter with the specialist in charge.
- The specialist in charge judges the patient's condition to conform to one or more of these medical criteria:
  - The patient has a diagnosis with grave prognosis.
  - The burdens of therapy outweigh the benefits from a patient's perspective.
  - The outcome is likely to be unacceptable to the patient.

Civetta[2] described a concept of assessing the appropriateness of care based on a model developed by Chaplain Ernle Young. In this model, an individual life is considered as a continuum between birth and death. At the beginning of life, the preservation of life has the highest priority; sanctity of life has precedence over quality of life. As the end of life approaches, the priorities alter. Alleviation of suffering to preserve quality of life may take precedence over the preservation of life for its own sake. Thus, for each individual life, there comes a time when the priorities change to a focus where alleviation of suffering becomes the major goal. In helping to determine when the main focus should be on palliation, there are two major considerations:
- Objective medical data concerning likely outcome.
- Subjective assessment of quality of life.

Objective assessment of survival probability

While objective assessment of the probability of survival in ICUs should appear easier to determine than other subjective values, the fundamental problem with the application of predictive data is that virtually every study provides a range of probabilities of death (e.g. 10–20%) or survival. For patients or relatives not fully cognizant of the suffering and loss of dignity related to treatment and not in the least concerned about the costs to the community of treatment, any chance may be worthwhile. Medical consensus and consensus within the broader ICU team about prognosis should be achieved prior to initiating family discussions. If individual doctors do not agree with the decision, they should be given the option of providing supporting opinions from their peers or withdrawing from the case.

Subjective assessment of value of treatment
When the objective chances of a successful or unsuccessful outcome are determined as far as can be, the subjective aspects should be considered. This involves:
• The assessment of the quality of life of the patient prior to illness.
• The suffering consequent upon treatment.
• The likely quality of life and longevity if treatment is associated with a successful outcome.

The only person who has the experience and standards to evaluate the quality of a patient's life is the patient and others may need to speak for them. When the patient can be involved in the process, the patient's assessment of quality of life is paramount, with the proviso that the effects of stress and pain and psychological disturbances, which may be remedied, may give the patient an inappropriate perspective at a particular time. When the patient cannot be involved in the decision-making process, discussion between health care providers and relatives should endeavour to determine the patient's values, and not inflict those of others upon the patient.

Scientific studies of such decision-making emphasize the value of an informed surrogate or 'person responsible'.

Integrating subjective and objective data determines the plan to be adopted. The benefit of any uncertainty should be given to the patient. Where doubt exists, treatment should be instituted and reconsidered later when more information becomes available.

The negotiation process
Nursing and ancillary staff, as deliverers of care, should also be involved prior to family discussions. The nursing staff will be the continuing providers of bedside care to the patient and family. Efforts should be made to contact any nurse who has shown particular interest in the patient and family or expended considerable energy in the patient's care, although shift work may make this difficult. Sternburg has emphasized the importance of nursing participation in the decision-making process, and notes the frustration experienced by nurses who are required to participate in care they may feel is inappropriate. The importance of group involvement is two-fold:
• Individual bias may be balanced.
• Support can be enlisted for the major participants, both providers and receivers.

When the providers are in agreement, the discussions with the family should begin.

Factors minimizing conflict with families
- The decision to withdraw treatment evolves. It is not a single event.
- Involvement of clinicians, nurses, and the family is a progressive undertaking in the course of the patient's illness.
- Several factors are likely to be associated with harmonious end-of-life negotiation.

The ICU as an environment for palliative care
Good management of death and dying has value to staff as well as to patients, relatives, and society, and should be as much a part of quality care as curative medicine. For the staff, such management produces feelings of a job well done rather than failure, and produces the benefits of realistic expectations, better interpersonal relationships, and improved teamwork. The rewards to clinicians provided by a well-managed death may be as great as those provided by a cure.

For families
- An atmosphere of quiet competence and efficiency that engenders confidence.
- Any interpersonal hostility among staff, noise, and drama provoke anxiety and hostility among families.

Ways to humanize the ICU
- Noise reduction.
- Windows with a view.
- Pictures.
- Privacy.
- Allow personal items such as picture, clothes, books, or toys (all helps to ameliorate the technological hostility of the environment).
- Keep the dying patient in the unit, wherever possible, although we explain that ICU is a limited resource and it may become necessary to transfer the patient. If transfer is necessary:
  - Maintain contact with the family and patient (who usually accept the changed circumstances).
- Minimize things that make us different from the patients and families. For example, in Sydney, Australia, these include uniforms, white coats, and scrubs. We introduce ourselves by first names, thereby giving patients and families the opportunity to choose between using a name or a title. We wait to be invited by patient or family to use first names with them.

Ethnicity and religion
It is important to show respect for cultural and religious beliefs, particularly to minority groups.
- Early involvement of religious or tribal leaders is important. This is an important issue in many parts of the world.
- Do not assume that members of any group have homogeneous views.
- Increasing liberalism and the presence of diverse sects in religions mean inconsistency. Religious and cultural attitudes may be modified over generations, particularly after immigration into another society. Cultural and religious beliefs may place a doctor in conflict with a family.

- Conflicts arise with families who believe it is wrong to inform the patient that they are at the end of life.
- This belief is in contrast to the western ethic which dictates that the patient has an absolute right to information.
- We believe that the beliefs of the family and patient should have priority and that the provider whose beliefs do not permit acquiescence should withdraw from the process.

Earning trust
- The person orchestrating discussions with either the patient or family must be someone identifiable as being significantly involved in the active care of the patient.
- It is extremely important that this key person has earned trust and credibility before embarking on discussions to withdraw active therapy.
- Trust is earned by early communication and being seen at the bedside.
- Discussions about limited treatment should ideally be introduced progressively at a timescale dictated by the disease process and the preparedness of the participants to deal with the issues under discussion.
- To avoid any seeming conflict of opinions, it is preferable that a single resource person fills this role, even if this person is no longer nominally on-call.
- Changes in the person leading the discussion are a source of confusion and anxiety in families.

The language of the end-of-life conference
- It is important that the discussions proceed in a language that is understood by all the participants.
- Our social worker or nurse remains with the family after the doctor leaves to ensure that the conversation is understood.
- Constantly and gently reinforce the fact that in these discussions, we are endeavouring to determine what is best for the patient and what the patients' wishes would be if he or she were able to participate in the discussion, and that what the family and providers want is of secondary importance.
- Economic realities and demand for beds that clearly impact on the availability of health care have no place in end-of-life negotiations.
- The family is concerned for their loved one and rightly regards triage and cost as a unit problem, not their problem.

Leadership
Where a palliative care option is under consideration, the lead physician should:
- Present the necessary information to patient and/or relations.
- Present an opinion and provide time for discussion.
- Then embark on a management plan involving the entire family unit.

It is our perception that few relatives wish to take the responsibility for making the decision to withdraw treatment. Making decisions that lead to the inevitable death of a loved one likely constitutes an unwelcome burden. Physician-guided consensus is the approach followed.

Should relatives want to take responsibility for the decision to withdraw treatment, it is probable that the appropriate response would be to provide them with sufficient information to enable them to feel comfortable with that decision if there is medical consensus that it is the correct option. In our practice, we have not met such a relative.

Conclusion

- I have presented our philosophy of and experience in the management of the dying patient in ICUs, and practical aspects of implementation.
- The concept of death as a medical failure is outdated.
- Doctors need to be more involved in the care of the dying patient and be aware of the issues that arise.

References

1. Angus DC, Barnato AE, Linde–Zwirbie WT, et al. (2004). Use of intensive care at the end of life in the United States: an epidemiologic study. *Crit Care Med* **32**, 638–43.
2. Intensive Care National Audit and Research Centre, www.icnarc.org/documents/summarystatistics 2006–7.pdf
3. Civetta JM (1981). Beyond technology: intensive care in the 1980s. *Crit Care Med* **9**, 763–7.

Further reading

1. The SUPPORT Investigators (1995). A controlled trial to improve care for seriously ill hospitalized patients. The study to understand prognoses and preferences for outcomes and risks of treatment (SUPPORT). *JAMA* **274**, 1591–8.
2. Prendergast TJ, Luce JM (1997). Increasing incidence of withholding and withdrawing of life support from the critically ill. *Am J Respir Crit Care Med* **155**, 15–20.

Care of the dying patient in the ICU, part 2: some current challenges

There are a number of reasons why end-of-life care seems to me to be getting harder:
- Rising consumer expectations.
  - When we give them the options of survival vs death.
  - And/or they want us 'to do everything'.
- Consumer awareness of evidence-based medicine.
- Issues of trust.
- Uncertainty of prognosis.
- Increasing primacy of protocols and clinical pathways.
- Treatment is initially an easier option than withholding treatment.

Consumer expectations

This is fostered by the media (especially TV) and greater internet access. The media highlights:
- Major breakthroughs.
- People who survived 'against the odds'.
- Survivors despite hospital teams saying it was hopeless. (In the latter instance, following up the case usually reveals a dichotomy between the information as it was given and as it was received.)
- Fictional hospital TV shows high success and survival rates have been shown to influence the views of both patients and doctors.

In contrast, the highlighting of medical errors in the media fosters mistrust of hospitals and doctors.

The internet provides easy access to descriptions of miracles such as awakening after long periods of coma, and 'treatments which the medical profession has ignored', all of which may bolster peoples' hopes. These hopes are often reinforced by the language of medicine where there are attempts to try 'just one more additional treatment.'

The options of survival or death are often put to consumers in a very simplified fashion.
- Not surprisingly given a simple choice, choice is often made for survival.
- It is often difficult for consumers to accept the concept of suffering in a patient who is sedated, and to all intents and purposes, looks comfortable.
- While the medical profession focuses on evidence-based medicine, non-medical consumers have little grasp of this concept.
- Internet information has often not been subject to critical review or is outside the mainstream, and maybe merely misleading.
- It is important to be tolerant of families who bring internet-based information to meetings, to read it, and to, wherever possible, explain any fallacies.

Palliative care physicians emphasize goals of care and this language can help. The options can be explained in terms of degrees or intensity of treatment (that is now not working) and the need for increasing the palliative care component—the latter being defined as making the patient's life as dignified, peaceful, and comfortable as possible. This should be followed by a discussion of various treatment modalities in terms of those which will and will not allow new or changing goals of care to be achieved.

Wanting everything done

There seems something absurd about the question often posed to patients and families, 'Do you want everything done?' The question inevitably invites a positive answer. This isn't surprising if there's a perception that 'everything' can be done. Most of us would think 'Do you want us to do nothing?' to be an unacceptable alternative. Families would perceive this as an invitation to abandonment. The expression 'no reasonable chance', albeit leading to the ethical dilemma of who decides what is reasonable, is a preferable approach to 'Do you want everything done?' Meanwhile, when families state without being asked (and often do) that they want everything done, it is important to explore what they mean by everything. This can be done by:

- Stepping back.
- Refocusing on the patient as a human being with values and needs.
- Then exploring whether current or proposed care is in alignment with this additional knowledge.
- It is essential to:
  - Assess the overall clinical situation prior to initiating discussions with the family.
  - And to discuss possibilities of adverse outcomes and suffering prior to any discussions about limiting treatment.
- It is also very important to emphasize to the family that the goal of discussions is to determine the patient's wishes rather than the wishes of the family or the carers.
- It is useful to point out that 'everything' is not an option. I begin that discussion with heart transplantation and then follow to explain that ventilation or dialysis is equally likely to be unsuccessful.

One of the problems that compound any difficult discussion about withholding/withdrawing life support treatment is that the patient is a stranger to the providers. Sometimes medical records are available and sometimes not. It is helpful to contact early someone who is known to the patient and family, particularly the family doctor, and involve them in the discussion processes.

Trust

When active treatment is to be withdrawn in the ICU after a period of treatment, a relationship has been established with patient and family.

- If there is confidence in the team and trust has been established, discussions focused on what is best for the patient are usually harmonious.
- In the emergency unit or wards, where the medical team is strangers, establishing trust is difficult.

This may be a particular problem with patients undergoing treatment for malignancy (where there is often repeated emphasis on cure). When the focus needs to change because cure is not possible, it is usually helpful to contact early a medical practitioner who is known to the patient and the relatives, and involve them in the discussion processes, in person, if possible, or by telephone, if not.

Uncertainty of prognosis

Uncertainty can be a problem in both family discussions and in the practitioner's confidence that the treatment plan is the optimal one. Nevertheless, patients and families seem comfortable with admissions of uncertainty. Mathematical scoring systems have many weaknesses and in general do not help in individual cases.

- Where there is hard outcome data for a particular condition, make this available to those involved in the discussion.
- Many factors influence the prognosis that is given to patients including:
  - Knowledge, beliefs, and motives of the practitioner.
  - Knowledge, beliefs, and motives of the family.

There will always be a few 'miracle' patients who defy predictive algorithms, wisdom, and experience, and who survive in spite of enormous odds. Mostly, this does not happen. Giving odds of say 1 in 10 chances of survival means little to people who buy lottery tickets. It is better in practical terms to use the expression 'No reasonable chance'. The best option to minimize the possibility of error is to engage a number of experienced clinicians and seek medical consensus regarding prognosis prior to initiating discussions.

Protocols and clinical pathways

While intuitively attractive, my personal view is that over-application of algorithms and pathways runs a risk of reducing patient care to impersonal menu-driven treatment in which the patient falls into the hands of the doctor technician. Finding A might lead to intervention B with little consideration of appropriateness or the patient's wishes. Where speed becomes essential, the wishes of the patient are rarely considered.

It is easier to treat than not to treat

The clinical settings where end-of-life care decisions need to be made are, by definition, complex. It may be an over-simplification, but it is true, nevertheless, that intubation and stabilization of a patient can almost always be achieved with more alacrity than any complex family discussions. Furthermore, it is, and should be, a reasonable use of ICU resources to provide a short period of intensive care, even to patients unlikely to survive, while families come together and are given time to accept the impending loss.

Conclusion: it all comes down to communication

Many advocate new paradigms where we accept the fallibility of medical predictions and the need to refocus care in terms of patients' values and preferences in the best interests of both individual patients and society. However, ultimately, the most important way in which we could reduce the problems associated with surrogate decision-making is adequate end-of-life planning earlier in disease trajectories, particularly the nomination of an informed surrogate.

Triage in the ICU

Introduction

The purpose of admission to the ICU is to diagnose, monitor, prevent, and treat multiple organ failure in severely ill patients. Given that mortality in an adult medical/surgical ICU often approaches 10–20%, ICUs play a vital role in end-of-life care for many patients.

The overall benefits of ICU admission remain unclear; although intensive care increases the number of survivors in the short term, it can merely prolong the dying process for some patients who have fatal underlying diseases. Moreover, studies like SUPPORT underpin the fact that in the past, many patients have been admitted to ICUs for treatment that was often unwelcome and ultimately, not of benefit.

ICUs offer specialized and costly medical services to a minority of patients. This creates three main challenges:

- How do intensivists make choices to use scarce resources for those patients who are most likely to benefit?
- How do we avoid mistakes in the classification of who might benefit if the patient is inappropriately refused or to unnecessary suffering (if the patient is inappropriately admitted)?
- How do ICUs and ICU teams justify either acceptance or refusal of patients for whom the focus of care becomes more predominantly palliative rather than potentially curative?

The selection procedure: 'triage'

Triage is a complex procedure that is based largely on non-scientific factors, some of which are arbitrary. This lack of sound objective data for triaging explains why triage practices vary widely across countries, institutions, as well as across physicians in a given institution. This selection procedure:

- Depends on a myriad of factors.
- Often involves a single physician who has not had the opportunity to build a relationship with the patient previously.
- Is often not supported by written criteria for ICU admission and discharge.
- Must often be conducted without detailed information on the patient's past and present health problems.
- Must often be conducted without the knowledge of the patient's preferences regarding ICU admission or treatment modalities or for levels of care.

Triage includes three phases:

- The pre-ICU phase (pre-triage) is conducted by the emergency physician or other clinicians who identify patients meeting the criteria for referral to the ICU. Several factors induce reluctance to refer patients to the ICU:
  - Advanced age, severe illness, poor prognostic factors.
  - Experience with similar patients being consistently refused ICU admission.
  - Apprehension about being judged incompetent by the intensivists or previous acrimonious interactions with the ICU team.
  - Extent of prior consideration/documentation of palliative issues.

- Triage, strictly speaking (ICU triage), is conducted jointly by the referring physician and the ICU physician. These two physicians may disagree about the appropriateness of ICU admission for individual patients, including those who ultimately might not survive, and friction may also arise with the family regarding the triage decision.
- The post-ICU phase is influenced by bed availability in ICUs and wards.
  - Whether intermediate care beds are available has a major influence on practices regarding patient discharge from the ICU. Patients who would be eligible for intermediate care, but are too close to death or too severely ill to be discharged to a ward, remain in the ICU if there is no intermediate care unit.
  - In some countries, patients without organ dysfunction cannot be transferred to the wards if they require specific types of life-supporting care, such as mechanical ventilation or a tracheostomy.

The population referred to intensivists for triage to the ICU may represent only a small proportion of patients who meet criteria for ICU referral. In a study conducted in the Paris area, France, only 25% of patients aged 80 years or over, who met ICU admission criteria defined in the Society of Critical Care Medicine guidelines, were referred to the ICU.

What criteria do physicians use for triage?

Studies available for triage have been conducted in only a few countries (France, Hong Kong, Israel, and Jamaica). ICU admission practices vary across countries.

- In some European countries and in several institutions in Canada, patients are triaged by the ICU physician, who often makes the decision alone and refuses patients deemed too sick or too well to benefit from ICU admission.
- In the UK, triage is also undertaken by senior critical care outreach nurses or medical emergency teams (MET). METs or rapid response teams (see 📖 Ch. 6) are operational in approximately 50% of UK hospitals and are used increasingly in Australia and Canada.
- In the US, nearly all patients with life-threatening illnesses are admitted to the ICU, regardless of their prospects for recovering from their acute illness or surviving their underlying disease with acceptable quality of life, unless the patient or surrogate declines ICU admission. Thus, refusal of ICU admission is uncommon, and when no beds are available, a patient is moved out to make room for the new patient, a strategy known as bumping. Triage decisions are usually made by a single physician.
- Guidelines for ICU admission and discharge have been developed using models based on prioritization, diagnosis, projected prognosis, or objective parameters. Unfortunately, these guidelines rest chiefly on expert opinion, as opposed to objective scientific data. In a study of patients aged 80 years or over, only 25% of patients who met the criteria set forth in the guidelines were referred for ICU admission.
- Triage is usually based largely on subjective factors related to the triaging physician. As a result, considerable variability occurs regarding triaging decisions for a given patient.
- These differences in triaging practices across countries hinder comparisons of reported ICU refusal rates.

- The rate of ICU refusal varied from 24% to 53%. In the only study that focused on the 80 and over age group, 72% of referred patients were refused.
- The refusal rate was strongly centre-dependent, with a range of 7% to 63% in a study of 11 ICUs in France.
- Both organizational and patient-related criteria influence the triage decisions made by intensivists.
- Organizational factors:
  - Circumstances of triage: triaging over the phone or after examining the medical file without seeing the patient is associated with higher ICU admission rates.
  - Time of referral.
  - Status of the triaging intensivist.
  - Bed availability.
  - Centre effect.
- Patient-related factors:
  - Severity of the acute illness.
  - Age older than 65 years is associated with ICU refusal in the overall population of referred patients. In the only study of patients aged 80 or over, being older than 85 was associated with refusal.
  - Comorbid conditions such as chronic respiratory or heart failure.
  - Medical conditions likely to cause death in the very short term such as metastatic cancer.
  - Self-sufficiency before admission.
  - Quality of life before admission is not widely used as a triage criterion, perhaps because there is no time for a reliable assessment of quality of life.

Of the patient-related criteria that influence triage decisions, all but one—the severity of the acute illness—are present before the acute illness arises. Therefore, patients should be encouraged to discuss their preferences regarding ICU admission at a time when they are still relatively healthy and free of life-threatening events.

Criteria considered important for triage in several consensus statements include the following:

- Risk of death due to the acute disease.
- Expected quality of life of the patient after ICU discharge.
- Wishes of the patient or surrogate regarding ICU admission.
- Burden that ICU admission may cause for the family or surrogate.
- Health needs and other needs of the community.
- Individual, institutional, ethical, and religious values.
- These criteria are rarely used as they are extremely difficult to assess in an emergency.

How can we evaluate triage?

Studies of triage have described procedures for selecting patients to ICU admission, but have failed to quantify lost opportunities associated with ICU refusal. Many studies failed to accurately adjust for confounding factors during the triage phase. Consequently, mortality rates in admitted and refused patients are difficult to interpret.

Triage should be evaluated based on comparisons of not just hospital mortality in both admitted and refused patients, but also on the quality of life after hospital discharge in admitted patients.

Quality of life after discharge

Survival to discharge from the ICU or hospital may not be the best end point for evaluating the impact of ICU admission. The traditional goal of critical care is to restore the pre-admission functional status and to return the patient to his or her previous living arrangements.

Therefore, the most appropriate end point may be the quality of life as assessed by the patient or the patient's answer to the question 'Was your ICU stay worth it?'

The best time after ICU discharge for evaluating quality of life is unclear. However, 6 to 12 months seem reasonable. However, in trauma patients, a longer interval may be preferable. Serial quality-of-life evaluations may be desirable to capture the dynamics of recovery over time.

Quality of life depends on several factors: age, severity at admission, reason for admission, pre-admission status, and events acquired in the ICU. Quality of life can be evaluated quantitatively or qualitatively.

- Quantitative evaluations rely on specific validated scales that explore domains such as social isolation, pain, energy, psychosocial issues, sleep, and physical mobility. The answers are weighted and the global quality-of-life score is computed. This approach permits comparisons of the study cohort and the general population.
- Qualitative evaluations are based on interviews with the patients. They are time-consuming, but are often better than scales when exploring issues that are influenced by personal values and beliefs, particularly in the psychosocial domains.

Studies performed in the overall ICU population showed that most patients were satisfied with their quality of life six months after hospital discharge and that their status was roughly unchanged compared to before their admission. Patients reported a faster recovery from the psychosocial effects of ICU admission than from the physical effects. In the elderly, similar results were obtained with a good perceived quality of life. However, these older patients reported more depression, more isolation, and less mobility compared to same age individuals with no history of ICU admission.

Conclusions

- Considerable heterogeneity in refusal rates exists across countries and within a given country.
- ICU refusal is associated with both organizational factors and patient-related factors.
- The most significant patient-related factor is the pre-admission status.
- The lost opportunity associated with ICU refusal is difficult to assess, although intuition suggests that it may exist.
- Evaluations of triaging should rely on adjusted ICU mortality and quality of life in admitted patients to determine whether the triage process reliably identifies those patients who have a substantial chance of recovery.

Further reading

1. Azoulay E, Pochard F, Chevret S, *et al.* (2001). Compliance with triage to intensive care recommendations. *Crit Care Med* **29**, 2132–6.
2. Sprung CL, Geber D, Eidelman LA, *et al.* (1999). Evaluation of triage decisions for intensive care admission. *Crit Care Med* **27**, 1073–9.
3. Garrouste–Orgeas M, Montuclard L, Timsit JF, *et al.* (2005). Predictors of intensive care unit refusal in French intensive care units: a multiple-centre study. *Crit Care Med* **33**, 750–5.
4. Sinuff T, Kahnamoui K, Cook DJ, Luce JM, Levy MM (2004). Rationing critical care beds: a systematic review. *Crit Care Med* **32**, 1588–97.
5. Carlet J, Thijs LG, Antonelli M, *et al.* (2004). Challenges in end-of-life care in the ICU. Statement of the 5th International Consensus Conference in Critical Care, Brussels, Belgium, April 2003. *Intensive Care Med* **30**, 770–84.

Older patients in the ICU

Introduction

Worldwide, there are 70 million people aged 80 or over, most of whom live in industrialized countries. The 'over 80' population is expected to grow five-fold by 2050. Lower birth rates and longer lifespans are increasing the proportion of older individuals in the general population.

The increasing number of older people will raise challenges for critical care providers. Medical advances made over the last few decades have had a considerable impact in ICU. However, when used inappropriately, modern treatments technologies may merely prolong the dying process, and divest patients of their dignity.

There are challenges at three major levels:

- For ICU physicians, the challenge is to identify those older patients who are likely to benefit from ICU admission.
- For hospital managers, the challenge is to create care systems that help frail, elderly patients recover after ICU discharge.
- For society, the challenge is to allow patients to express their wishes regarding involvement in making decisions about their own care.

Who is old?

In the medical literature, fixed chronological age ranges are widely used to define groups of elderly patients: 75–79 years for the 'young old', 80–85 years for the 'old old', and more than 85 years for the 'oldest old'.

This type of classification fails to take into account:

- Changes in life expectancy that occur within populations.
- Marked inter-individual heterogeneity that characterizes organ reserve, responses to treatments, and self-sufficiency.
- Physiological age, which reflects changes in organ function over time, is more informative than chronological age.
- The terms 'frail' and 'vulnerable' that are often used to distinguish old people who are in poor general condition or at high risk of death from people who are in the same chronological age group, but who are doing well.

Who is admitted to the ICU and who is not?

The challenge for ICU physicians is to recognize which older patients may benefit from ICU admission. Older patients are often refused ICU admission, and age has been a consistent independent risk factor for refusal of admission in studies of triaging to the ICU.

- Among patients aged 80 years or over, 70% are refused ICU admission (vs 24% to 50% in a general population of patients).
- The decision about ICU admission depends on a myriad of medical and organizational factors.
- Surgical patients are less likely to be refused ICU admission.
- Bed availability, local factors, time in the 24-hour cycle, and ICU experience of the physician can all influence the decision to grant or to refuse ICU admission.

ICU characteristics of admitted patients once admitted to an ICU:

- ICU and hospital lengths of stay and the proportion of mechanically ventilated patients are similar in the younger and older age groups.
- Workloads (as assessed using specific tools) are similar or lower in older patients.
- After adjustment for the severity of illness, treatment is less aggressive in patients older than 80 years than in patients aged 65 to 75 years; more specifically, mechanical ventilation, dialysis, and tracheotomy are less often used.

What defines successful critical care?

While a goal of critical care is to restore a patient to the pre-admission level of function and to return the patient to his or her pre-admission social setting:

- Many older ICU patients are discharged to long-term care facilities.
- Age over 80 is an independent factor for discharge from the hospital to a long-term care facility.
- Post-discharge self-sufficiency and quality of life six months or one year after ICU discharge are likely to be more important than ICU or hospital mortality for assessing the impact of ICU admission in elderly patients.

Mortality in the ICU

ICU mortality is related to a combination of multiple factors, including age, severity of illness at admission, admission diagnosis, comorbid conditions, self-sufficiency, and conditions acquired in the ICU (iatrogenic events, nosocomial infections, and pressure sores). When these factors are assessed by multivariate analysis, the strongest independent risk factor for mortality is the severity of illness at admission.

- Age per se makes a very small contribution to mortality compared to organ failure and disease severity.
- Age alone is not a reason to refuse ICU admission since older age has little independent impact on ICU mortality.

Admission rates among older patients referred to the ICU show considerable centre-to-centre variability, with a range of 14% to 30%. Mortality rates in the elderly vary widely, from 20% to 50%, suggesting a role for case mix. Cardiopulmonary resuscitation prior to ICU admission carries a grim prognosis in older patients. As with other age groups, older patients who die in the ICU usually have prior treatment limitation decisions. The rate of treatment limitation decisions in older ICU patients worldwide is unknown.

Mortality after hospital discharge

After hospital discharge, mortality is consistently higher in older than in younger patients. Post-hospital mortality depends on age, function before ICU admission, and comorbid conditions.

- Mortality is highest within the first three months after ICU discharge, when the proportion of deaths is considerably higher than in same age individuals with no history of ICU admission.

- Other factors, such as patient preferences and differences in practice patterns across physicians, may have a greater impact on mortality in older than in younger patients.
- One year after ICU discharge, 30% to 40% of older patients are still alive.
- The influence of ICU admission one, two, or three years after ICU discharge is minimal compared to the effect of age, comorbid conditions, and self-sufficiency.

Quality of life

Quality of life (QoL) is a multidimensional personal concept that covers all aspects of life considered important by the individual. These aspects may include a variable combination of the following:
- Physical function.
- Ability to perform daily activities.
- Mental health.
- Social function.
- Pain, fatigue, and energy.
- Sleep.
- Sexual function.

These aspects of health are influenced by many factors. Although they are not age-dependent, the relative importance of each aspect may vary across age groups. Specific scales for ageing are being introduced. There is a complex relationship between declining function, which is an inevitable concomitant of ageing, and QoL.

QoL is best evaluated during a face-to-face interview with the patient, at a time when the patient is doing well and can express personal feelings and opinions. QoL assessments will be suboptimal:
- During ICU triage.
- If dependent only on interviewing the family or proxies (though inevitably, this will occur in settings where patients lack decisional capacity).

Few studies have addressed QoL in the elderly and, more specifically, in the 'over 80' age group.
- Quantitative studies based on scales are heterogeneous (single centre, prospective or retrospective, different case mixes).
  - Perceived QoL in older patients is not different from that in younger groups and increases over time despite a decrease in the ability to perform activities of daily living.
  - Compared to the general population, QoL is worse regarding isolation, mobility, and physical function.
- Qualitative studies based on in-depth interviews are very few.
  - QoL is the ability to maintain self-image, self-esteem, and the meaning of life.
  - The most important factor is maintaining social relations, activities, health, and projects for the future.
  - Some patients would be unwilling to exchange any time spent living in their current state of health for a shorter life in excellent health. Life is precious, even for frail elderly people.

Independent living or self-sufficiency

Older patients are at risk for subsequent poor functional status:
• As a result of failure to recover the ability to perform activities of daily living to the same extent as before admission.
• As a result of impairments acquired during the ICU stay.

Self-sufficiency can be evaluated based on the ability to perform activities of daily living, such as dressing, bathing, maintaining sphincter control, toileting, transferring, and eating. The ability to perform activities of daily living can be reported by the patient and by the family at any time during the hospital stay.

There are few studies on self-sufficiency in the elderly, and more specifically, in the 'over 80' age group.
• Activities of daily living are unchanged one or two years after ICU discharge compared to the pre-admission status.

Patient preferences

Patient-centred care is a cornerstone of quality healthcare. Patient-centred care involves allowing the patient to participate in decisions about his or her health care and placing emphasis on the patient's needs and preferences.

Efforts to promote participation of older patients in their care have met with limited success for the following reasons:
• Older patients often feel it is not their place to participate in their care.
• Patients may feel that the details of their everyday life are too intimate to be discussed with their physician.
• The patient may feel ready to discuss the issue of participation at a time when the physician is under too much work pressure to have time for an in-depth interview.

Physicians are often unaware of the patient's preferences regarding ICU admission and whether ICU admission and mechanical ventilation or other treatments would be welcomed, even when the underlying condition is chronic and has progressed slowly over several years.

Findings from the few studies on consent to care in elderly patients showed the following:
• Consent to ICU admission is not influenced by previous quality of life. Therefore, QoL, as estimated by the physician at the time of triage, is not a reliable marker for the patient's willingness to be admitted.
• Physicians overestimate the willingness of patients to consent to mechanical ventilation, dialysis, or surgery.
• Senior intensivists are not better at predicting patients' wishes than are intensivists in training.

Conclusions

Providing high quality care to the very old will be a major challenge for intensivists over the next few decades. In the future, ICUs specifically for the elderly may need to be created.

Research on older patients should pursue two goals:
• Development of a general scoring system that takes into account all the determinants of hospital mortality in the elderly to quantify the loss of chance associated with refusal of ICU admission.

- Education of the general population about participation in health care decisions and the need to express health care-related wishes before the development of immediately life-threatening events.

Further reading

1. Garrouste-Orgeas M, Timsit JF, Montuclard L, et al. (2006). Decision-making process, outcome, and 1-year quality of life of octogenarians referred for intensive care unit admission. *Intensive Care Med* **32**, 1045–51.
2. Walke LM, Gallo WT, Tinetti ME, Fried TR (2004). The burden of symptoms among community-dwelling older persons with advanced chronic disease. *Arch Intern Med* **164**, 2321–4.
3. Fried TR, Bradley EH, Towle VR, Allore H (2002). Understanding the treatment preferences of seriously ill patients. *N Engl J Med* **346**, 1061–6.

Complications of cancer and ICU admission decisions

Introduction

For many years, it was assumed that cancer patients who required ICU admission had a very poor prognosis, raising the question of the justification of intensive care in this setting. Many intensive care physicians became reluctant to admit such patients to the ICU, despite requests from colleagues in haematology and oncology who had invested so much in the care of these patients. Fortunately, the overall mortality from cancer has dropped by 20% over the last two decades as a consequence of advances in treatment of malignancies and in supportive care. Within this same time frame, numerous studies have reported improved outcomes of ICU cancer patients with actual survival rates of 35–50%. In this chapter, we will discuss current indications for ICU admission for patients who have complications of cancer within the context of providing justifiable uses of ICU resources and avoidance of unnecessary suffering.

What factors account for improved outcomes for cancer patients in the ICU?

Advances in the treatment of malignancies

- Over the last two decades, new therapeutic approaches have translated into improved disease-free and overall survival, either through enhanced anti-tumoural activity, early detection of relapse, or through decreased treatment-related toxicity. For example:
  - Monitoring of residual disease through the detection and quantification of transcript fusion (e.g. bcr-abl in chronic myeloid leukaemia) in patients with clinically undetectable disease.
  - Use of high-dose chemotherapy and total body irradiation, followed by autologous haematopoietic stem cell transplantation (HSCT).
  - Allogeneic HSCT: better selection of donors, non-myeloablative conditioning regimens, prophylaxis and treatment of graft-versus-host disease (GVHD), donor lymphocyte infusion in case of relapse.
  - New treatments directed against specific molecular targets: rituximab (non-Hodgkin lymphoma), herceptin (breast cancer), imatinib (chronic myeloid leukemia), all-trans retinoic acid and arsenic (acute myeloid leukemia (AML)-3), thalidomide and bortezomib (multiple myeloma), sunitinib and sorafenib (renal cell carcinoma).
- As a consequence, some patients with advanced disease or in poor general condition, who would have been considered for palliative care a few years ago, might actually be eligible for new treatment strategies that prolong survival.

Advances in surgical care

- For example, partial hepatectomy for liver metastases, radical trachelectomy, robotic prostatectomy, laryngeal surgery, and oesophagogastrectomy.

Advances in supportive care (availability may vary from country to country)

- Prevention and treatment of complications imposed by the disease itself or by treatments are major issues in the management of cancer patients.
- Prompt control of metabolic disorders (e.g. rasburicase for hyperuricaemia) in tumour lysis syndrome.
- Prevention and empirical and pre-emptive treatments of infections
  - Accelerated recovery from neutropaenia by G-CSF.
  - New tools for early diagnosis of infectious complications: PCR for virus detection such as cytomegalovirus (CMV) and enzyme-linked immunosorbant assay (ELISA) for Aspergillus galactomannan antigen detection.
  - New antifungal drugs that are less toxic and possibly more efficient (liposomal amphotericin B, caspofungin, voriconazole).
- Prevention (ursodeoxycholic acid) and treatment (defibrotide) of sinusoidal obstruction syndrome (hepatic veno-occlusive disease)

Advances in ICU care

- Acute respiratory failure and septic shock are the two main reasons for ICU admission in cancer patients. Improvements in outcome reflect:
  - Close collaboration between haematologists/oncologists and intensive care physicians.
  - Early identification of high-risk patients who could benefit from early aggressive management of organ failures.
  - Improved management of organ failures.
- Acute respiratory failure is a feared complication that frequently requires endotracheal intubation and mechanical ventilation in cancer patients.
  - Although numerous studies have reported a significant improvement in the outcome of mechanically ventilated cancer patients with actual survival rates of 35–50%, avoiding endotracheal intubation remains a major issue for cancer patients.
  - Non-invasive ventilation was shown to decrease the intubation rate and finally to improve survival in immunocompromised patients with acute respiratory failure. In addition, non-invasive ventilation applied during, and/or after fibreoptic bronchoscopy can improve the tolerance of the procedure and avoid the subsequent need for endotracheal intubation.
  - When endotracheal intubation is required, mechanical ventilation with low tidal volumes has been shown to improve survival rates in patients with acute lung injury and acute respiratory distress syndrome.
- The outcome of severe sepsis and septic shock is highly dependent on early and adequate treatment of infection, and on rapid and aggressive restoration of haemodynamics (early goal-directed therapy). In addition, although their true benefits remain questionable, some adjuvant therapies have been associated with better outcomes.
  - Low-dose corticosteroids.
  - Intensive insulin therapy.

- Drotrecogin alfa (activated protein C—although thrombocytopaenia will be a limiting factor for many patients).
- In cancer patients with septic shock, early admission to the ICU for aggressive management of organ failures and implementation of adjuvant therapies has been associated with improved outcome.

Malignancy-related characteristics and the triage decision

- **Characteristics** (type, nature, extent, and grade) of the underlying malignancy do not influence the short-term outcomes (28 days, ICU and hospital survival), but determine long-term outcomes (six months, one year) after recovery from acute illnesses. Because short-term survival is a necessary, but simplistic end point, the expected long-term outcome and future therapeutic options (if any) should be key components of the decision-making process. Accordingly, ICU admission is strongly advocated in the setting of complete remission or during the first line of treatment, while patients with end-stage diseases (expected lifespan <6 months) are poor candidates.
- **Newly diagnosed malignancies** may be complicated by life-threatening disorders that require prompt control of the underlying disease:
  - Tumour lysis syndrome (hyperleukocytic acute leukaemia, Burkitt lymphoma).
  - Coagulation disorders (AML-3).
  - Disseminated intravascular coagulation.
  - Pulmonary leukaemic infiltration (AML-4 and AML-5).
  - Bulky mediastinal tumours and superior vena cava obstruction.
  - Carotid artery rupture in head and neck cancers patients.
  - Chemotherapy-induced capillary leak syndrome.
  - Spinal cord compression.
  - Complications of use of trial drugs, e.g. neutropaenic sepsis.
  - Macrophage activation syndrome.

In this setting, chemotherapy is feasible in the ICU along with aggressive management of organ failures, even in the presence of concomitant infection, and can be lifesaving in a significant proportion of cases.

- **Allogeneic haematopoietic stem cell transplantation** still carries a poor prognosis in the ICU. Mechanical ventilation is associated with nearly 85% overall mortality. However, patients with complications occurring within the first 30 days following HSCT (engraftment period) fare better. Conversely, the value of mechanical ventilation is questionable for patients with extensive GVHD requiring high-dose corticosteroids and who sustain profound immune suppression.
- **Functional capacity**, as assessed by the Performance Status (PS), is an independent predictor of outcome for mechanically ventilated cancer patients. Thus, patients with major restriction (PS 3–4) are unlikely to benefit from intensive care.

Limits of ICU triage decisions

- Although cancer remains an independent risk factor for refusal of ICU, the spectrum of diseases is wide and heterogeneous, and cannot be considered as a single entity. The triage decision should take into account the relevant prognostic factors of each disease: type, extent, grade, and future therapeutic options.

- Even in centres in which ICU triage policies are based on an extensive experience with care of cancer patients, outcome predictions at ICU admission are inaccurate in a high proportion of patients.
- Indications for and timing of ICU admission substantially differ between haematologists/oncologists and intensive care physicians.
- The short-term outcome in the ICU is mainly related to the nature and extent of organ failures which may not be reliably assessed at ICU admission:
  - Severity scoring systems rely on variables collected during the first day of ICU stay, but are poor predictors of outcome in cancer patients and are not sufficiently accurate to be used in routine triage decision on an individual level.
  - In contrast, the time course of organ dysfunctions in the ICU, including the response to optimal management or further acquisition of additional organ failures, reliably refines the prediction of outcome.
- Advance directives are rarely utilized in Europe.

The benefit of the doubt: towards a broad ICU admission policy (see Fig. 1.1)

The ICU admission decision should be made by both the intensive care physician and the referring haematologist or oncologist, and involves consideration of accurate information regarding the disease status, a delineation of the goals of intensive care, and clear communication with patients and their relatives.

At the time of an ICU referral, some criteria can be used to more clearly support ICU admission or refusal:

- Newly diagnosed malignancy (first-line treatment) and complete remission are formal criteria for ICU admission and unlimited life-sustaining interventions.
- Major restriction should be considered when:
  - Patients are bedridden prior to an acute crisis.
  - Patients have end-stage disease (uncontrolled disease without treatment options and lifespan expectancy <6 months).
- These are situations where we feel it is appropriate to encourage palliative care.

In all other situations (good functional capacity, availability of lifespan-extending anticancer treatments), the patients should be offered the benefit of the doubt on the basis of the following considerations:

- The aforementioned limits of ICU triage and the more reliable prediction of outcome after a brief ICU stay justify a wide admission policy with maximal organ supports.
- A broad admission policy is conditional on subsequent reappraisals of the benefits of intensive care through the time course of organ dysfunctions over 3–7 days (see Fig. 1.1).
- Changes of organ failure scores (logistic organ dysfunction score (LOD) or sequential organ failure assessment score (SOFA)) after 3–7 days are more accurate predictors of outcome than admission

scores. However, some physicians may feel uncomfortable basing their decision-making process on scores.
- A more pragmatic approach at the bedside is to consider the initiation or the weaning of life-sustaining treatments. Thus, the requirement for initiation of mechanical ventilation, vasopressors, or renal replacement therapy after three days in the ICU is almost constantly associated with mortality.

End-of-life decisions to withhold or to withdraw life supports should always be taken collectively by members of the ICU and haematology/oncology staff when all participants are convinced that maintenance or increase in life-sustaining therapies is without benefit and that death in the short term is inevitable.

Whether or not patients can be transferred back to the haematology or oncology ward after withdrawal of life support should depend on where the best palliative care can be provided.

Psychological issues that can occur in the care of ICU cancer patients

- Critically ill cancer patients commonly experience distressing symptoms such as pain, discomfort, anxiety, sleep disturbance, or unsatisfied hunger and thirst during their stay in the ICU. While many cancer patients in the ICU are actively dying, particular attention should be paid to the prevention, detection, and treatment of these symptoms:
  - Improve communication between patients and ICU staff.
  - Be highly sensitive to patients' comfort needs.
  - Extend the visiting hours.
  - Minimize noise and lighting during night time.
  - Premedication with sedatives and/or analgesics for interventions expected to cause pain and discomfort.
- During the course of a malignant disease, patients often experience major fear and anxiety towards death, disability, and suffering, while hoping for cure and restoration of normal function and life expectancy. When there is a mismatch between hope for cure and the reality of probable death in the ICU, care of cancer patients can impose a significant moral burden on members of the ICU team (physicians or nurses). Assistance from the referring haematologist/oncologist or from a psychologist can be helpful for patients as well as for the ICU staff. Moral distress is discussed in more details in Ch. 6.
- Beyond vital status, the outcomes of interest should be expanded towards quality of life among survivors (and the bereaved) by considering post-traumatic stress disorders and disability that requires prolonged rehabilitation after discharge and/or affects the continuation of optimal anticancer treatment.

Conclusion

We have highlighted multidimensional issues that should be involved in the decision-making process for ICU admission of patients who have complications of cancer or of its treatment. Over the last two decades, haematologists/oncologists and intensive care physicians have increasingly collaborated to overcome the reluctance for ICU admission of

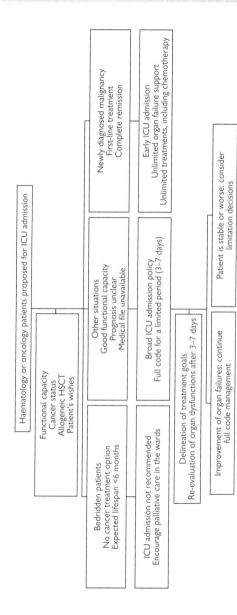

Fig. 1.1 Indications and limitations of ICU admission in cancer patients (data adapted from: Azoulay E, Afessa B (2006), *Intensive Care Med* **32**, 3–5).

cancer patients. While a broader admission policy appears acceptable and reasonable in most cases, individual decisions remain complex and are based upon case-by-case clinical judgement at the bedside.

Further reading

1. Thiery G, Azoulay E, Darmon M, *et al.* (2005). Outcome of cancer patients considered for intensive care unit admission: a hospital-wide prospective study. *J Clin Oncol* **23**, 4406–13.
2. Pène F, Aubron C, Azoulay E, *et al.* (2006). Outcome of critically ill allogeneic haematopoietic stem cell transplantation recipients: a reappraisal of indications for organ failure supports. *J Clin Oncol* **24**, 643–9.
3. Hilbert G, Gruson D, Vargas F, *et al.* (2001). Non-invasive ventilation in immunosuppressed patients with pulmonary infiltrates, fever, and acute respiratory failure. *N Engl J Med* **344**, 481–7.
4. Soares M, Salluh JI, Spector N, Rocco JR (2005). Characteristics and outcomes of cancer patients requiring mechanical ventilatory support for >24 hrs. *Crit Care Med* **33**, 520–6.
5. Pène F, Percheron S, Lemiale V, *et al.* (2008). Temporal changes in management and outcome of septic shock in patients with malignancies in the intensive care unit. *Crit Care Med* **36**, 690–6.
6. Azoulay E, Afessa B (2006). The intensive care support of patients with malignancy: do everything that can be done. *Intensive Care Med* **32**, 3–5.
7. Lecuyer L, Chevret S, Thiery G, Darmon M, Schlemmer B, Azoulay E (2007). The ICU trial: a new admission policy for cancer patients requiring mechanical ventilation. *Crit Care Med* **35**, 808–14.

Improving palliative and end-of-life care

Barriers to high-quality ICU palliative care *42*
Judith E Nelson
Evaluation of palliative care quality *46*
Judith E Nelson

Barriers to high-quality ICU palliative care

Although ICU palliative care has been prioritized for quality improvement, the pace of progress remains slow. A number of impediments can be identified, including:

- Attitudes toward the relationship between palliative care and critical care.
- Systems and structures for organization of care.
- Other factors related to clinicians, patients, and families.

Recognizing these barriers is an essential step toward overcoming them.

The 'comfort vs cure' dichotomy

Although attitudes are gradually changing, the view that palliative care is a mutually exclusive alternative to 'aggressive' critical care is still widely prevalent among clinicians as well as patients and their families. This 'comfort vs cure' dichotomy is probably the single most significant barrier to high-quality palliative care for critically ill patients and their families as it generally operates to postpone attention to palliative needs until death is imminent—or after, when it is too late. Patients come to the ICU precisely because they are at high risk of death or serious morbidity and, despite our sophisticated prediction models, we continue with prognostic uncertainty. Even if we could, it would not make sense to limit palliation to a subpopulation of patients who are obviously dying since comfort, communication, and other palliative needs are nearly universal in the ICU, regardless of vital status at discharge. Palliative care can, and ideally should, be integrated from the beginning into comprehensive critical care for all ICU patients, including those receiving life-prolonging therapies. To clear this biggest barrier, specialists in both intensive care and in palliative medicine need to embrace this integrative approach rather than presenting patients, families, and themselves with a wrenching 'either or' choice that doesn't need to be made.

Fragmentation of care of the critically ill

High-quality palliative care includes coordination of the efforts of multiple caregivers, consistent communication about prognosis, treatment and goals, and continuity of care during transitions among settings. However, this kind of care is a special challenge in the ICU, where the patient is often approached not as a whole person, but as the sum of multiple organs in various stages of dysfunction. Isolated specialists come and go with minimal interaction among themselves and with limited, often inconsistent communication with patients and their families. Caregivers in different disciplines, physicians, nurses, and others, are separated in 'silos'. There is often even a disconnect in the approach to patients and families, whereas the most appropriate model of palliative care would approach them as a unit. Although fragmentation of care is not limited to the ICU, the consequences are particularly problematic for patients with very complex, high-acuity illness as well as for their families and for clinicians themselves. Neither palliative care nor critical care can be optimized in the absence of a collaborative, interdiscplinary approach to the whole patient and the family.

Empirical evidence about barriers to better ICU palliative care: the US ICU Director Survey and others

In a large-scale survey of a random, nationally representative sample of nursing and physician directors of US ICUs, a diverse group of almost 600 respondents representing 468 ICUs (78% of sample) rated barriers to optimal palliative care in the ICU. The survey questionnaire classified potential barriers in three categories: institutional/ICU factors, clinician factors, and patient/family factors. Half the respondents reported that 'unrealistic patient/family expectations' and the 'inability of patients to participate in discussions' were large or huge barriers. Important barriers in the 'clinician' category (which were each rated separately with respect to physicians and nurses) related to communication by physicians, with one third of directors reporting 'insufficient training of physicians in communication about end-of-life issues' and 'inadequate communication between the ICU physicians and patients/families about appropriate goals.' A lack of regularly scheduled meetings between senior ICU physicians and patients/families was identified by respondents as another important barrier. Nurse and physician directors generally agreed about the magnitude of barriers, with respondents from both disciplines reporting that physicians posed greater barriers than nurses, particularly in the area of communication.

Other recent surveys of critical care professionals in the US provide additional evidence about barriers to better ICU care. Important barriers that have been repeatedly identified across these studies are summarized as follows:

- Unrealistic patient and family expectations about prognosis or effectiveness of ICU treatment.
- Unrealistic expectations by physicians about prognosis or effectiveness of ICU treatment.
- Insufficient training of ICU physicians in palliative medicine, including communication skills.
- Inadequate financing and insurance coverage for palliative care.

Across continents

International comparisons show major differences in the organization of health care in general and specifically, in legal frameworks for end-of-life care. Heterogeneity exists within Europe as well as between Europe and the US, particularly with respect to authority for decision-making about limitation of life-sustaining therapies and the relative roles of physicians and patients and families in this process. However, interestingly, there are many common, transcontinental themes in the perspectives of critical care professionals on barriers to high-quality ICU palliative care. The 'European perspective' is one where these barriers are 'mainly related to our ability to inform and communicate with family members, to 'poor communication within the ICU team and with non-ICU professionals', to the use of an 'organ failure-orientated strategy' rather than a 'patient comfort-centred strategy', and to the prevalence of the 'rule of rescue culture' in contrast to a 'culture of comfort care'. Such observations are familiar to those practising and researching critical care elsewhere, as are concerns expressed from the European perspective about the 'lack of palliative medicine training in schools of medicine', about the 'inadequate knowledge and misconceptions about the ICU', and about the paucity of 'families [who] discuss their beliefs and wishes related to death, organ donation, decisions to forgo life-saving treatments, surrogate designation, and advance directives'. Like the US, Europe has also been described as a 'death-denying society'.

Common threads: internationally recognized barriers to high-quality ICU palliative care
• Poor communication (among clinicians, patients and families).
• Care fragmentation.
• Rescue culture of ICU.
• Inadequate ICU professional knowledge and skills in palliative medicine.

Overcoming barriers

Knowledge and skills in palliative medicine can be taught more effectively to intensivists and others involved in treating the critically ill and their families; recent educational initiatives are designed for this purpose. The ability to communicate in a clear, candid, and sensitive way and to ensure comfort for patients and families while advanced technology is used to restore health would be among the most important topics for further education of health care professionals. For the public, education about what can be expected from critical care treatments and what should be expected from critical care professionals would be especially valuable. A broad range of other strategies have also been endorsed as effective and a growing body of empirical evidence as well as clinical experience and consensus of expert opinion supports their use. These concrete efforts in education and clinical practice will help to overcome existing obstacles to high-quality palliative care in the ICU. However, significant and sustained quality improvement will also require a shift in the basic paradigm, with increasing acceptance of the integral role of palliative care for all critically ill patients, regardless of prognosis and their families. Palliative care is not an optional alternative to critical care; it is part of critical care as much as mechanical ventilation and haemodynamic support. From this basic premise, better ICU palliative care quality will ultimately follow.

Further reading

1. Nelson JE (2006). Identifying and overcoming the barriers to quality palliative care in the ICU. *Crit Care Med* **34**(Suppl), 324–31.
2. Nelson JE, Angus DC, Weissfeld LA, *et al.*, for the Critical Care Peer Workgroup of Promoting Excellence in End-of-Life Care (2006). End-of-life care for the critically ill: a national ICU survey. *Crit Care Med* **34**, 2547–53.
3. Fassier T, Lautrette A, Ciroldi M, *et al.* (2005). Care at the end of life in critically ill patients: the European perspective. *Curr Opin Crit Care* **11**, 616–23.
4. Kirchhoff KT, Beckstrand RL (2000). Critical care nurses' perceptions of obstacles and helpful behaviours in providing end-of-life care to dying patients. *Am J Crit Care* **9**, 96–105.

Evaluation of palliative care quality

Why measure ICU palliative care quality?

Palliative care is increasingly accepted as an essential element of comprehensive intensive care for all patients in the ICU and their families. Although many strategies have been suggested to improve the quality of ICU palliative care, important opportunities for improvement still exist for each key component of this care: symptom control, timely and compassionate communication, alignment of treatment with patient preferences, and continuity across care settings. Quality improvement depends on the ability to assess and monitor performance. As they go forward to optimize palliative care, ICU clinicians, administrators, and researchers will need to evaluate their efforts using appropriate measures.

How is quality of care measured?

Quality of health care, including palliative care, can be evaluated in terms of structure (how care is organized), process (what providers do), or outcome (what happens to patients and families) (Table 2.1). Recent initiatives for ICU performance improvement have relied mainly on process measures, which have several important advantages:
- Focus on activities that are actionable by professional caregivers.
- Suitable for providing feedback to these caregivers.
- Practical.
- Minimally burdensome for patients and families.

Table 2.1 Three ways to measure quality of care: the structure-process-outcome model

Structural measures (how care is organized)
- Material resources and organizational or operational aspects of health care.
  - E.g. presence or absence of a palliative care consultation service; care model (open or closed) of the ICU.

Process measures (what caregivers do)
- Clinical and non-clinical processes and procedures.
  - E.g. identification of a surrogate decision-maker for a patient lacking capacity.

Outcome measures (what results are achieved)
- Consequences of care for patients, families, and resource use.
  - E.g. patient outcomes, including mortality and specified morbidities; family outcomes, including satisfaction with care or psychological symptoms; utilization outcomes, including length of ICU stay.

In addition, although outcomes are intuitively important targets, process measures are generally more sensitive to improvement efforts and less dependent on adjustment for patient characteristics and preferences. Key attributes of an appropriate quality measure are: importance, validity, reliability, responsiveness, interpretability, and feasibility (Table 2.2). Importance and validity depend on scientific foundation and for process measures, on strong association with outcomes that are valued by patients, families, and clinicians. The perspectives of the ICU manager, hospital administration, and community may also be relevant.

Table 2.2 Key attributes of quality measures

• **Important**	Addresses a common, clinically significant issue.
• **Valid**	Serves the measurement purpose, as reflected in comparison to a gold standard (criterion validity) or to other measures or constructs along the same lines (construct validity). For a process measure, validity depends ultimately on evidence that variations in the process are associated with outcomes of importance.
• **Reliable**	Yields the same result across different raters (inter-rater reliability) and repeated measurements (intrarater reliability).
• **Responsive**	Sensitive to change through quality improvement efforts.
• **Interpretable**	Readily understood by those involved, including caregivers and managers.
• **Feasible**	Practical and relatively easy to implement in a busy ICU.

What are appropriate domains for measurement?

Domains of ICU palliative care quality have been defined as follows, based on research evidence and expert consensus: symptom management and comfort care, patient and family-centred decision-making, communication within the team and with patients and families, emotional and practical support for patients and families, spiritual support for patients and families, continuity of care, and emotional and organizational support for ICU clinicians (Table 2.3). These domains are consistent with those defined as a framework for clinical practice guidelines and preferred practices for palliative care professionals.

Table 2.3 Domains of ICU palliative care quality

- Symptom management and comfort care.
- Patient- and family-centred decision-making.
- Communication within the team and with patients and families; emotional and practical support for patients and families.
- Spiritual support for patients and families.
- Continuity of care.
- Emotional and organizational support for ICU clinicians.

How do ICUs operationalize evaluation of palliative care quality?

For evaluation of care in clinical settings, domains are operationalized as measures, each with a numerator and denominator. The denominator defines the target population. While inclusion of all ICU patients and their families could be justified for the evaluation of palliative care quality, feasibility will usually require a selection of subgroups with special risks or needs, e.g. high severity of illness or prolonged ICU stay (Table 2.4), which are associated with higher rates of hospital mortality and functional impairment. Numerators for process measures should be selected on the strength of evidence that performance of the process by caregivers will lead to clinically important outcomes. This selection too must be limited by what is feasible and informed by the 'perfect can defeat good' principle; while addressing a wide range of care processes, an exhaustive measure set may collapse under its own measurement burden.

Table 2.4 Possible denominators for ICU palliative care quality measures

- Patients in the ICU for ≥ specified number of days (e.g. 3 or 5).
- Patients with high severity of illness (e.g. APACHE II score ≥ specified number).
- Patients with prolonged dysfunction of multiple organs.
- Patients with evidence of global cerebral ischaemia.

In a national survey of US ICUs, physician and nurse directors strongly endorsed quality monitoring as an effective strategy for optimizing ICU palliative care. The survey highlighted low utilization of this strategy, which was then available in only 26% of ICUs led by the responding director. More recently, a 'bundle' of process measures for routine monitoring, feedback, and improvement of the quality of ICU palliative care was published with detailed specifications and implemented in a broad, diverse, and growing group of ICUs. This abbreviated tool (Table 2.5) addresses established domains of ICU palliative care and specifically evaluates the following care processes:
- Identifying a medical decision-maker.
- Advance directive status and resuscitation status.
- Distributing a family information leaflet.
- Assessing and managing pain.
- Offering social work and spiritual support.
- Conducting an interdisciplinary meeting with the patient and family.

Time triggers (specified days after ICU admission) are included for prompt performance of important palliative care processes. Documentation in medical records is the source for data collection; direct observation of care may be more accurate, but less practical. ICUs can decide whether data will be collected prospectively or retrospectively, recognizing that target populations defined by the length of stay can only be identified in retrospect.

How are quality measures implemented to achieve performance improvement?

Meaningful implementation of quality measures involves more than collection of data. If the purpose is (as it should be) to improve palliative care, the process should begin with a discussion of what changes in clinical practice or clinician behaviour are needed to enhance performance on the measures and who within the ICU interdisciplinary team will have responsibility for effecting these changes. Another task is to determine whether current documentation practices should be modified to represent clinical performance more clearly. Educational efforts are needed to apprise staff of the purpose of the evaluation and to communicate knowledge (e.g. legal and regulatory standards for the limitation of life-sustaining therapies) and skills (e.g. delivery of distressing news) that are required for successful performance of measured processes. Finally, quality improvement depends on regular feedback to caregivers and collaborative planning to improve palliative care performance.

Further reading

1. Nelson JE, Mulkerin CM, Adams LL, Pronovost PJ (2006). Improving comfort and communication in the ICU: a practical new tool for quality improvement and performance feedback. *Qual Saf Health Care* **15**, 264–71.
2. Clarke EB, Curtis JR, Luce JM, *et al.* (2003). Quality indicators for end-of-life care in the intensive care unit. *Crit Care Med* **31**, 2255–62.
3. Care and communication bundle of ICU palliative care quality measures of the Voluntary Hospital Association, Inc. transformation of the ICU programme). Available from: http://www.qualitymeasures.ahrq.gov. Accessed July 15, 2009.

Table 2.5 Examples of process measures of palliative care quality
Unless otherwise specified denominator for each measure: total number of patients with an ICU length of stay >5 days.

Quality indicator	Numerator (N) and/or denominator (D)* for quality measure
Medical decision-maker Documentation of efforts to identify a medical decision-maker (family member or other appropriate surrogate) for the patient on or before day 1 in ICU.	**N**: number of patients who have documentation of ICU efforts to identify a health care proxy (or other appropriate surrogate decision-maker) on or before day 1 of ICU admission.
Advance directive Documentation on or before day 1 in ICU.	**N**: number of patients who have documentation of advance directive status on or before day 1 in ICU.
Resuscitation status Documentation on or before day 1 in ICU.	**N**: number of patients who have documentation of resuscitation status on or before day 1 in ICU.
Family information leaflet Documentation of distribution to family member on or before day 1 in ICU.	**N**: number of patients whose family was personally given a written information leaflet by an ICU team member on or before day 1 in ICU
Pain assessment Regular.	**N**: total number of 4-hour intervals (on days 0 and 1 in ICU) for which pain was assessed and documented. **D**: total number of 4-hour intervals (on days 0 and 1 in ICU) for patients with an ICU length of stay of ≥ 5 days.**

(Continued)

Table 2.5 (Continued) Examples of process measures of palliative care quality*

Quality indicator	Numerator (N) and/or denominator (D) for quality measure
Pain management Optimal.	**N**: total number of 4-hour intervals (on days 0 and 1 in ICU) for which the documented pain score was 3. **D**: total number of 4-hour intervals (on days 0 and 1 in ICU) with numerical pain values of 0 to 10, for patients with an ICU length of stay ≥ 5 days.**
Social work support Offered to ICU patients and/or families on or before day 3 in ICU.	**N**: number of patients who have documentation in the medical record that social work support was offered to the patient and/or family on or before day 3 in ICU.
Spiritual support Offered to ICU patients and/or families on or before day 3 in ICU.	**N**: number of patients who have documentation in the medical record that spiritual support was offered to the patient and/or family on or before day 3 in ICU.
Interdisciplinary family meeting Adequate clinician-patient/family communication on or before day 5 in ICU.	**N**: number of patients who have documentation in the medical record that an interdisciplinary family meeting was conducted on or before day 5 in ICU.

* Denominotor (D) for each measure: Total number of patients with an ICU length of stay ≥ 5 days

** This number cannot be greater than 12

Symptom control

Common symptoms in ICU patients at high risk of dying: an
    introduction *52*
Jennifer McAdam, Shoshana Arai, Kathleen Puntillo

Symptom relief for the imminently dying patient *54*
Kathleen Puntillo, Cathy Schuster

Pain *60*
Kathleen Puntillo, Shoshana Arai, Jennifer McAdam

Dyspnoea *66*
Shoshana Arai , Jennifer McAdam, Kathleen Puntillo

Anxiety *68*
Jennifer McAdam, Shoshana Arai, Kathleen Puntillo

Delirium in the critically ill patient at the end of life: issues and
    management *74*
Yoanna Skrobik

Sleep disturbances *78*
Shoshana Arai, Jennifer McAdam, Kathleen Puntillo

Thirst/dry mouth *80*
Shoshana Arai, Jennifer McAdam, Kathleen Puntillo

Common symptoms in ICU patients at high risk of dying: an introduction

ICU patients at high risk of dying are at an increased risk of suffering from physical and psychological symptoms. Despite this increased risk, there is limited research on the 'real time' symptom experiences of these patients. However, we do know that ICU patients may suffer from a variety of symptoms such as anxiety, restlessness, agitation, dyspnoea, thirst, and sleep disturbances.[1–3] In one study focusing on chronically critically ill ICU patients, investigators reported that:

- 90% of ICU patients complained of at least one symptom during their ICU stay.
- 75% of ICU patients had 10 or more symptoms during their ICU stay.
- The mean number of symptoms experienced by ICU patients was 8.62.

Anxiety, restlessness/agitation, dyspnoea, thirst, sleep disturbances, pain, and delirium are the key symptoms that we explore in this section.

Optimal assessment and management of symptoms in ICU patients at high risk of dying should be a high priority for clinicians. With the appropriate use of medications, treatments, and non-pharmacologic techniques, we can reduce the amount of symptom burden for our patients and improve the quality of care given in the ICU.

'Although some patients may be willing, they may not need to suffer to survive a critical illness.'
Nelson (2001). p282.

References

1. Nelson J, Meier DE, Oei EJ, et al. (2001). Self-reporting symptom experience of critically ill cancer patients receiving intensive care. *Crit Care Med* **29**, 277–82.
2. Nelson J, Meier DE, Litke A, Natale DA, Siegel RE, Morrison SR (2004). The symptom burden of chronic illness. *Crit Care Med* **32**, 1527–34.
3. Li DT, Puntillo K (2006). A pilot study on coexisting symptoms in intensive care patients. *Appl Nurs Res* **19**, 216–9.

Symptom relief for the imminently dying patient

'The heart-wrenching decision to withdraw life support on Mrs T had just been made. After the family meeting, Mrs T's daughter and I hugged by her mother's bedside, both in tears. I was Mrs T's 'continuity of care' nurse for the three weeks she was in our ICU. Mrs T was dying from septic shock and multiple organ failure. Her family had looked to me for clarification, guidance, and comfort during her ICU stay. They were anxious for their mother to be comfortable and were ready for the withdrawal of life support process to begin. My goal was to spend time with Mrs T's family to explain the 'how and why' of care that I would be providing to their mother and to answer their many questions. But when I opened the chart to read the withdrawal of life support orders, I couldn't believe it. The orders for pain and anxiety relief and discontinuation of treatments were incomplete. While the orders included a morphine infusion, they did not address the potential episodic pain. Anxiety relief medications were not prescribed. The surgery team had written to stop antibiotics and blood tests, but the medications that maintained the patient's blood pressure and continuous renal replacement therapy were not discontinued. This contradictory plan was going to make my patient's living and dying difficult. I needed to leave the bedside multiple times to consult with two teams in order to obtain complete orders. Then, I traversed ten floors to the pharmacy to obtain the comfort medications in a timely manner. All this time spent away from Mrs T was stressful for both the patient and family. All of this 'hunting and gathering' to ensure complete orders and assemble medications and supplies had to happen before I could ensure Mrs T a death free of pain, anxiety, dyspnoea, nausea, and any other discomforts.'

ICU nurse

Preparing for a comfortable death

As in the story above, ICU patients are often too ill to participate in care decisions. When professionals and family members believe that the best care for the patient is to provide comfort during the patient's dying period, the focus changes from the more curative therapeutic interventions and approaches of the earlier phases of the ICU admission to a focus on palliation. At this point, the aim of care should be to make dying as smooth and comfortable as possible for both patient and family. In order to minimize patient symptoms, the following should be considered:

• Routine procedures such as taking vital signs, drawing blood for laboratory tests, repositioning, and endotracheal suctioning should be re-evaluated from the perspective of the imminently dying patient. These procedures are unlikely to contribute to the patient's comfort and indeed, may cause unnecessary discomfort.[1]

- Thoughtful consideration should be given to the discontinuation of procedures, interventions, and medications that are not directly related to the provision of comfort to the dying patient.
- Some patients may wish to remain awake and alert for as long as possible. The critical care team needs to manage the difficult balance between having a patient awake, but not suffering.

Symptom relief

Managing patient symptoms during the dying period is one of the most important aspects of care that a critical care team can provide. Effective symptom control may be one of the last interventions offered to dying patients and their families. The most frequent symptoms experienced by the imminently dying patient may be pain, dyspnoea, and anxiety/agitation.[2] Table 3.1 outlines some pharmacological interventions for these symptoms. Selection of these interventions must be preceded by an assessment of the patient for the presence of symptoms (see other sections within this chapter regarding specific symptom assessment).

Table 3.1 Pharmacological symptom management*

Symptom	Drug type most frequently used	Method of administration	Usual dose**
Pain	Opioids (e.g. morphine, fentanyl, hydromorphone)	Continuous IV infusions*** with use of intermittent boluses for procedure-related pain or during treatment withdrawal	Continuous infusion (morphine equivalents): 1–10mg/h Bolus: 1–10mg IV slow push, titrate to effect
Anxiety, agitation	Benzodiazepines (e.g. midazolam, lorazepam, diazepam)	Same as opioids	Continuous infusion (midazolam): 2–25mg/h or titrate to effect Bolus (midazolam): 5–10mg IV to augment. continuous infusion
	Propofol	Continuous IV infusion	Continuous: 50–300mg/h Bolus: 10–50mg
Dyspnoea	Oxygen	Multiple methods (e.g. nasal cannula, mask, ventilator)	Concentration as needed
	Opioids (e.g. morphine)	Continuous IV infusion and/or IV bolus or via nebulizer	See above for IV doses. Via nebulizer: 2.5mg in 3mL NaCl (preservative-free) or sterile water every 4h
	Benzodiazepines	See above	See above

* Data adapted from: Prendergast TJ, Puntillo KA (2002). Withdrawal of life support: intensive caring at the end of life. *JAMA* **288**, 2732–40.

** Drug doses are general recommendations. Dosing should be individualized to a particular patient. Under usual circumstances, start with low doses, wait for effect, and titrate to desired effect.

*** When titrating infusions, consider the dying patient's previous exposure to opioids since tolerance to opioids may have developed. For patients in general, an increase of infusion rate less than 25% is not usually noticeable to the patient. In the absence of research data, dose escalation recommendations are as follows: 25–50% if the pain is thought to be mild to moderate in intensity, 50–100% if the pain is thought to be moderate to severe in intensity (Source: www.eperc.mcw.edu. Fast Fact and Concept #020: opioid dose escalation).

Ethics of symptom management in the imminently dying patient

The generous use of medications, when carefully titrated to control refractory symptoms, is well established in medical practice and is rooted in the doctrine of 'double effect.' This doctrine identifies the important difference between the aggressive palliation of pain (and of other symptoms) and the active hastening of death. Palliation of symptoms in the dying patient is ethically justifiable as long as the caregiver's primary intent is to alleviate suffering.[3] In other words, there is no limit to the doses of medications that can be used to manage the patient's symptoms as long as their administration is based on assessments of signs of distress from symptoms and the intent is to relieve the symptoms, not cause death. However, the risk of hastened death as a consequence of use of necessary analgesia and/or sedation is legally[4] and morally[5] acceptable in these circumstances. Documentation of symptom assessment and reasons for administration and titration of medications is imperative. It is also important for health care providers to communicate to families their rationale for administering medications lest families have concerns about the motivation for using large doses of medications.

Non-pharmacological comfort measures

Comfort measures administered by critical care nurses, such as positioning, eye care, and mouth care, may augment pharmacological interventions. Family members may be encouraged to participate in providing this comfort care.[6] Care-giving activities can include:

• Assisting with face washing.
• Hair combing.
• Gently massaging hands or feet with the use of lotion.

This may provide family members a sense of comfort, intimacy, and involvement when they might otherwise feel helpless.

Guidelines for symptom assessment and management in the imminently dying patient

Like many other procedures performed in ICUs, procedures for managing symptoms during the withdrawal of life-sustaining therapies can be protocolized. See 📖 Appendix, p 360 for one such set of guidelines developed for the adult ICUs at the University of California, San Francisco Medical Centre. These guidelines are comprehensive, yet simple to navigate. The use of such guidelines helps to avoid similar scenarios to the one we presented at the beginning of this chapter. Their use allows clinicians to focus on the most important aspects of patient care, i.e. to provide comfort to the patient while meeting family needs during their loved one's dying.

Recommending the introduction of a practice intervention such as the development of guidelines for the withdrawal of life-sustaining therapies requires a thoughtful plan. The following steps were taken by the nurse whose quote began this chapter:

• Identify a need by documenting the instances when current withdrawal practices were inferior.
• Identify the unit leaders and stakeholders and solicit their support.
• Convene an end-of-life interdisciplinary committee.

- Develop drafts of a 'withdrawal of life support' protocol, order set, and educational reference after reviewing best practices from other hospitals and literature.
- Work with pharmacy colleagues to improve the availability of medications commonly used during end-of-life care in the ICUs.
- Finalize document and share with other experts or opinion leaders (e.g. the hospital's palliative care team) for their input.
- Introduce the guidelines during educational sessions with staff.
- Have committee members serve as resources during the initial stage of guideline implementation.
- Validate the effectiveness of the guidelines by conducting a 'before and after' survey of ICU nurses.
- Make necessary changes to guidelines and implement in practice.

Summary

When patients are actively dying, the care priority is provision of comfort. This can be attained through the thoughtful use of pharmacologic and non-pharmacologic interventions accompanied by ongoing (re)assessments and documentation of symptoms being treated. Family members who are apprised on the rationale for caregivers' practices and who are invited to provide and/or participate in provision comfort measures may have fewer painful memories after the patient's death.

> 'How people die remains in the memory of those who live on'
> Dame Cicely Saunders

References

1. Nelson JE, Meier DE, Oei EJ, et al. (2001). Self-reported symptom experience of critically ill cancer patients receiving intensive care. *Crit Care Med* **29**, 277–82.
2. Desbiens NA, Wu AW, Broste SK, et al. (1996). Pain and satisfaction with pain control in seriously ill hospitalized adults: findings from the SUPPORT research investigations. For the SUPPORT investigators. Study to understand prognoses and preferences for outcomes and risks of treatment. *Crit Care Med* **24**, 1953–61.
3. Beauchamp TL, Childress JF (2001). *Principles of biomedical ethics*, 5th edn. Oxford University Press, Oxford.
4. Cruzan vs Director (1990). Missouri Department of Health 497 US 261.
5. Sulmasy DP, Pellegrino ED (1999). The rule of double effect: clearing up the double talk. *Arch Intern Med* **159**, 545–50.
6. McAdam JL, Arai S, Puntillo KA (2008). Unrecognized contributions of families in the intensive care unit. *Intensive Care Med* **34**, 1097–101.

Pain

'Pain finds its way everywhere, into my vision, my feelings, my sense of judgement; it's an infiltration … You have to die so many times before you die.'
Alphonse Daudet (1840–1897), *In the land of pain*.

The assessment and management of pain are essential components of high-quality end-of-life/palliative care in the ICU. Pain is common, occurring in 40–63% of ICU patients at moderate to severe levels.[1,2] Diagnosing and treating pain can promote patient comfort, improve outcomes, relieve suffering, and can prevent further tissue injury. If untreated, pain can be associated with many other symptoms such as anxiety, disturbed sleep, confusion, delirium, paranoia, post-traumatic stress, and chronic pain.

Definition

A physiologic definition of pain is of an 'unpleasant sensory and emotional experience associated with actual or potential tissue damage or described in terms of such damage.'[3] A more clinical definition recognizes that pain is invariably subjective. Pain is 'whatever the experiencing person says it is, existing whenever he/she says it does.'[4] However, neither definition is helpful if the patient is not able to communicate with ICU clinicians.

Pain assessment

'She is not a complainer. Even when she is in pain. I can just look at her facial expressions and tell just how she feels … I will ask her 'Are you in pain?' … I don't know if she is aware, but may be she just recognizes my voice. I just assumed that something is hurting her, but you don't really know because she can't speak. I had asked the nurse 'Do you think she might be having pain?' You know, she just had a big operation, she's been poked and prodded, and she [nurse] said she can get a little more, whatever they are giving her.'
Source: mother of a 43-year old woman with toxic shock syndrome and multiple organ dysfunction who died after ten days in ICU.[5]

The following are important considerations regarding pain.

Assessment

• Pain should be assessed routinely in ICU patients. If the patient is able to talk, the clinicians can obtain the patient's self-report of *pain intensity* using a validated pain scale such as a numerical rating scale (NRS) and *pain location* using a body outline diagram. Both have been shown to be useful and usable for many ICU patients, even those who are intubated (see Fig. 3.1 for a copy of a bedside pain assessment tool).
• Assessing pain in a patient unable to communicate or in a cognitively impaired ICU patient can be more of a challenge. Clinicians can use several techniques noted in Table 3.2. Pain assessment instruments are available to determine *indicators of* pain presence in ICU patients

unable to verbalize their pain or discomfort. Their validity and reliability testing are ongoing.

Types of pain

Consideration should be given to the different, sometimes overlapping, types of pain that ICU patients could be experiencing. See Table 3.3 for types, comments, and suggested interventions.

Procedural pain

'I found that before, they turned and bathed her and did a lot of big things … Because her body is so sore, they give her medication before they even start doing it, and I appreciate that. It helps me.'
Source: mother of a 43-year old woman with toxic shock syndrome and multisystem failure who died after ten days in ICU.[5]

Procedural pain is ubiquitous in the ICU environment. It is induced by health professionals during diagnostic or treatment-related procedures. Careful attention to good analgesic practice can minimize procedure-associated pain. See Table 3.4 for pain information on commonly performed procedures. Clinicians can monitor and assess how frequently these procedures/treatments are needed, and try to reduce or eliminate any that are unnecessary, especially if the patient's death is inevitable.

Non-pharmacological interventions for pain

'**Interviewer:** What are other people doing, we are kind of talking about her pain now. Other things you are seeing being done by physicians or by the family for her pain?
Nurse: Specifically for her pain? I'm not seeing anything else being done other than the provision of analgesics, occasional touch. There is a tape recorder at the side [of the bed]. The family keeps music going. That could be distracting as far as pain goes. That's pretty much it, music, touch, talking to her, distraction. Trying to minimize interventions. Suctioning as little as possible. Things like that.'
Source: nurse caring for a 43-year old woman with toxic shock syndrome and multiple organ dysfunction who died after ten days in ICU.[6]

Non-pharmacological interventions for pain can augment medications or be used alone if shown to be effective for a particular patient.
- **Physical interventions** such as acupuncture, cutaneous stimulation through rubbing or massage theoretically block transmission of noxious stimuli. Peripherally applied heat promotes circulation, while cold application decreases release of pain-inducing chemicals.[7]
- **Cognitive behavioural interventions** can influence the pain experience through activation of pain inhibitory pathways.
- **Music interventions** for acute pain have been reviewed recently. In a meta-analysis of 51 randomized clinical trials, Cepeda and colleagues[8] found lower pain intensity scores, a higher likelihood of pain relief, and

the need for less opioid among patients who did vs those who did not receive a music intervention.
- Relaxation techniques to supplement the use of analgesics have been shown to decrease pain intensity and distress in a group of post-operative patients.[9]

Non-pharmacologic interventions for pain usually cost little, are safe and easy to provide, and can be easily implemented by clinicians and even family members in many circumstances. These interventions may help to alleviate the suffering as well as the pain of ICU patients.

General guidelines on analgesic practices for dying patients in ICU
- Clear documentation of:
  - Pain assessment (for patients who can and cannot communicate).
  - Intent of an analgesic intervention.
  - Intervention itself promotes clarity, provides justification, and fosters clinician-to-clinician communication and understanding of the patient's situation.
- Since analgesic needs differ from person to person, consider initial doses with the following in mind:
  - Patient's age.
  - Patient's current level of consciousness.
  - Patient's previous opioid exposure.
  - Patient's underlying organ dysfunction (to assess pharmacokinetics of drug to be administered for pain and thus, the likelihood of positive effect).
  - Patient's wishes regarding level of consciousness.
- Consider any type of analgesics that will relieve the patient's pain.
- Titrate doses according to effect on the patient's pain, not on physiological parameters.
- Provide any amount of drug that is needed to relieve the patient's pain. There is no maximal dose for pain relief unless patients are experiencing toxic effects from the drug.
- Pre-emptive dosing in anticipation of and to relieve subsequent pain from a pending procedure known to cause pain is good palliative care.
- See 📖 in 'Symptom relief for the imminently dying patient' p54 for guidelines specific to that time period.
- Liverpool Pathway (LCP) (see 📖 'The Liverpool Care Pathway for patients dying in intensive care in the UK p276. Additional information on the LCP is available from:

http://www.mcpcil.org.uk/liverpool_care_pathway/non-cancer/lcp_intensive_care_unit).

A few words about suffering
As noted earlier, pain is both a sensory and emotional experience and should be treated as such. However, pain and suffering in ICU patients are different. Suffering is multidimensional and may include:
- Physical.
- Psychological.

- Social.
- Spiritual/existential aspects.

Suffering may be even more difficult to assess and treat since the causes of suffering are so individualized, and ICU clinicians are not well trained in assessing and treating suffering. When pain and suffering coexist, clinicians can use multimodal methods of alleviation:

- Analgesics to reduce sensory pain.
- Non-pharmacologic therapies to help to control pain and existential distress.
- Call upon spiritual counsellors who can assist with the patient's and family's suffering, if such an intervention is acceptable to them.

Suffering is by no means a privilege, a sign of nobility, a reminder of God. Suffering is a fierce, bestial thing, commonplace, uncalled for, natural as air. It is intangible; no one can grasp it or fight against it; it dwells in time—is the same thing as time; if it comes in fits and starts, that is only so as to leave the sufferer more defenseless during the moments that follow …
Cesare Pavese (1908–1950) Italian poet, critic, novelist, and translator

Table 3.2 Techniques for assessing pain in patients unable to communicate verbally*

Technique	Source of evidence
Non-verbal behaviour cues (i.e. grimacing, rigidity, wincing)	Research-based
Physiological signs (e.g. increased heart rate, blood pressure)	Not research-based; these signs change for many reasons; however, used by clinicians
Family or caregiver proxy reports	Research-based: evidence equivocal; useful in situations where other techniques not helpful
Anticipation	Logic (i.e. if a procedure or diagnosis seems painful, one can assume it is painful)

References

1. Puntillo KA (1990). Pain experiences of intensive care unit patients. *Heart Lung* **19**, 526–33.
2. Nelson JE, DE Meier, *et al.* (2001). Self-reported symptom experience of critically ill cancer patients receiving intensive care. *Crit Care Med* **29**, 277–82.
3. International Association for the Study of Pain (1979). Pain terms: a list with definitions and notes on usage. *Pain* **6**, 249–52.
4. McCaffery M (1979). Nursing management of the patient with pain. Lippincott, Philadelphia.
5. Puntillo K. Unpublished interview.
6. Puntillo K, Smith D, Arai S, Stotts N. Critical care nurses provide their perspectives of ICU patients' symptoms. *Heart Lung* (in press).
7. Mobily PR (1994). Non-pharmacologic interventions for the management of chronic pain in older women. *J Women Aging* **6**, 89–109.
8. Cepeda MS, Carr DB, Lau J, Alvarez H (2006). Music for pain relief. *Cochrane Database Syst Rev* **2**, CD004843.
9. Good M, Stanton–Hicks M, Grass JA, *et al.* (1999). Relief of post-operative pain with jaw relaxation, music, and their combination. *Pain* **81**, 163–72.

* Further reading for pain behaviour in patients who cannot communicate verbally

1. Payen JF, Bru O, Bosson JL, et al. (2001). Assessing pain in critically ill sedated patients by using a behavioural pain scale. Crit Care Med **29**, 2258–63.
2. Gelinas C, Fillion L, Puntillo KA, Viens C, Fortier M (2006). Validation of the critical-care pain observation tool in adult patients. Am J Crit Care **15**, 420–7.
3. Aissaoui Y, Zeggwagh A, Zekraoui A, et al. (2005). Validation of a behavioural pain scale in critically ill, sedated, and mechanically ventilated patients. Anesth Analg **101**, 1470–6.
4. Young J, Siffleet J, Nikoletti S, Shaw T (2006). Use of a behavioural pain scale to assess pain in ventilated, unconscious and/or sedated patients. Intensive Crit Care Nurs **22**, 32–9.
5. Puntillo KA, Morris AB, Thompson CL, Stanik–Hutt J, White CA, Wild LR (2004). Pain behaviours observed during six common procedures: results from Thunder Project II. Crit Care Med **32**, 421–7.

Table 3.3 Types of pain and suggested interventions

Types	Comments	Interventions
Acute Abrupt in onset due to surgical or trauma-related tissue injury.	Experienced by most ICU patients who have pain.	ICU patients in acute pain are most often treated with opioids. Use of IV fentanyl, morphine, or hydromorphone is recommended.
Chronic Usually considered to have been ≥3 months in duration. Tissue injury not always confirmed.	Many patients in ICUs can have chronic and/or persistent or intermittent cancer-related pain in addition to the current acute pain. It is essential to ascertain the patient's pre-ICU analgesic regimen, either from the patient or family.	Consider continuing patient's pre-ICU analgesic regimen that could include NSAIDs, antidepressants, or antiepileptics that have analgesic properties; add opioids for new onset pain. Assess for opioid tolerance and dependence if patient has been taking long-term opioids or continues on them for longer than a few days in ICU.
Nociceptive Initiated by a stimulus that activates normal pain processing system.[1]	Acute pain is most often nociceptive.	See above interventions for acute pain.
Neuropathic Pain that occurs as a result of nervous system injury or dysfunction.[1]	Chronic pain is often, but not always, neuropathic. Note: ICU patients can have acute-on-chronic pain.	See above interventions for chronic pain.
Breakthrough Pain that is initiated during a time when analgesics are being administered.	A pain 'flare' that occurs as a result of loss of effectiveness of the analgesic and/or onset of a new pain (e.g. procedural pain).	Consider using 'rescue doses' in addition to current analgesic regimen. Fentanyl is often a good choice because of its fast onset and offset.

Further reading

1. Puntillo KA, Miaskowski C, Summer G (2003). Pain. In: Carrieri–Kohlman V, Lindsey A, West CM (eds.) *Pathophysiologic phenomena in nursing*, 3rd edn, pp 235–54. Harcourt Health Sciences, Philadelphia.
2. Desbiens NA, Mueller–Rizner N (2000). How well do surrogates assess the pain of seriously ill patients? *Crit Care Med* **28**, 1347–52.
3. Jacobi J, Fraser GL, Coursin DB, *et al.* (2002). Clinical practice guidelines for the sustained use of sedatives and analgesics in the critically ill adult. *Crit Care Med* **30**, 119–41.
4. Hawryluck LA, Harvey WR, Lemieux–Charles L, Singer PA (2002). Consensus guidelines on analgesia and sedation in dying intensive care unit patients. *BMC Med Ethics* **3**, E3.
5. American Pain Society (2003). *Principles of analgesic use in the treatment of acute pain and cancer pain*, 5th edn. American Pain Society, Glenview.

Table 3.4 Pain associated with procedures for adults

Procedure	Nelson et al.*	Puntillo et al.**	Siffleet et al.**
Arterial blood gas puncture	32%		
Arterial catheter insertion	30%		
Central catheter insertion	30%	2.7	
Chest tube removal		6.6^2; 4.7^3	
Endotracheal suctioning	34%	4.9^2; 3.9^3	4.4
Endotracheal tube in place	28%		
Indwelling urethral catheter	8%		
Mechanical ventilation	8%		
Moving from bed to chair	19%		
Nasogastric tube insertion	22%		
Nasogastric tube in place	25%		
Peripheral IV insertion	30%		
Turning	33%	4.9	4.1
Wound care		4.4	
Wound drain removal		4.7	6.5

* Prevalence at moderate to severe intensity. ** Intensity per 0–10 NRS

Further reading

1. Nelson JE, Meier DE, Oei EJ, *et al.* (2001). Self-reported symptom experience of critically ill cancer patients receiving intensive care. *Crit Care Med* **29**, 277–82.
2. Puntillo K (1994). Pain: its mediators and associated morbidity in critically ill cardiovascular surgical patients. *Nurs Res* **43**, 31–6.
3. Puntillo KA (1996). Effects of interpleural bupivacaine on pleural chest tube removal pain: a randomized controlled trial. *Am J Crit Care* **5**, 102–8.
4. Puntillo KA, White C, Morris AB, *et al.* (2001). Patients' perceptions and responses to procedural pain: results from Thunder Project II. *Am J Crit Care* **10**, 238–51.
5. Siffleet J, Young J, Nikoletti S, Shaw T (2007). Patients' self-report of procedural pain in the intensive care unit. *J Clin Nurs* **16**, 2142–8.

Dyspnoea

'Dyspnoea is a form of suffering and is probably the most important symptom that must be relieved for patients dying in ICU.'[1]

Dyspnoea is the subjective awareness of unpleasant and difficult breathing. Dyspnoea is the result of a complex interaction of signals arising from the central nervous system, upper airways, lungs, and chest wall. Dyspnoea can exhaust and tire the patient, and can be very upsetting for family members to observe. A high percentage of ICU admissions result from respiratory failure where dyspnoea is a presenting symptom. Moreover, dyspnoea is a very common symptom in high-risk ICU patients, especially those receiving mechanical ventilation. The prevalence of dyspnoea ranges from 34% to 60% at a moderate to severe level.[2]

Risks/causes[3,4]

Patients most at risk are those with pulmonary disease (i.e. acute respiratory distress syndrome (ARDS), COPD, asthma) or cardiac disease (i.e. congestive heart failure (CHF)) as well as those who have underlying anxiety, fear, and depression.
- Heightened ventilatory demand (due to some excessive stimulus, i.e. hypoxia, acidosis).
- Abnormal resistance to ventilation (i.e. airflow obstruction, stiff lungs).
- Respiratory muscle weakness.
- Abnormal central perception of dyspnoea.
- Dyspnoea may be caused by anxiety and panic or it may be a cause of anxiety and panic, leading to distress that might be disproportionate to the underlying lung disease or ongoing need for mechanical ventilation.

Assessment[3,4]

- A patient's self-report of dyspnoea is the most reliable measure.
- Clinicians can use several reliable and valid tools to assess the intensity of dyspnoea such as the horizontal visual analog scale (VAS) or the vertical analog dyspnoea scale (VADS), both of which are scored on a scale ranging from 0='no dyspnoea' to 100='severe dyspnoea', or clinicians can use NRS (commonly used to assess pain) which ranges from 0='no shortness of breath' to 10='worst shortness of breath'. All of these tools work in assessing dyspnoea in mechanically ventilated patients.
- The following information should also be assessed: onset, associated symptoms, precipitating/relieving factors.
- If the patient is unable to speak or is cognitively impaired, the clinicians can assess behavioural and objective indicators of dyspnoea (see Table 3.5).

Non-pharmacological management[5]

- Simple repositioning: sitting upright or resting on an overbed table with pillows can be effective.
- 'Air hunger': use a cool air fan, open window, or a cool moist towel placed on the cheeks or forehead to increase airflow to the trigeminal nerve dermatomes.
- Try guided imagery techniques.
- Identify activities associated with increased dyspnoea; provide anticipatory symptom relief in advance of interventions likely to result in worsening dyspnoea.

- Family members' anxiety can exacerbate a patient's sense of dyspnoea; laboured breathing or tachypnoea may not be distressing to the patient, but they become anxious because others around them appear anxious.
- Mechanical ventilation strategies to manage dyspnoea and optimize comfort, for example pressure support ventilation.

Pharmacological management[5,6]

- Oxygen therapy may provide symptom relief and reduce dyspnoea in advanced cancer patients and patients with advanced COPD or CHF, although this approach is not supported by a recent systematic review.[7]
- Opioids are effective via oral/nasogastric, subcutaneous, and parental routes.
- There is not sufficient evidence to support the use of nebulized opioids.
- Benzodiazepines used for dyspnoea were ineffective in four out of five RCTs.
- Corticosteroids: prednisolone improves dyspnoea scale scores in patients with COPD.
- If airflow obstruction is present, bronchodilator therapy may be indicated.

References

1. Truog RD, Cist AF, Brackett SE, et al. (2001). Recommendations for end-of-life care in the intensive care unit: the Ethics Committee of the Society of Critical Care Medicine. Crit Care Med **29**, 2332–48.
2. Nelson J, Meier DE, Litke A, Natale DA, Siegel RE, Morrison SR (2004). The symptom burden of chronic illness. Crit Care Med **32**, 1527–34.
3. Campbell ML (2004). Terminal dyspnoea and respiratory distress. Crit Care Clin **20**, 403–17, viii–ix.
4. Powers J, Bennett SJ (1999). Measurement of dyspnoea in patients treated with mechanical ventilation. Am J Crit Care **8**, 254–61.
5. Dahlin C (2006). It takes my breath away end-stage COPD. Part 2: pharmacologic and non-pharmacologic management of dyspnoea and other symptoms. Home Healthc Nurse **24**, 218–224; quiz 225–6.
6. Dahlin C, Lynch M, Szmuilowicz E, Jackson V (2006). Management of symptoms other than pain. Anesthesiol Clin **24**, 39–60, viii.
7. Cranston JM, Crockett A, Currow D (2008). Oxygen therapy for dyspnoea in adults. Cochrane Database Syst Rev **3**, CD004769.

Table 3.5 Objective signs that may be associated with dyspnoea*

• Stridor	• Restlessness	• Diaphoresis
• Agitation	• Cyanosis	• Increased respiratory rate
• Use of accessory muscles	• Abnormal ABG assessment	• Decreased O_2 saturation
• Respiratory dyssynchrony	• Abnormal breath sounds	• Audible snoring in non-ventilated patient

* Data adapted from:
Campbell ML. Terminal dyspnea and respiratory distress. Crit Care Clin. Jul 2004;20(3): 403–417, viii–ix.
Kuebler K. Dyspnea. In: Kuebler K, Berry P, Heidrich D, eds. End of Life Care: Clinical Pratice Guidelines. Philadelphia: W.B. Saunders Company; 2002:301–315.

Anxiety

Anxiety is a common experience in ICU patients at high risk of dying. It occurs in 53–63% of ICU patients at a moderate to severe level.[1] ICU patients are at an increased risk of anxiety due to unfamiliar surroundings, uncertainty regarding prognosis, and exposure to many unfamiliar faces.[2] In addition, mechanically ventilated patients are especially at risk because of difficulties with communicating and/or expressing their fear.[2]

Definition

Anxiety is a subjective experience of diffuse apprehension or uneasiness accompanied by feelings of uncertainty and helplessness.[2] It is associated with an increase in autonomic arousal, myocardial workload and coagulability, and a reduction in the patient's immune response.[2]

Causes/risk factors[2,3]

Anxiety may be associated with:
- Unrelieved pain or dyspnoea, particularly in mechanically ventilated patients. They have difficulty communicating their respiratory distress and the resultant excess motor activity is often interpreted as anxiety.
- Underlying somatic processes (i.e. hypoxia, sepsis) and diagnoses such as cardiovascular and pulmonary disease.
- Situational stressors.
- Medications such as steroids, anticholinergic agents, theophylline, bronchodilators, amphetamines, and alcohol or benzodiazepine withdrawal.

Assessment

- Anxiety should be routinely assessed in all ICU patients; it is often severe and is associated with adverse sequelae.
- If the patient can speak, the clinicians can obtain the patient's self-report of their anxiety intensity using a validated scale such as NRS.
- Clinicians can also simply have patients rate their anxiety as either mild, moderate, severe, or extreme (panic).
- If the patient is unable to communicate verbally, the clinicians can assess for anxiety by using behavioural, observable, and physiologic signs (see Table 3.6). Clinicians can also use a single item Faces Anxiety Scale to assess anxiety. The Faces Anxiety Scale also works in assessing anxiety in mechanically ventilated patients.[3]

Restlessness/agitation

It is common for the terms restlessness, agitation, and anxiety to overlap, but they do have slightly different features. Restlessness has been defined as the inability to relax or be still, along with feelings of uneasiness and worry.[4]

Agitation is considered further along the continuum than restlessness and anxiety. Agitation is characterized by four features:[4]
- Physically aggressive behaviours: hitting, punching.
- Physically non-aggressive behaviours: pacing, disrobing.
- Verbally agitated behaviours: cursing, screaming, calling out.
- Hiding/hoarding behaviours.

Agitation occurs in approximately 52% of ICU patients.[4] It may interfere with the patient's care and is associated with a poorer prognosis than non-agitated patients.[4] Agitation has the potential to increase oxygen consumption, the patient's heart rate, respiratory rate, and blood pressure. Agitated patients are at risk of removing lines and tubes along with possible self-extubation. Agitation is also associated with a higher rate of nosocomial infections and a longer duration in ICU and hospital length of stay.[4]

Causes/risks
There are multiple causes or risk factors associated with an increase in agitation in ICU patients. See Table 3.7 for a list of causes.

Assessment
- Agitation is often under-diagnosed and may lead to multiple problems for ICU patients; therefore a systematic evaluation of this problem is needed. Clinicians can use several reliable and valid tools to assess for agitation. (See Figs. 3.1, 3.2, 3.3).
- Clinicians can also assess behaviours in agitated patients such as fidgeting, constant motion, combativeness, kicking, fighting the ventilator, pulling tubes, and restraints.[5]

Pharmacologic management of anxiety/agitation[5]
- Anxiolytics may help patients gain control over anxiety; monitor for excessive sedation and motor and sensory impairment or signs of ICU delirium (see 📖 in 'Delirium in the critically ill patient at the end of life: issues and management' p74).
- Scheduled dosing is more effective; rebound anxiety may occur if given on an 'as needed' basis to patients.
- Monitor all anxiolytics for effectiveness, dependency, abuse, and the possibility of withdrawal symptoms when discontinued.
- Lorazepam is relatively unaffected by liver disease, age, or concurrent use of specific serotonin reuptake inhibitors (SSRIs). Drawbacks include amnesic episodes, and more frequent dosing may be required to reduce interdose anxiety caused by its short half-life.
- Cyclic antidepressants, if used to treat anxiety in depressed critically ill patients, must be carefully monitored for potentially deleterious side effects which include excessive sedation, anticholinergic effects, and orthostatic hypotension.
- Restlessness and agitation can be treated with neuroleptics such as haloperidol (0.5–2mg PO 2–3 times per day) and increase doses based on response. Acute agitation: initially 2–10mg IM or IV, with the doses repeated at one hour intervals, if needed. Convert to oral therapy as soon as possible. Disadvantages include extrapyramidal symptoms and prolonged QT interval at high doses.
- Restlessness and agitation can also be treated by the judicious use of benzodiazepines.
- Caution: sedatives are not to be used as a means for coercion, discipline, convenience, or retaliation by staff.

Non-pharmacological management[6]

- Exclude reversible physical causes of anxiety or restlessness/agitation; assess if pain is the cause of acute agitation.
- Provide frequent gentle re-orientations.
- Anticipate related symptoms such as pain, dyspnoea (particularly in mechanically ventilated patients), and fatigue.
- Provide the patient and family members with information that is clear and easily understood.
- Encourage the presence of supportive persons and listen to patients' feelings, doubts, and fears.
- Use a calming presence and acknowledgement to help the patient manage panic.
- Use relaxation and, if possible, self-hypnosis techniques.
- Teach breathing, imagery, visualization, and focusing techniques or try music therapy.

Environmental management

- Reduce external stimuli such as noises; adjust 24-hour lighting.
- Familiarize surrounding with photos of family, close friends, pets.
- Minimize changes in staff.
- Reduce sensory deprivation by providing calendars and clocks visible to patient.

References

1. Nelson J, Meier DE, Oei EJ, et al. (2001) Self-reporting symptom experience of critically ill cancer patients receiving intensive care. *Crit Care Med* **29**, 277–82.
2. Szokol JW, Vender JS (2001). Anxiety, delirium, and pain in the intensive care unit. *Crit Care Clin* **17**, 821–42.
3. McKinley S, Stein–Parbury J, Chehelnabi A, Lovas J. Assessment of anxiety in intensive care patients by using the Faces Anxiety Scale. *Am J Crit Care* **13**, 146–52.
4. Jaber S, Chanques G, Altairac C, et al. (2005). A prospective study of agitation in a medical-surgical ICU: incidence, risk factors, and outcomes. *Chest* **128**, 2749–57.
5. Jacobi J, Fraser GL, Coursin DB, et al. (2002). Clinical practice guidelines for the sustained use of sedatives and analgesics in the critically ill adult. *Crit Care Med* **30**, 119–41.
6. Lang EV, Benotsch EG, Fick LJ, et al. (2000). Adjunctive non-pharmacological analgesia for invasive medical procedures: a randomized trial. *Lancet* **355**, 1486–90.

Table 3.6 Subjective, observable, and physiologic descriptors of anxiety*

Subjective	Observable	Physiologic
• Apprehension	• Tense posture	• Changes in vital signs
• Nervousness	• Fidgeting	• Diaphoresis
• Fear	• Dryness and licking the lips	• Flushing or pallor
• Irritability	• Insomnia	• Dry mouth
• Restlessness	• Trembling	• Dilated pupils
• Difficulty concentrating	• Frequent sighing	• Urinary frequency
• Headaches		• Fatigue
• Nausea		• Diarrhoea

* Adapted from:

Frazier SK, Moser DK, Riegel B, et al. Critical care nurses' assessment of patients' anxiety: reliance on physiological and behavioral parameters. Am J Crit Care. Jan 2002; 11(1): 57–64.
Pasacreta J, Minarik P, Nield-Anderson L. Anxiety and Depression. In: Ferrell B, Coyle N, eds. Textbook of Palliative Nursing. New York: Oxford; 2001: 269–289.
Kuebler K, Heidrich D. Anxiety. In: Kuebler K, Berry P, Heidrich D, eds. End of Life Care: Clinical Practice Guidelines. Philadelphia: W.B. Saunders Company; 2002: 199–212.

Table 3.7 Causes of agitation*

- Excessive stimulation.
- Inability to communicate.
- Hypoxaemia.
- Alcoholism and regular use of antipsychotic medicines.
- Abuse of sedation.
- Untreated hyponatraemia and hypernatraemia.
- Invasive procedures.
- Metabolic imbalance.
- Sleep deprivation.
- Use of sedatives and/or analgesics 48 hours preceding onset of agitation.
- Neglected hyperthermia >38°C.

* Adapted from:

Kuebler K, English NK, Heidrich D. Delirium, Confusion, Agitation, and Restlessness. In: Ferrell BR, Coyle N, eds. Textbook of Palliative Nursing. New York: Oxford; 2001: 290–308.

Level	Description
1	Patient anxious and agitated, restless, or both.
2	Patient cooperative, orientated, and tranquil.
3	Patient awake, responds to commands only.
4	Patient asleep, brisk response to a light glabellar tap.
5	Patient asleep, sluggish response to a light glabellar tap.
6	Patient asleep, no response to a light glabellar tap.

Fig. 3.1 Agitation assessment scale: the modified Ramsay scale (scored from 1=patient anxious to 6=no response to light glabellar tap). Adapted from: Ramsay MA, Savege TM, Simpson BR, Goodwin R (1974). Controlled sedation with alphaxalone-alphadolone. *Br Med J* **2**, 656–9.

Level	Behaviours
7	Dangerous agitation, immediate threat to safety. Examples: pulls at endotracheal tubes and catheters, climbs over bed rails, strikes out at staff.
6	Very agitated. Examples: unable to calm down to verbal reminders, requires physical restraints, bites at endotracheal tube.
5	Agitated, anxious. Examples: attempts to sit up in bed, calms down with verbal reminders.
4	Calm and cooperative.
3	Sedated. Examples: difficult to awaken, drifts off easily, follows simple commands.
2	Very sedated. Examples: arouses to physical stimuli, but no communication or following of commands.
1	Unarousable. Examples: minimal to no response to noxious stimuli.

Fig. 3.2 Agitation assessment scale: sedation-agitation scale—SAS (scored from 1=unarousable to 7=dangerous agitation). Adapted from: Riker RR, Fraser GL (2001). Monitoring sedation, agitation, analgesia, neuromuscular blockade, and delirium in adult ICU patients. *Semin Respir Crit Care Med* **22**, 189–98; Riker RR, Picard JT, Fraser GL (1999). Prospective evaluation of the Sedation-Agitation Scale for adult critically ill patients. *Crit Care Med* **27**, 1325–9.

Score	Description
+4	Combative. Examples: violent behaviour, immediate danger to staff.
+3	Very agitated. Examples: pulls or removes tubing, catheters, aggressive behaviour.
+2	Agitated. Example: frequent, non-purposeful movements.
+1	Restless. Example: anxious movements, not aggressive.
0	Alert and calm.
−1	Drowsy. Examples: not fully alert, can stay awake for more than 10 seconds, has eye contact to voice.
−2	Light sedation. Example: awakens briefly (less than 10 seconds) to voice.
−3	Moderate sedation. Examples: movement, but no eye contact to voice.
−4	Deep sedation. Examples: no response to voice, movement to physical stimuli.
−5	Unarousable. Examples: no response to voice or physical stimuli.

Fig. 3.3 Agitation assessment scale: the Richmond agitation sedation scale—RASS (scored from +4=very combative and dangerous to −5=non-responsive and unarousable; score 0=calm and cooperative). Adapted from: Sessler CN, Gosnell MS, Grap MJ, et al. (2002). The Richmond Agitation-Sedation Scale: validity and reliability in adult intensive care unit patients. *Am J Respir Crit Care Med* **166**, 1338–44.

Delirium in the critically ill patient at the end of life: issues and management

A 60-year old patient with end-stage lymphoma agreed to intubation and maximal support in the context of a potentially reversible bacterial pneumonia. Now that she has ARDS and is developing renal failure, she makes it clear that she no longer wishes aggressive therapy and requests to be removed from mechanical ventilation. Her family and friends gather around her in what they hope to be an emotional, but peaceful accompaniment to her death. The patient makes no eye contact with anyone in the room and is clearly frightened; her eye movements seem to follow moving targets on the ceiling. Her clinical picture is compatible with delirium. What is your approach?

Definition of delirium
- The diagnostic and statistical manual of mental disorders (DSM) IV criteria (presence of a medical illness, disturbance of consciousness, change in cognition, and sudden onset/fluctuation in time) are the standard clinical features for identifying delirium.
- Delirium can manifest in one of two subtypes (agitated, hypoactive; most often, both manifestations are present).[1] Neither is associated with prognosis, but agitation in subsyndromal delirium is a poor prognostic sign.
- Underlying neurologic pathology should be eliminated in the differential diagnosis.
- Standardization of use of the term delirium, within the spectrum of acute brain dysfunction in the ICU, was the subject of a recent international initiative.[2]

Incidence
- Adult ICU patients commonly develop delirium. A range of 22–45% is often quoted[3] (although 11–89% is described) in the ICU literature. Critically ill children seem to develop delirium less commonly (5% or less).[4]
- A disease spectrum exists: both children and adults can have full-blown delirium clinical symptoms or transient delirium features. In adults, the percentage of incidence for developing delirium, subsyndromal delirium,[5] and remaining cognitively normal are roughly 33% each. In children, the subsyndromal delirium type appears to exist as well, but descriptions of incidences do not exist in the paediatric ICU population.
- The presence of subsyndromal and full-blown delirium are associated with longer ICU and hospital lengths of stay, and with higher mortality.

Risk factors for delirium
- Risk factors for delirium in adults include prior alcohol consumption, prior hypertension, and severity of illness on admission to ICU. Once admitted to ICU, the most significant associated risk factor is iatrogenic coma (i.e. excessive sedation), attributable to opiates or benzodiazepines regardless of administered drug doses.

- In children, only the severity of illness has been shown to correlate with delirium incidence.
- Cancer or the presence of terminal illness is not associated with a delirium diagnosis in the ICU, in contrast with medical or hospice patients. There may be differences in baseline vulnerability (e.g. cognitive status) and the timing of delirium symptoms in relation to death among terminally ill cancer and non-cancer patients.

Impact of delirium

- Delirium is distressing for family members and patients, and burdensome for caregivers.[6] Patients are frightened as many experience paranoid delusions. Families can experience severe stress if their loved ones' behaviour is something they don't recognize or that they find disturbing. In addition, they will worry they may not get the opportunity to communicate with family members who are nearing death.
- Informing patients and families of delirium manifestations prior to and during its occurrence may be helpful and may reduce delirium symptomatology.

Tools to measure delirium

- Delirium **screening** can be conducted using two screening scales that are commonly used in the ICU: the intensive care delirium screening checklist (ICDSC) and the ICU-adjusted Confusion Assessment Method (CAM-ICU). Both are validated in mechanically ventilated patients.
- ICDSC allows for the identification of eight clinical features whereas CAM-ICU is a 'binary' (presence/absence of delirium) scale (available from: http://www.icudelirium.org). Thus, the ICDSC allows for the identification of three categories of patients: the cognitively intact, those with delirium, and those with subsyndromal delirium in the ICU, an intermediate category of both disease severity and poor outcomes (where patients manifest some, but not all symptoms of delirium). Comparative publications suggest ICDSC may be preferred by nurses and somewhat easier to use.
- Delirium **severity** should be measured with validated tools specific for that purpose, such as the delirium rating scale (DRS). All such tools require verbal responses and are thus difficult to apply in the critical care setting.
- Teaching nurses and other critical care caregivers to identify delirium[7] with validated scales helps to:
  - Screen for and thus identify delirium early (before worsening psychomotor agitation sets in).
  - Reassure patients. Patients describe that it is comforting to experience reorientation, and receive explanations that they are not irretrievably psychiatrically ill and that their symptoms are common complications among the critically ill.
  - Differentiate psychomotor agitation stemming from delirium from, for instance, pain, to medicate patients more appropriately.

Prevention and treatment: non-pharmacological approaches

- Many non-pharmacologic approaches have been proposed. None of them have been tested; intensive care clinicians have not reached a consensus on what is useful and what is not.[8]
- Hand restraints, for instance, are alternatively used or limited in delirious patients; their recent association with a higher auto-extubation rate has not been stratified based on whether patients were delirious or not.
- Patients able to recall delirium symptoms describe intense fear and distress.
- Patient symptoms appear modifiable by staff reassurance and personalized interaction with the patient.
- Non-pharmacologic approaches (reducing noise level, ambient light, offering music for relaxation) should, therefore, be centred on what the individual patient finds reassuring.
- Fear should be addressed directly and palliated when possible.
- Families may take some reassurance in the knowledge that delirium symptoms are frequent and that they have an important role in reorienting and reassuring the patient.[6]

Pharmacological approaches

- Titrating and minimizing medications for sedation and analgesia for adequate pain relief with a minimum of opiate analgesia (with co-analgesics and dose titration) may be helpful and probably reduces the incidence of subsyndromal delirium.
- Rotating opiates when they are administered in high doses (e.g. alternating 24 hours of fentanyl and morphine).
- Meperidine has more excitatory effects on the central nervous system than other opioids and should be avoided, where possible, in favour of alternative opioids.
- Treating delirium has traditionally been proposed with antipsychotics such as haloperidol. Most haloperidol recipients will experience a reduction in psychomotor agitation regardless of whether their delirium symptoms abate or not. Other delirium features (such as hallucinations or delusions and the fear associated with them) should be 'tracked' to monitor appropriate response to pharmacologic intervention.
- Overall, antipsychotics may reduce psychomotor agitation and hallucinations, but their general benefit is not clearly established. In clinical descriptions of critically ill children, haloperidol is considered effective and on occasion, 'proof' (particularly in very young children) that agitation is attributable to delirium.
- Haloperidol is problematic in patients with extrapyramidal symptoms and prolonged QT intervals. Maximal antipsychotic doses are 2–20mg/day range; if the patient is not better after 24–48 hours at this dose, he/she should be considered a haloperidol 'failure'. Many (up to 50–60%) of adult ICU patients do not respond to haloperidol.
- Alternative antipsychotics should be considered such as olanzapine, risperdal, and seroquel. Their benefit is equivalent to that of haloperidol. Some patients may respond to one antipsychotic, but not another. Others derive benefit from either combining sedatives (benzodiazepines, small doses of propofol, or, where available, dexmetomidine) with

antipsychotics or to using sedatives alone. Regular assessments of and communication with patients as to symptoms severity and frequency are the mainstay of treatment response evaluation.

- In regular high alcohol consumers (purportedly 20% of the population), withdrawal should be considered in the differential diagnosis of agitation. These patients should be managed specifically and probably exclusively with benzodiazepines. Better symptom control and lower complication rates are associated with strictly adjusting drug administration to alcohol withdrawal symptoms, which can be monitored for alcohol withdrawal scales modified for ICU use such as the Clinical Institute Withdrawal Assessment for Alcohol scale. Although alcohol can be administered to patients suspected or known to have alcohol withdrawal, it is probably preferable to add a sliding scale of benzodiazepines to this regimen as regular alcohol consumers can develop withdrawal even when getting oral or intravenous alcohol in the ICU. Chronic benzodiazepine users should also be managed with benzodiazepines as a first-line drug, and antipsychotics such as haloperidol added to control symptoms such as hallucinations or delusions once adequate sedation has been established.

The 60-year old patient with lymphoma was initially managed with small doses of intravenous haloperidol. Opioids were changed from fentanyl to morphine. Her nurse reoriented her systematically and taught the family how to reassure her when she was fearful. She improved with this non-pharmacological approach combined with 0.5–1mg of intravenous haloperidol every 2–4 hours and small doses of short-acting benzodiazepines. She died in comfort and was aware of her family's presence to the end.

Key points

Non-pharmacological approaches, compassion, and hands-on caring that supplement effective pharmacological strategies can go a long way to ease the burden of delirium for patients, families, and the ICU team.

References

1. Marquis F, Ouimet S, Riker R, Cossette M, Skrobik Y (2007). Individual delirium symptoms: do they matter? *Crit Care Med* **35**, 2533–7.
2. Morandi A, Pandharipande P, Trabucchi M, *et al.* (2008). Understanding international differences in terminology for delirium and other types of acute brain dysfunction in critically ill patients. *Intensive Care Med* **34**, 1907–15.
3. Ouimet S, Kavanagh BP, Gottfried SB, Skrobik Y (2007). Incidence, risk factors and consequences of ICU delirium. *Intensive Care Med* **33**, 66–73.
4. Schieveld JN, Leroy PL, van Os J, *et al.* (2007). Paediatric delirium in critical illness: phenomenology, clinical correlates, and treatment response in 40 cases in the paediatric intensive care unit. *Intensive Care Med* **33**, 1033–40.
5. Ouimet S, Riker R, Bergeron N, *et al.* (2007). Subsyndromal delirium in the ICU: evidence for a disease spectrum. *Intensive Care Med* **33**, 1007–13.
6. Breitbart W, Gibson C, Tremblay A (2002). The delirium experience: delirium recall and delirium-related distress in hospitalized patients with cancer, their spouses/caregivers, and their nurses. *Psychosomatics* **43**, 183–94.
7. Devlin JW, Marquis F, Riker RR, *et al.* (2008). Combined didactic and scenario-based education improves the ability of intensive care unit staff to recognize delirium at the bedside. *Crit Care* **12**, R19.
8. Cheung CZ, Alibhai SM, Robinson M, *et al.* (2008). Recognition and labeling of delirium symptoms by intensivists: does it matter? *Intensive Care Med* **34**, 437–46.

Sleep disturbances

'Sleep is that golden chain that ties health and our bodies together.'
Thomas Dekker (1577–1632)

Sleep disturbances are very common for patients at risk of dying in the ICU and affect around 42–68% of patients at a moderate to severe level.[1] ICU patients recalling their ICU experience reported that lack of sleep was a major stressor for them.[1]

Definition

Sleep consists of two distinct states: rapid eye movement (REM) and non-rapid eye movement (NREM). REM sleep consists of 25% of sleep time where the patient has bursts of REM, irregularly respirations and heart rate, and paralysis of the major muscles, except muscles used for breathing. NREM sleep consists of four stages that are progressive in nature and range from light sleep to deep sleep. Stage 4 is considered to be the most restorative. REM and NREM sleep cycles occur about every 90 minutes throughout the night with clustering towards early morning hours.[2]

Causes/risks of sleep disturbance[2,3]

- ICU environment (i.e. noise, light).
- Patient care activities (i.e. vital signs, medication administration, diagnostic testing).
- Mechanical ventilation (especially with ventilator dyssynchrony).
- Medications (i.e. sedatives, hypnotics, analgesics, antipsychotics, stimulants, and antidepressants) that affect the sleep cycle adversely, generally diminishing REM sleep.
- Pain or underlying illness.

Adverse effects[2–4]

Various studies show that sleep deprivation can:

- Alter immune function.
- Alter psychological functioning (i.e. causing symptoms such as irritability, memory loss, inattention, ICU delirium, delusions, hallucinations, slurred speech, incoordination, and blurred vision).
- Lower the quality of life for ICU patients.
- Increase morbidity and mortality.

Sleep patterns common in ICU patients[2,5]

- Increased fragmented sleep and decreased duration.
- Long sleep onset.
- Poor sleep efficiencies.
- Increase in stage 1.
- Decrease in stages 2–4 and REM.
- Increase arousal and awakenings.

Assessment[2,3]

' … a medicated state of sleep may resemble sleep on the surface, but may not provide the physiological benefits associated with true sleep.'
Parthasarathy & Tobin (2004). p 200

- Sleep quality and quantity are very difficult to assess in ICU patients because of their critical conditions requiring sedation.
- Polysomnography (the most accurate way to measure sleep) is not practicable in most ICUs due to complex interpretation and because of electrical interference and muscle contraction of agitated, restless patients.
- It is important to note that patients' total sleep time may be normal, but the actual quality of their sleep is compromised, and that patients may perceive their quality of sleep to be poor even after receiving high doses of sedatives that achieved adequate levels of sedation.

Non-pharmacological management[5]

- Minimize unnecessary interruptions.
- Do not bathe patients between 9 p.m. and 6 a.m. or, if necessary, give a warm bath that may promote sleep afterwards.
- Cluster activities to provide extended blocks of uninterrupted sleep.
- Review nocturnal care interventions and the practice protocols that require assessments every two hours. Nocturnal interventions at 3 a.m. correspond to the physiological nadir in sleep, temperature, and alertness rhythms for both the patients and nurses.

Pharmacological management[6]

- Benzodiazepines, opioid analgesics, and propofol are frequently used to sedate critically ill patients.
- Benzodiazepines can improve some aspects of sleep by decreasing the time to fall asleep, decrease the number of awakenings, increase sleep duration and sleep efficiency.
- Benzodiazepines, however, alter the normal sleep patterns and suppress REM and slow wave sleep, the most restorative stage of sleep.

Environmental management[2]

- Control noise through the use of earplugs to increase REM sleep, turn down alarms to the lowest audible level possible, or use light alarms instead of sound alarms on monitors.
- If possible, decrease room lighting levels at night and open window shades during the day.

References

1. Nelson J, Meier DE, Oei EJ, et al. (2001). Self-reporting symptom experience of critically ill cancer patients receiving intensive care. Crit Care Med **29**, 277–82.
2. Parthasarathy S, Tobin MJ (2004). Sleep in the intensive care unit. Intensive Care Med **30**, 197–206.
3. Gabor JY, Cooper AB, Crombach SA, et al. (2003). Contribution of the intensive care unit environment to sleep disruption in mechanically ventilated patients and healthy subjects. Am J Respir Crit Care Med **167**, 708–15.
4. Eddleston JM, White P, Guthrie E (2000). Survival, morbidity, and quality of life after discharge from intensive care. Crit Care Med **28**, 2293–9.
5. Tamburri LM, DiBrienza R, Zozula R, Redeker NS (2004). Nocturnal care interactions with patients in critical care units. Am J Crit Care **13**, 102–12; quiz 114–5.
6. Friese RS, Diaz–Arrastia R, McBride D, Frankel H, Gentilello LM (2007). Quantity and quality of sleep in the surgical intensive care unit: are our patients sleeping? J Trauma **63**, 1210–4.

Thirst/dry mouth

Thirst and dry mouth are very common symptoms in ICU patients at risk of dying, with 40–78% of patients reporting it at moderate to severe levels.[1,2]

Definition
In general, thirst is an indication of a lack of fluids in the body or of an increase in osmolarity of the blood. When patients are fluid-depleted, saliva production is reduced, making the mouth feel dry and cottony.[3]

Cause/risk factors[3]
- Mouth breathing.
- Medications (e.g. diuretics, anticholinergics, opioids, and steroids).
- Blood loss.
- Sweating/fevers.
- Vomiting and diarrhoea.

Assessment[3–5]
- Self-report is the gold standard.
- Often the patient will report feeling weak, lightheaded, and/or complain of headaches.
- If the patient is unable to verbalize their thirst, clinicians can assess the mouth area routinely for dry lips and tongue and assess blood biochemistry that may indicate dehydration.
- The role of dehydration/rehydration in the cause and relief of the thirst sensation in terminal cancer patients remains unresolved in palliative care practice.
- Cancer patients receiving morphine were approximately four times more likely to have a dry mouth than patients taking a weak opioid, non-opioid, or no analgesic.
- Assessment may reveal thick, ropey secretions or absent saliva.

Non-pharmacological management for xerostomia (oral dryness)[6]
- Meticulous oral care is essential; frequent cleaning using a soft toothbrush and moistened foam swabs.
- Consider using oral cleansing agents: chlorhexidine oral rinse, sodium bicarbonate, and fluoride.
- Administer ice chips to reduce mouth dryness.

Pharmacologic management for xerostomia (oral dryness)[6]
- Assess medications for possible sources of dry mouth.
- Artificial saliva or saliva substitutes may be used: pilocarpine 5mg orally, three times daily (not to exceed 10mg per dose); bethanechol 25mg, three times daily; methacholine 10mg, once daily; or cevimeline spray or mouthwash (not available in the UK).

References

1. Nelson J, Meier DE, Oei EJ, *et al.* (2001). Self-reporting symptom experience of critically ill cancer patients receiving intensive care. *Crit Care Med* **29**, 277–82.
2. Nelson J, Meier DE, Litke A, Natale DA, Siegel RE, Morrison SR (2004). The symptom burden of chronic illness. *Crit Care Med* **32**, 1527–34.
3. Kedziera P (2001). Hydration, thirst, and nutrition. In: Ferrell BR, Coyle N (eds) *Textbook of palliative nursing*, pp 156–63. Oxford University Press, New York.
4. Morita T, Tei Y, Tsunoda J, Inoue S, Chihara S (2001). Determinants of the sensation of thirst in terminally ill cancer patients. *Support Care Cancer* **9**, 177–86.
5. White ID, Hoskin PJ, Hanks GW, Bliss JM (1989). Morphine and dryness of the mouth. *BMJ* **298**, 1222–3.
6. O'Reilly M (2003). Oral care of the critically ill: a review of the literature and guidelines for practice. *Aust Crit Care* **16**, 101–10.

Caring for families in the ICU

Families of dying patients: an introduction to meeting their
    needs 84
Alexandre Lautrette, Élie Azoulay

From admission to bereavement: the patient- and family-centred
    care approach 88
Heather MacDonald

Relationships and iatrogenic suffering: part 1 94
David Kuhl

Conducting an ICU family conference: a VALUES approach 104
J Randall Curtis

Decision-making for patients who lack capacity to decide: the
    surrogate in the ICU 112
Alexandre Lautrette, Élie Azoulay, Jeffrey Watts, Bertrand Souweine

Observational studies of families of patients who died in the
    ICU 118
Élie Azoulay, Graeme Rocker

Families of dying patients: an introduction to meeting their needs

Introduction

Most deaths in the ICU occur after decisions to withhold or withdraw life-sustaining treatments. Family members of dying patients have specific needs related to distressing emotions, a tendency toward denial of death, difficulties in understanding medical information, and being unprepared for surrogate decision-making. Several studies describe the specific needs of bereaved relatives, identifying the following needs from questionnaires and interviews:

- Clear, timely, consistent, and easy to understand information.
- Intimacy with caregiver's team.
- Being convinced that the dying patient is not in pain or anxious.
- That the patient's preferences and values will be fully respected.
- To be useful to the dying person.
- To find meaning in the death of a loved one.

These specific family needs should be among treatment targets of ICU nurses and physicians as they manage dying patients.

Data from observational studies

Findings from observational studies have highlighted specific needs of relatives from dying patients that influence family satisfaction, symptoms of anxiety or depression, and those related to post-traumatic stress disorder (PTSD).

The main sources of family dissatisfaction are:
- Poor communication with caregivers.
- Insufficient, unclear, or contradictory information.
- Discussion with the 'doctor in charge' in a waiting room.
- Low frequency of physician communication.
- Conflicts between the family members and the ICU team.
- Financial difficulties.
- Suboptimal visitation policies.

The main sources of family satisfaction are:
- Respect and compassion from caregivers.
- Completeness of information on the diagnosis, prognosis, and treatment.
- Information on the process of withholding and withdrawing life-sustaining therapies.
- Conversation with 'doctor in charge' in a quiet place.
- Discussion of the patient's preferences with medical staff.
- Family ability to voice concerns, to express emotions.
- Feeling that the patient seems to be comfortable at all times during end-of-life care.
- Opportunity to have pastoral care or psychological support.

The main sources of family anxiety/depression or of symptoms related to PTSD are associated with:
- Receiving incomplete or contradictory information.
- The guilt of having made the bad decision.
- The nature of their role in end-of-life decision-making.

The provision of sufficient information is the determining factor of satisfaction with care and the extent of psychological disorders among relatives of dying patients. Information exchange and communication are strongly linked. Improving communication between the ICU team and the families about end-of-life care is both a major challenge and a crucial step towards improving patient and family outcomes, most notably when decisions are made to limit treatment. When this occurs, the feeling of guilt of sharing an end-of-life decision may be the cause of complicated grief.

Interventions to improve the care of families of dying patients

Several interventions can improve communication with family members of patients dying in the ICU. These include:
- Interventions by nurses or social workers to enhance patient-family autonomy and to prevent conflicts (see 📖 in 'Conflicts, negotiations, and resolution: a primer' p202).
- Implementation of clinical ethics programmemes (see 📖 in 'The ethics consultant and clinical ethics committee' p208).
- Intensive communication with therapeutic goals (see also 📖 in 'Relationships and iatrogenic suffering: part 1' p94 and 📖 'Conducting an ICU family conference: a VALUES approach' p104).
- A family information leaflet and active participation of physicians in family information initiatives.
- Earlier and proactive palliative care intervention.

Intensive communication about therapeutic goals allows the patient, family, and ICU staff to discuss patient preferences, the care plan, patient goals, and criteria to determine whether those goals are met. When goals are not met, additional meetings should occur to discuss a predominant focus on palliative care. This intensive communication strategy results in a shorter length of ICU stay and earlier access to palliative care, with no increase in mortality.[1]

Family information leaflets increase the comprehension of diagnosis and treatment, improve the effectiveness of information exchange, and satisfaction with care, but only for family members with adequate comprehension of the information.[2] Junior physicians perform as well as senior physicians in terms of families comprehending them, family satisfaction, and effect of symptoms of anxiety and depression on family members. Collectively, a proactive communication strategy, characterized by an early and intensive communication between family members and caregivers, improves the care of families of dying patients in the ICU. In relatives of patients dying in the ICU, a proactive communication strategy that includes formal end-of-life family conferences alleviates symptoms of stress, anxiety, and depression.[3] These conferences provide ICU clinicians with a unique opportunity to meet point by point each of the family needs. In particular, listening to the relatives and making every effort to elicit questions and to respond to questions helps families to cope with the distress of bereavement and alleviates the feeling of guilt of having shared an end-of-life decision.[4]

Conclusions

ICU staff members must be aware of the specific needs of relatives of dying patients. Structured and planned family conferences increase decision-making potential, improve communication between physicians and families of patients who are unable to make decisions, and help to alleviate the family's emotional burdens. These strategies should be included in communication training programmes aimed at improving both global communication and the quality of dying and death in the ICU. These issues are explored further in other chapters.

References

1. Lilly CM, De Meo DL, Sonna LA, *et al.* (2000). An intensive communication intervention for the critically ill. *Am J Med* **109**, 469–75.
2. Azoulay E, Pochard F, Chevret S, *et al.* (2002). Impact of a family information leaflet on effectiveness of information provided to family members of intensive care unit patients: a multicentre, prospective, randomized, controlled trial. *Am J Respir Crit Care Med* **165**, 438–42.
3. Lautrette A, Darmon M, Megarbane B, *et al.* (2007). A communication strategy and brochure for relatives of patients dying in the ICU. *N Engl J Med* **356**, 469–78.
4. Curtis JR, Patrick DL, Shannon SE, Treece PD, Engelberg RA, Rubenfeld GD (2001). The family conference as a focus to improve communication about end-of-life care in the intensive care unit: opportunities for improvement. *Crit Care Med* **29**(2 Suppl), N26–33.

From admission to bereavement: the patient- and family-centred care approach

What is patient- and family-centred care?

The philosophy of patient- and family-centred care (PFCC) offers a vision of health care based on the belief that patients and families have unique knowledge and expertise to improve service delivery. Its fundamental principles are grounded in partnerships, collaboration, informed choice, decision-making, communication, healing, dignity, and respect.[1] The demands for PFCC are growing in recognition of its capacity to improve outcomes, enhance patient safety, and increase satisfaction of staff, patients, and families.

In Halifax, Nova Scotia, Canada, we created a patient and family council to enhance the development of PFCC locally and describe this initiative in more detail below. It is our belief that the creation of similar councils in ICUs around the world can only improve the provision of more widespread PFCC.

The critical care PFCC advisory council

The patient and family advisory council is an innovative and effective strategy for involving patients and families in transformational change. First established by the Institute for Family-Centred Care, these councils typically include members of the multidisciplinary team along with patients and families as health care consumers. Because patients and families see care through a different lens, their perspective is important to facilitate health care providers' understanding and insight into their experience. The invitation to include ICU patients and families as advisors and partners in care signifies willingness for ICUs to be more collaborative and transparent.

The primary goal of the council is to incorporate the patients' and families' perspective and expertise into redesign and process planning that will improve the health care experience. Advisors serve as 'listening posts' for staff and administration, allowing an open dialogue and creative problem-solving between the organization, patients, and family members.

Responsibilities

The council responsibilities may include:
- Advocacy and involvement of patients and families to provide information about their needs, expectations, and experiences.
- Participation in programme planning, development, implementation, and evaluation, i.e. ICU family support programme, pager programme, communication devices for voice-disabled patients, bereavement aftercare).
- Engage in patient safety discussions, quality improvement initiatives, and policy review, i.e. (visitation, infection control, advance directives, signage).
- Staff selection, hiring, recruitment, orientation, and in-service training programmes.

- Participate in the renovation planning and redesign of family waiting rooms, buildings, services.
- Group facilitator and co-chair leadership role.
- Advocate for quality end-of-life care.
- Generate change concepts and ideas.
- Assist with the redesign of resources, tools that support team relationships, communication, documentation, and family meeting records.
- Participate in needs assessments.
- Advocacy for health resources and community services.
- Reviewer of patient and family handbooks, grant proposals.
- Participate as guest speakers in education seminars, i.e. 'telling their story through the patient's eyes'.
- Communication of council activities: PFCC newsletter, storyboards such as 'family matters'.

Getting started

Initially, it is a good idea to start your patient and family advisory council with members recommended and recruited by the ICU team, either through direct contact or a specific recruitment strategy, i.e. a focus group or patient representative.
- The composition of the council will depend on the size of your organization or if your council will be a unit-based (ICU) patient and family advisory council. Usually between a total of 10–20 members that includes a diverse group including support staff, unit clerks, dietary, and housekeeping.
- Health care consumer membership should include former ICU patients, family members of ICU survivors, and non-survivors.
- Recruitment should involve an interview process and general application.
- Call for an 'expression of interest'.
- Post on the inpatient units or via newsletter.
- Members join in a volunteer capacity; a stipend can be offered for travel, meals, etc. based on hospital policy.
- They must be in telephone contact.
- They should be articulate and comfortable speaking, and actively participating in team discussion and teamwork.
- Context of the meetings are based on conversations asking crucial questions about 'what matters'.
- Council work is 'action-orientated' and geared toward implementation.
- Time commitment is two to four hours monthly, scheduled at convenient times for consideration of workload, employment, and childcare responsibilities.
- Request a minimum of a one-year term commitment.
- A signed letter of agreement.
- Adhere to confidentiality and privacy legislation.
- Embrace the role as a learner, teacher, coach, and mentor.
- Commit to a full orientation and training.
- Willingness to **share their story** in a respectful, constructive, no-blame manner.

Consideration of others' roles

The patient and family advisory council needs to work diligently to understand the perspective of everyone involved in planning and service delivery. However, at times, professional boundaries overlap and create tension based on different or conflicting motivations. Council members offer simple, economical suggestions that are not legislated by rules or ulterior motives.

The experiences of a council

Real life stories are an important component of a PFCC, offering a tool for change and an opportunity to make the 'human connection'. These stories are usually scripted in the context of 'what matters most' to patients and families, and how 'small things make a difference' and what appears to be 'the defining moments in peoples lives.' The PFCC advisory council is a forum for storytelling and story gathering. Patients and family members tell us they need:

• Unlimited and unrestricted access to their loved one.
• A compassionate presence.
• Respectful relationships that honour their value and beliefs.
• To be listened to.
• Consistent honest information.
• Family meetings: opportunities to ask questions.
• Healing environment privacy: non-clinical family rooms.
• Bereavement aftercare.
• Hope, acceptance, and grace in the midst of dying.
• Meaning making, finding meaning and purpose in critical illness and death.
• Dignity and choices.

Bereavement: innovative practices in ICU

Through the work of the advisory council and a PFCC model, health care providers are able to promote a positive health care experience using innovation and shared learning.

Journals

One day in the ICU family crisis room, we discovered a bible, torn and withered, the back cover ripped away, but underneath, we found handwritten scripts by ICU families, journaling about their experience, facing death, uncertainty, and the unfamiliar, technological world of ICU. They wrote about hope, faith, spirituality, and healing.

High tech/high care in an adult ICU

In the midst of technology, families strive to make sense of their loss. We have learnt to focus on creating memories (remembering) and crafting an experience by the following:

• Memory boxes (meaning making).
• Handprints.
• Ceramic hearts, placed on the dying patient, symbolizing the reunion of hearts.
• Locks of hair.
• Teddy bear programme—angel and hope bears given to young children.

- Books related to bereavement, explaining death and loss.
- Rituals and leaving a legacy of organ and tissue donation, honouring their lived one's wishes.
- Healing environment.

Bereavement aftercare

The ultimate goal of bereavement care following the death of a loved one in the ICU is to let the family members know that they are not alone. How this is accomplished is unique to each family, each individual, and staff member. Improvements in this area can significantly affect the grieving process and strongly influence the bereavement experience for family members and staff. Complicated grief and negative health outcomes for family members and staff can be affected by changes made in the ICU approach to holistic bereavement care. Overall themes from family members and staff include:

- A preventative approach to complicated bereavement. Many ICU family members of deceased ICU patients convey their need for psycho-/social/spiritual support to facilitate their overall capacity to cope and grieve. Many feel a sense of abandonment once they leave the ICU.
- Hospital and programme-based bereavement follow-up.
- Staff bereavement care/education.

Recommendations

- Compassionate supportive presence and behaviour from staff—this is one of the most appreciated aspects of ICU service.
- The need for information and communication from the team that is free of jargon. This allows the family the comfort of knowing that the right decisions were made.
- Unrestricted and unlimited visits at the bedside.
- Improved care before, during, and after the dying process.
- Advance directives and knowledge of their loved one's wishes in many ways can alleviate family members' anxiety, and these issues should be addressed as soon as appropriate.
- Follow-up with the bereaved families can involve:
  - Cards sent at certain intervals (anniversary, birthday, set periods of time).
  - Phone calls from trained individuals.
  - Referral to a mental health professional for those at risk for complicated grief.
  - Connection to therapeutic support groups education.
  - Staff education seminars and training to illuminate barriers to effective palliative care. Some highlights include the need for staff to grieve and the difficulty in 'switching gears' (from curative to palliative). Some research has explored grief support groups for staff to address bereavement related issues.

Hope

Many families tell us the importance of sustaining hope regardless of the outcome. They view hope as their 'life jacket' and ask that hope be maintained, not stripped or eroded.

Children visiting dying family members in ICU

Many families tell us about the need to be more open to children being present in the ICU. Strategies to engage children's presence at end of life in the ICU include:

- All ages—preschool to adolescent age-appropriate interventions.
- Using books that provide guidance to explaining critical illness throughout all the developmental ages.
- Must be a controlled situation with adequately trained support staff as a resource.
- Preplanning involving family members who know the children and their ability to cope with this situation.
- Conceal head trauma incisions with an operating room sterile hat.
- Preparing the environment by concealing the technology (machines, monitors) with sheets, placing a scarf over the 'trach' site: this allows the child to fully concentrate on being with their family without distraction.
- Obtaining an ECG strip: draw a heart on it.
- Debrief with the child and the family members afterwards.
- Colouring books, stickers, encouragement cards, and picture boards.

Education

- Interprofessional education is recommended, focusing on a PFCC curriculum.
- Use reflective practice.
- Celebrate the council's successes with recognition and praise.
- Scripting conversations for breaking bad news, role play, including organ and tissue donation with end-of-life discussions.

Evaluation

Critical care programmes and health care organizations in general must find systemic effective methods to ask patients and families what they need, experience, and expect from us. One method to solicit feedback involves surveys, conversations, committees, and storytelling. This information is then used to implement improvement projects within the ICU.

- Measurement: ICU family satisfaction surveys,[2] measure three important domains—communication, decision-making, and end-of-life care.
- Benefits for patients and families: improve services, opportunity to bring about meaningful change, improve satisfaction, enhance patient safety, expands new knowledge and skills, and networking.

Reflecting on a personal role: giving voice to a family member

My role is to give families a voice in trying to change the way we treat patients and family members in the ICU. It is important to make sure the health care provider considers the importance of family members. When we need to, we shouldn't be afraid to say 'I know you are busy, doctor, but you need to talk to us' or 'We need your attention because we/they are scared'. This kind of supportive role is satisfying and worthwhile. What matters to me is that our council is making a genuine effort to improve health care.

References

1. Gerteis M, Edgman–Levitan S, Daley J, Delbanco TL (eds.) (1993). *Though the patient's eyes: understanding and promoting patient-centred care.* Jossey–Bass Publishers, San Francisco, CA.
2. Dodek PM, Heyland DK, Rocker GM, Cook DJ. Translating family satisfaction data into quality improvement. *Crit Care Med.* 2004 Sep; **32**(9): 1922–7.

Further reading

1. Jeppson ES, Thomas J (1997). *Families as advisors: a training guide for collaboration.* Institute for Family-Centred Care, Bethesda, MD.
2. Webster PD, Johnson B (2000). *Developing and sustaining a patient and family advisory council.* Institute for Family-Centred Care, Bethesda, MD.
3. Frampton SB, Gilpin L, Charmel PA (2003). *Putting patients first: designing and practising patient-centred care.* Jossey–Bass. San Francisco, CA.
4. Institute of Medicine (2001). *Crossing the quality chasm: a new health system for the 21st century.* Washington, DC, National Academy Press.
5. Johnson, BH (1999). Family-centered Care: Creating Partnerships in Health. *Group Practice Journal.* **48**(9): 18–21.

Relationships and iatrogenic suffering: part 1

> 'The dying need the friendship of the heart—its qualities of care, acceptance, vulnerability; but they also need the skills of the mind—the most sophisticated treatment that medicine has to offer. On its own, neither is enough.'
> Dame Cicely Saunders, founder of St. Christopher's Hospice in London, England

Experiencing an illness or receiving care in a hospital is more than a physical event. It is a human, social, and spiritual process for the patient as well as for the health care provider. The essence of the work that is done by health care providers is based on relationship(s)—relationship with oneself, colleagues, patients/families and, perhaps, even with one's sense of the spiritual.

In the next few sections, I will provide an overview of the causes and effects of suffering that relate not to illness or disease itself, but more to the manner in which clinicians relate to patients, families, and colleagues.

Scenario[1,2]

A 78-year old woman with a long-standing history of cancer is asked about receiving her diagnosis of cancer. She states that while she received the diagnosis a decade ago, she remembers it as though it were yesterday, the familiar sound of her surgeon's voice from the doorway of her room. Unlike the other visits when they had discussed her 'lump', this time he did not greet her by name, he did not ask her how she was doing, nor did he ask if there were any family members with her or that he might call on her behalf. He simply blurted out 'Oh by the way, we were wrong, it is cancer. I have made an appointment for the oncologist in a few days.' His voice sounded particularly cold and distant, and after those few words, the surgeon walked away. No discussion, no touch, no empathy. The woman was left with her many unanswered questions, her concerns about how her family would receive this message, the thoughts of 'if only … ', and her rage at how she had just been told that she had cancer. 'The way in which the doctor spoke with me was more painful than the disease itself.'

Causing suffering

Despite all the good that is done in the context of medical interventions, poor communication can render ineffective much of that goodness. Poor communication has the potential to increase the suffering of the patient and their family. Many physicians have strong communication skills that make them very effective in the work they do. There are many others, who, without being aware of it, contribute to the suffering of their patients and/or patients' families because of the manner in which they communicate. This can be thought of as iatrogenic suffering—'The way in which the doctor spoke with me was more painful than the pain from the disease itself'; the healer (namely the physician) is the source of the suffering experienced by the patient. The suffering results from the activity, namely the communication skills, of the physician.[1]

How does iatrogenic suffering occur?

There are two fundamental issues:
- Issues that are systemic to health care.
- Issues that pertain to personal/professional issues.
  - Some old traditions of medical practice.
  - Diminishing the impact of information that is being given to the patient.
  - Limited communication skills.
  - Doctors' own emotional, psychological, and spiritual issues.
  - Time pressures.
  - Vicarious trauma/compassion fatigue.
  - Moral distress, burnout.
  - Death anxiety, grief.
  - Identifying with the patient.
  - Shame.

In the case of iatrogenic suffering, who suffers? Is it only the patient and/ or the patient's family, or might it also be the health care provider? How do we reduce the likelihood of causing iatrogenic suffering? It is my sense that iatrogenic suffering is reduced when the physician knows him/herself, understands expressed empathy, and has effective communication skills.

Communication as the cornerstone and foundation of every relationship

Communicating a diagnosis of a serious or terminal illness is a challenge to the most experienced and highly skilled physician. It is best if a message of a life-altering illness is given in the context of a close relationship between the physician and the patient, characterized by mutual trust, respect, and honesty. It is often difficult to develop such a relationship in an acute care setting, let alone in an ICU. Nevertheless:
- Pay attention to what you say and how you say it.
- Not communicating is not an option, i.e. you cannot not communicate.
- Remember that 60% of communication is non-verbal (facial expression, posture, hand gestures, tone of voice, silent pause).
- It is easy to hide behind medical jargon.
- Be aware of what it is that you are saying as well as what it is that you are not saying.
- Truth and hope are not mutually exclusive!

What you say and what they hear

Another important feature of communication has to do with differentiating between that which is spoken and that which is heard. One's intent cannot determine the effect! Generally when people hear words like 'cancer', 'AIDS', 'ALS', 'we've reached the end of the options available to you' or worse, 'there is nothing more we can do for you,' they hear nothing more. One of the greatest risks at that time is that the clinician will address an emotional need with a cognitive response. In so doing, the intent of the clinician is to decrease the patient's anxiety with information. However, the effect may be one of estrangement and isolation because the patient is experiencing strong emotions such as fear and anxiety, and would best respond to an empathic response at that time, whatever that might be, e.g. 'this may be difficult to hear', 'often people are unable to take in a lot of new and detailed information at this time', 'often people who receive information like this feel numb'. The most effective way of making an intention known is by being explicit about the intention, and the most effective way of learning about the effect one's message might have on the person who receives it is by being explicit in inquiring about the effect the message has on the individual—'What do you feel regarding the information I have just given to you?'

Family meetings, family stress, and ways to minimize iatrogenic suffering[1,2]

Hospitalization, serious illness, uncertainty about health outcomes and terminal illness often exacerbate and exaggerate family stress, distress, and dysfunction. And in that context, there are often many topics to discuss, decisions to make, and business to attend to. Health care professionals may feel that the most urgent decisions pertain to code status, interventions, and treatment plans specific to a hospital setting. The context of the patient's life is much broader and may provide valuable information regarding decisions that need to be made while in the hospital.

Family members who disagree, who are estranged from one another, and/or have not seen each other for many years are often called to the bedside of a family member who is very sick and may not be able to make his/her wishes known (often the case in the ICU). All the hurt and estrangement that has been present in a family for years is present even when one of their loved ones is very sick. When speaking with families or facilitating a family meeting, there are some important features to remember and guidelines to follow:

- Remember: ICU physicians and staff work with many patients and their families while the patient usually only goes through the process once.
- Every clinical situation has its own context and its own set of relationships.
- Some family members are estranged from one another or are in the middle of active disagreements that cannot be set aside even in the face of serious illness or impending death.
- Some families may be too fragile or disintegrated for the group process to be helpful or effective.
- Patients and families may ask that a particular staff member attends or in some cases, that a particular staff member does not attend the family meeting.
- It is important to remind the participants that patients' wishes take priority over that which others would want for the patient.

Conducting a meeting

- Conduct the meeting in a quiet and private room where interruptions to the meeting will be the exception.
- Set the time and space in advance, if possible, so that those people who need to be there are able to make arrangements to forgo their other obligations in order to attend the meeting.
- Begin on time and end on time.
- Explain the purpose of the meeting and the process of decision-making to the patient (if the patient is able to participate) and to

the participants. Speak in a way that is understood by the patient and everyone else who is attending the meeting.
- Include the appropriate staff members in the process.
- Some meetings may be set to provide information to the patient and family.
- Other meetings will be set to make a decision or to develop a plan of care. In those instances, the goal is to work toward a consensus via interaction, cohesiveness, and inclusion.
- Make certain all the participants are comfortably seated and that each participant is able to see every other participant (recall that non-verbal communication may be 'louder' than verbal communication).
- Have the participants introduce themselves by name and by their relationship with the patient. (Work to understand who the patient is in the context of the other people present. If the person is the leader ('patriarch' or 'matriarch') in the family, the illness or impending death may be significant in a different way than if that is not the case. How will this family be able to function when the patient is no longer present? Understanding the answer to that question may help you to understand perspectives and opinions of the people present. It may also help you to understand the emotional response of the family members and friends who are present.).
- Be aware that as the group size increases, the more anxious, forceful, and aggressive members will likely be the first to express their ideas unless the leader provides opportunity and periodically invites each member to speak.
- People are encouraged to speak directly to the issues and concerns raised by other members of the group (patient, professional, family, and friends) and to raise their own concerns, i.e. they are encouraged to make 'I' statements.
- Expression of feelings and ideas are welcome.
- It may be helpful to record the information on a flip chart.
- Once the group is gathered, it may be valuable to discuss some of the essential ingredients of the group process, primarily those of respect of self and others in the group, confidentiality, suspending judgement of what others are saying, equal opportunity to speak, equal air time (as best as is possible), and people speaking for themselves.
- Emphasize the significance of non-verbal communication such as raised eyebrows, a smirk, a frown, or even an extended period of silence. Any of these could alter the sense of safety and degree of trust that is necessary for the process to proceed to conclusion and in a comfortable manner.
- In some instances, it may be necessary to invite the silent person to speak.
- It may also be important that the person who speaks a lot and is highly anxious be asked to give others an opportunity to speak.
- Encourage participants to be present through the entire process. If someone leaves, ask if they are returning. If not, invite them to share opinions and concerns before they leave.

A decision-making process (important questions and topics of discussion)[3,4]

Medical indications (what is the reason for being here? What are my options with regard to medical treatment?):

- What are the facts of the medical history? What is the reason for the person being in the hospital or the ICU/coronary care unit (CCU)?
- What is/are the specific diagnosis(es)? What is the prognosis?
- What are the treatment options? What has been done? What is being done? What are the risks and benefits of treatment, of not providing treatment, of maintaining present treatment?
- Is the patient experiencing any pain? What about other symptoms? Are they being well controlled? Are there other options still available with regard to the pain and other symptoms?
- What is the past experience of 'using' the health care system? How much waiting was there? What were the relationships with health care providers like on previous hospital admissions—either those of the patient or those of family members?
- What are the patient's expectations with regard to treatment plans, resuscitation (if medical TV shows are a reference, the success rate of resuscitation attempts is very high), or other interventions?
- What does resuscitation mean to this person?
- What was the functional level prior to admission? How has that changed during the hospital stay?
- How would this person regard suffering? What does suffering mean to them? How are they experiencing suffering (physical, emotional, spiritual) at this time?
- Are there any curative components of this illness? Is the disease process or are the effects of the disease process reversible?

Patient preferences (if I could have anything I wished for, what would it be?)

- Is the patient competent? Does he or she comprehend the situation and the reason for the family meeting?
- Does the patient have a health care proxy and/or a living will? Who is best able to act as the patient's advocate?
- What are the patient's goals/wishes/desires regarding treatment? What is the patient's understanding of the treatment options available to them at present?
- What are the patient's goals, wishes, and desires (physical, psychological, spiritual) pertaining to their lives in general, especially in the context of a limited life expectancy? Who are the important people in this person's life? Is there any unfinished business, any conversations that need to occur?
- What is the patient's understanding of end-of-life care, comfort care, and/or hospice/palliative care?
- If the patient could 'shoot for the moon', what would they most want at present?
- How has this person made decisions through their lifetime? Is it possible to follow a similar process at present?
- Who has the authority to decide on behalf of the patient? What are the ethical and legal limits of that authority?

Quality of life (what is the reality of my wishes being fulfilled?)

- What does quality of life mean to this person? How might this be interpreted in the context of the present illness?
- How do people other than the patient perceive the patient's quality of life and of what ethical relevance are their perceptions?
- What gives this person meaning? Consider physical, social, psychological, and spiritual issues?
- Are there circumstances under which the patient would consider stopping all medication and/or other treatments?
- What sustains the patient at present (sense of self, relationship with others, spirituality, etc.)
- What is achievable with regard to the patient's preferences? (That which is not achievable may result in grief and loss on the part of the patient and his/her family.)

Contextual features

- Where will the patient receive care or be cared for during the course of this illness or perhaps for the remainder of his/her life? In the hospital (which unit, which ward?), at home (what supports are necessary in order for that to happen?), residential care facility, or in a hospice?
- Is it possible to develop a treatment plan given the information that was gained through this process? If not, what is missing? If so, who is affected by the plan and how?
- What is necessary to actualize the plan? What are the available resources: economic/fiscal, physical, emotional, societal? Remember that most resources are limited and the limitation may have a profound effect on the patient and/or family members.
- What does the law say about the plan?
- Are the people who participated in this process comfortable with the treatment plan? (If family members and friends have made a commitment of support for the patient, especially with regard to anything that requires a considerable amount of time, energy, or money, suggest that the group resumes in to review the implementation of the plan at a time suited to the context of the illness).

Respect, truth, honesty, and creativity are believed to contribute significantly to the success of the decision-making process discussed above. When all participants are treated respectfully and their contributions encouraged and affirmed, the process generally moves quickly and is beneficial. This method enables the participants to connect with one another in ways that support and strengthen the relationships.

References

1. Kuhl D (2002). *What dying people want.* Doubleday Canada, Toronto.
2. Kuhl D (1999). *Exploring spiritual and psychological Issues at the end of life. A doctoral dissertation.* University of British Columbia.
3. Kuhl D, Wilensky P (1999). Decision-making at the end of life: a model using an ethical grid and principles of group process. *J Palliat Med* **2**, 75–86.
4. Jonsen A, Siegler M, Winslade WJ (1992). *Clinical Ethics*, 3rd edn. McGraw-Hill, New York.

Giving life-altering/bad news

Before you enter the room to give someone life altering/bad news, to discuss resuscitation/code status, or to inform a patient that they have a terminal illness, stop and think about your own feelings about the person, the message, and the process that is about to happen. To know and understand your own emotional response to your patients and their families is an important feature of reducing iatrogenic suffering.

Remember:

- How you speak is usually based on how you feel.
- How you speak is a louder message than the words you say.
- Be honest about your own emotions such as sadness, frustration, discomfort about the topic, dread, feelings of ineptitude, and, perhaps, even a desire to run away from this difficult task, leaving it for someone else.
- Simply, be aware of whatever emotions your feel.
- If your emotional response is a strong one, it would be valuable for you to speak to someone about the emotion before speaking to the patient.
- It is particularly important to be aware of feelings that the patient or someone in the patient's family reminds you of your own family.
- It is equally important to differentiate yourself from the patient/ patient's family. That may be difficult if someone in the family asks questions like 'if this were your mother, father, sister, brother or you, what would you do?' While that may be a flattering question, it is a distraction as the patient is not likely any of those people.
- Make recommendations on the basis of your knowledge of the patient, the patient's desires, and the medical assessment that has been completed. There is a fine line between empathy and identification. Identification presupposes no separation between me and the patient, that which is good for me or my family is good for this person. That may not be true. Empathy works to understand the experience of another person from that person's perspective.

A: Attend[1,2]

- Attend to your own experience.
  - What am I experiencing?
  - What am I aware of within myself?
  - What is the emotion I am experiencing as I approach the patient with whom I am about to have a difficult conversation?
  - What is my relationship to serious or terminal illness?
  - How do I understand dying and death?
- Attend to possible interruptions.
  - Turn off your pager, Blackberry®, and/or cell phone (or leave them with someone else).
  - Let people know not to interrupt you for a period of time (usually a minimum of 10 to 20 minutes).
  - Turn off any radios, CD players, or televisions in the room. Ask for permission from the patient before doing so.

- Attend to the patient.
  - Sit down (preferably on a chair; if you sit on the bed, ask for permission to do so before you sit down). Use active listening skills (SOLER) as follows:
    1. **S**: face the patient **SQUARELY** to indicate interest in the exchange.
    2. **O**: adopt an **OPEN** body posture.
    3. **L**: **LEAN** towards the patient.
    4. **E**: use **EYE CONTACT** to show you are paying attention.
    5. **R**: maintain a **RELAXED** body posture to decrease the patient's anxiety.
  - Make certain that the patient and other people present in the room are comfortable.
  - What is the patient experiencing?
  - What do you know about the patient and/or the patient's family?
  - What information does this person already have regarding the diagnosis/prognosis? Does she/he understand the purpose of tests and investigations that have taken place?

B: Bridge
- Let the person know they are about to hear something that may be difficult for them to hear.
  - 'I have some information that may be difficult to hear.'
  - 'I have something to say to you that is difficult for me to do.'
- Ask whether the person would like to hear the information that you have to give to them.
  - 'We have some things to discuss with regard to your health. Would you like to talk about your health and well-being now or would you prefer to wait?'
  - 'Do you want to hear this information on your own or would you prefer that a family member or a friend be present?'
  - 'Would you prefer that I speak with you directly or that I speak to a family member or a friend about your health?'
  - 'I am wondering whether you would like to have that conversation now or whether you would prefer to wait until you have a family member or a friend with you.'
- Introduce the topic.
  - 'Do you remember the tests and investigations that have been completed over the past days and weeks?'
  - 'What is your understanding about the purpose of those tests/investigations?'
  - 'What do you think might be going on with regard to your health (or with regard to the specific symptoms you are experiencing at present)?'
- Listen very carefully to every response the patient makes. The response and the way in which it is given to you will give you a great deal of information about the patient and the understanding the patient has of the present situation.
  - Use the same type of language and concepts to explain what is going on with regard to the patient's health. (Remember that you are very familiar with medical terms—the patient likely does not

share that familiarity). At times, it is easy to hide behind medical jargon. Keep the language simple, even when speaking with health care professionals who might be your patients.
• Remember that after words like 'cancer', 'ALS', 'AIDS', 'there is no further treatment to reverse any component of the disease process', the patient is not likely to hear a lot.

C: Comment
• Present the information.
  • 'I need to tell you that we have the results of the tests … Unfortunately, they are not what I/we hoped for.'
  • 'I am sorry to say that the results of those tests show that you have … '
  • 'I know that once people hear the word 'cancer', they usually don't hear anything else after that.'
• Invite a response.
  • 'What is your understanding of what I have just told you?' (Do not assume that silence on the part of the patient is an indication that the message you gave them was understood by them.)
  • 'Do you have any questions?'
  • 'Is there any other information you or your family might like to have at this time?'
• Watch for non-verbal response to information.

D: Develop a plan
• The present.
  • 'I invite you to stay in this room for a while. I will be seeing another patient, and then, I will return to see you.'
  • 'I have written the diagnosis on a piece of paper. I have added the times for your next appointments here as well as with other physicians.'
  • 'I am aware that many people are in a state of emotional shock after hearing news such as that I just gave to you. Often, they have difficulty concentrating and begin to think about the people they love.'
• The future.
  • 'How will you be spending the day? How did you get here? If you drove by yourself, it will be important for you to concentrate on driving. Would you like to call someone to be with you or to pick you up?'
  • 'Is there someone with whom you might spend the rest of the day?'
  • 'I would be pleased to see you again in the near future. I am certain that either you or your family will have some questions in the next while.'
  • 'I have set some time aside to meet with you in the near future. The dates are … (and I have written them on a piece of paper).'
  • 'I have made an appointment for you to see … '

As stated earlier, in considering iatrogenic suffering, one must ask who suffers? Is it only the patient and/or the patient's family and friends? Might it also be the health care providers who suffer? If so, how? Do we as health care providers know ourselves? What is our relationship to suffering, dying, death, difficult family dynamics, our sense of helplessness in the face of unfixable suffering, our inability to change the course of a disease process in a patient we really care about, our distress because we feel that it is not in the patient's best interest to fulfil the requests of family members for their loved one or the expectations of other team members.

References

1. Mak AS, Westwood MJ, Barker MC, Ishiyama FI (1998). Developing sociocultural competencies for success among international students: the EXCELL programme. *J International Educ* **9**, 33–8.
2. Westwood D, Pearson H (2000). *Sociocultural competencies: communication skills for career and employment success,* Log No. 1535). Centre for Curriculum Transfer and Technology, Victoria.

Conducting an ICU family conference: a VALUES approach

Most critically ill patients do not have decisional capacity. Consequently, family members frequently become involved with clinicians in discussions about the goals of care. In these situations, family members or surrogate decision-makers (a term used more often in the US and France) need to represent patients' values and treatment preferences in these discussions. Therefore, clinician-family communication is a central component of good, medical decision-making in the ICU. However, clinician-family communication in the ICU is often less than adequate. The goal of this chapter is to provide practical, evidence-based guidance on how to conduct an ICU family conference.

Why is communication with family members important?

• Studies demonstrate that almost half of all family members of critically ill patients experience significant symptoms of anxiety, depression, and PTSD. Despite the emotional burdens of being a family member and a surrogate decision-maker, many health care systems do not provide adequate support for family caregivers. Improved communication with family members in the ICU leads to significant reductions in symptoms of anxiety, depression, and PTSD in family members three months after a patient dies in the ICU.[1]

• Since family members are often serving as surrogate decision-makers, contributing to decisions about the care of the patient, these decisions depend, in part, on the family. To the extent that family members' burdens and symptoms of anxiety and depression have an effect on their ability to function as a surrogate decision-maker, these symptoms among family members may also interfere with patient care.

What is shared decision-making and why is it important?

Critical care physicians generally conceptualize their role in decision-making in one of three distinct ways:

• Parentalism, in which the physician makes the treatment decision with little input from the patient or family.

• Informed choice, in which the physician provides all relevant medical information, but withholds his or her opinion and places responsibility for the decision on the family.

• Shared decision-making, in which the physician and family each shares their opinions and jointly reach a decision.

While the prevalence of these decision-making styles varies from country to country, in 2005, five European and North American critical care societies issued a joint consensus statement advocating shared decision-making about life support in ICUs.[2] This consensus statement, created from expert opinion, characterizes a shared decision as one in which 'responsibility for decisions is shared jointly by the treating physician and the patient's family.'

However, it is important to realize that family members of critically ill patients vary in how involved they want to be in decisions about life support. The majority want the physician to provide a recommendation about whether to limit life support and then, share in the final decision. However, the spectrum of family preferences ranges from letting the physician decide to the family member assuming all responsibility for the final decision. Therefore, family-centred decision-making requires that clinicians assess the families' preferred role in decision-making and adapt their communication style accordingly.

High-quality shared decision-making is a process with a number of important components and not simply an agreement to allow family members to be involved in decision-making. Table 4.1 describes the components of shared decision-making based on prior theoretical models and empiric evaluation of communication during ICU family conferences.

What is a 'VALUES history' and why is it important?

- A 'VALUES history' is an important part of communication with family members. It is a careful investigation of the patient's treatment preferences and health-related values.
- Surrogate decision-makers face a substantial emotional burden when making decisions about life support for a family member, especially when that person has not completed an advance directive.
- It is important to help surrogates/family members understand and articulate the distinction between their own hopes for the patient and the patient's preferences. It is not uncommon for surrogates' own emotions to lead to a desire to continue life support, even when it is clear the patient would not choose ongoing treatment for themselves. Emphasizing the need to follow the patient's wishes may help alleviate some of the burden of surrogate decision-making.
- Shared decision-making requires physicians to be expert in helping family members understand and articulate patients' values. Exploring patients' preferences and the appropriate influence of those preferences on medical decision-making is one of the common missed opportunities during ICU family conferences.[3]
- Careful attention to the individual beliefs and uniqueness of the patient by the physician may help surrogates trust the physician enough to listen to their advice. This may be particularly important in situations in which the physician does not have a long-term relationship with the patient and family.
- Two specific techniques to elicit relevant values include asking open-ended questions that allow the family to describe what is important to the patient and inquiring about health states the patient would consider 'worse than death.'

An evidence-based approach to communication during the ICU family conference

- Specific features of ICU family conferences have been associated with improved family experience or with a better assessment of the quality of communication.
  - Improved family outcomes have been associated with having a private place for family communication and with consistent communication by all members of the health care team.
  - A 'pre-conference' may help ensure consistent communication from team members. These 'pre-conferences' allow the interdisciplinary

team to discuss the goals of the family conference and reach consensus on the prognosis and on what treatments are indicated.
- During the conference, family members are more satisfied with clinician communication when clinicians spend more time listening and less time talking.
- Other features of clinician communication that are associated with improved family experiences include assurances that the patient will not be abandoned prior to death, assurances that the patient will be comfortable and will not suffer, and support for a family's decisions about care, including support for family's decision to withdraw or not to withdraw life support.
- Evaluation by experts suggest categories of important missed opportunities during ICU family conferences, including the opportunity to listen and respond to family members' questions, the opportunity to acknowledge and address family emotions, and the opportunity to address basic tenets of palliative care, including the exploration of patient preferences, explanation of the principles of surrogate decision-making, and assuring non-abandonment by clinicians.[3]

- Table 4.2 summarizes the components of clinician-family communication that have been associated with increased quality of care, decreased family psychological symptoms, or improved family ratings of communication.
- Several of these findings have been combined into a mnemonic for five features to enhance clinician-family communication: VALUE. Fig. 4.1 describes this mnemonic. This mnemonic has been used as part of an intervention to improve clinician-family communication in the ICU that has been shown to significantly reduce family symptoms of anxiety, depression, and PTSD three months after the patient's death.[1]
- Table 4.3 provides an overview of the structure and one approach to conducting a family conference.
- Table 4.4 provides some additional suggestions to help families when making a decision to withdraw life-sustaining treatments.

Discussing prognosis
- Physicians have an important responsibility to share prognoses with patients and their families. However, studies suggest that many physicians do not discuss prognosis directly, and when they do, there is considerable variability in how this is done.
- Patients' willingness to consent to life-sustaining treatment declines substantially as the chances for death or severe functional impairment increase. Therefore, clear, empathic disclosure of prognosis is especially important as the prognosis worsens.
- There are limited data to guide discussion of prognosis in the ICU, but it is interesting that physicians in ICU family conferences are more likely to discuss prognosis for quality of life than they are to discuss prognosis for survival. Prognosis for quality of life is at least as important to patients and family members as is prognosis for survival. This also highlights the importance of current efforts to develop accurate predictors of functional outcomes after critical illness.

- Experts suggest that the use of numeric expressions of risk (e.g. '90% of people as sick as your mother do not survive') may lead to better comprehension than qualitative expressions of risk (e.g. 'your mother is very unlikely to survive').
- Since prognostic information applies to outcomes of groups of patients, experts recommend that prognostic information be framed as outcomes for populations rather than as individual outcomes (e.g. 'out of a group of 100 patients like your mother, I would expect about 90 would not survive this').
- Some experts also recommend describing both the probability of death as well as the probability of survival to improve understanding.
- In addition, because some individuals have strong cultural reasons for not wanting to receive prognostic information, and because all methods of communicating prognosis are fallible, experts recommend the 'ask-tell-ask' approach to discussing prognosis. Under this approach, physicians seek permission to discuss prognosis prior to doing so and ask families their understanding of the prognosis after the discussion to ensure comprehension.

Importance of interdisciplinary involvement in family conferences

- End-of-life care in most settings is delivered by an interdisciplinary team that includes nurses, physicians, and other clinicians. Patients and families report that interdisciplinary communication is a key component of good end-of-life care.
- Improving interdisciplinary communication is associated with improved patient outcomes, including:
  - Decreased length of stay and decreased readmission rates.
  - Decreased symptoms of anxiety and depression among family members.
  - Higher patient satisfaction and lower rates of ICU nurse and physician burnout.

The importance of protocols for communication

- One important feature of the interventions that have been shown to improve clinician-family communication in the ICU is the 'proactive' nature of the successful interventions, i.e. a protocol or standardized procedure ensured that communication with family occurred earlier in the ICU course than usual care. A reasonable conclusion is that some type of ICU protocol or procedure is likely to be necessary to replicate the successes seen in these studies.
- At the same time, it is also essential that communication be conducted in a way that adapts to the needs of individual patients and family members. Communication cannot become protocolized to the point of being robotic and thus, risk missing opportunities to respond to individual needs. It is possible to develop protocols or manuals for a communication intervention that allow a standardized intervention, but also allow the communication to respond to the needs of the individual. It is also important to allow individual clinicians to use their intuition and individual communication styles to respond in ways that are authentic.

Summary

Critical care is by nature complex, and high-quality critical care requires extensive training, interdisciplinary collaboration, implementation of protocols that ensure high levels of adherence to processes of care that are associated with improved outcomes, and adaptation of this care to the needs of the individual. In this way, communication with family members is no different than other aspects of critical care. Improvements in this aspect of critical care will require training, interdisciplinary teamwork, and implementation of effective and flexible protocols. We are beginning to identify the best ways to accomplish each of these tasks with the ultimate goal of improving the way we communicate with and care for critically ill patients and their families.

References

1. Lautrette A, Darmon M, Megarbane B, *et al.* (2007). A communication strategy and brochure for relatives of patients dying in the ICU. *N Engl J Med* **356**, 469–78.
2. Carlet J, Thijs LG, Antonelli M, *et al.* (2004). Challenges in end-of-life care in the ICU. Statement of the 5th International Consensus Conference in Critical Care, Brussels, Belgium, April 2003. *Intensive Care Med* **30**, 770–84.
3. Curtis JR, Engelberg RA, Wenrich MD, Shannon SE, Treece PD, Rubenfeld GD (2005). Missed opportunities during family conferences about end-of-life care in the intensive care unit. *Am J Respir Crit Care Med* **171**, 844–9.

V	Value the family's statements.
A	Acknowledge the family's emotions.
L	Listen to the family.
U	Understand the patient as a person.
E	Elicit the family's questions.

Fig. 4.1 VALUE: a 5-step approach for improving clinician-family communication in the ICU.

Table 4.1 Components of shared decision-making adapted to the ICU family conference*

Dimensions of shared decision-making	Example of physician behaviours
Providing medical information and eliciting patient values and preferences	Discuss nature of decision.
	What are the essential clinical issues we are addressing?
	Describe alternatives.
	What are the clinically reasonable choices?
	Discuss pros and cons.
	What are the pros and cons of the treatment choices?
	Discuss uncertainty.
	What is the likelihood of success of treatment and how confident are we in this estimate?
	Assess understanding.
	Is the family now an 'informed participant' with a working understanding of the decision?
	Explore the patient's values and preferences.
	What is known about the patient's medical preferences or values? What is important to the patient?
Exploring the family's preferred role decision-making	Discuss the family's role.
	What role should the family play in making the decision?
	Assess desire for others' input.
	Is there anyone else the family would like to consult?
Deliberation and decision-making	Explore 'context'.
	How will the decision impact on the patient's life?
	If the family is to participate in decision-making, elicit family opinion about the best treatment choice.
	What does the family think is the most appropriate decision for the patient?

* Adapted from: White DB, Braddock CM, Berknyei S, Curtis JR (2007). Toward shared decision-making at the end-of-life in intensive care units: opportunities for improvement. *Archives of Internal Medicine* **167**, 461–7.

Table 4.2 Additional communication components shown to be associated with increased quality of care, decreased family psychological symptoms, or improved family ratings of communication

- Identify a private place for communication with family members.

- Provide consistent communication from different team members.

- Increase proportion of time spent listening to family rather than talking.

- Identify commonly missed opportunities.[3]
  - Listen and respond to family members.
  - Acknowledge and address family emotions.
  - Explore and focus on patient values and treatment preferences.
  - Explain the principle of surrogate decision-making to the family (the goal of surrogate decision-making is to determine what the patient would want if the patient were able to participate).
  - Affirm non-abandonment of patient and family.

- Assure the family that the patient will not suffer.

- Provide explicit support for decisions made by the family.

Table 4.3 Suggestions for conducting an ICU family conference*

- Making preparations prior to a discussion about end-of-life care in the ICU.
  - Review previous knowledge of the patient and/or family.
  - Review knowledge of the disease, prognosis, and treatment options.
  - Plan the specifics of location and setting: a quiet, private place.
  - Conduct a 'pre-conference' with the clinicians involved in the conference.
  - Have advance discussion with the family to make sure all the important people are present if possible.

- Holding a discussion about end-of-life care in the ICU.
  - Introduce everyone present.
  - Find out what the patient or family understands in a non-threatening way.
  - Discuss the prognosis frankly in a way that is meaningful to family.
  - Avoid the temptation to give too much medical detail.
  - Make it clear that withholding life-sustaining treatment is NOT withholding caring.
  - Use active listening and provide the family adequate time to speak.
  - Acknowledge strong emotions and use reflection to encourage patients or families to talk about these emotions.
  - Respond empathetically to tears or other grief behaviour.
  - Tolerate silence.

- Finishing a discussion of end-of-life care in the ICU.
  - Achieve common understanding of the disease and treatment issues.
  - Make a recommendation about treatment.
  - Ask if there are any questions.
  - Ensure a basic follow-up plan and make sure the patient and/or family knows how to reach the team for questions.

* Adapted from Curtis JR (2004). Communicating about end-of-life care with patients and families in the ICU. *Critical Care Clinics* **20**, 363–80

Table 4.4 Helping families make decisions about withdrawing life support in the ICU*

- Focus the family on what the patient would want, not what the family wants.

- If life-sustaining therapy is to be withdrawn, emphasize that:
  - Life-sustaining therapy cannot reverse the underlying disease process.
  - Withdrawal of life-sustaining therapy allows the natural course of the disease to occur.
  - Aggressive palliative therapy will be used to ensure that the patient is comfortable.

- Some families need time to adjust to withdrawing life-sustaining therapy; such time can be an important use of ICU resources.

- Educate the family about what will likely happen after life-sustaining therapy is withdrawn:
  - Discuss the likely time to death as well as the variability and uncertainty.
  - Discuss agonal respirations and myoclonus.

- Educate and elicit family preferences about extubation.

- Mention organ donation, but leave the discussion to the 'professionals'.

* Adapted from Curtis JR (2004). Communicating about end-of-life care with patients and families in the ICU. *Critical Care Clinics* **20**, 363–80.

Decision-making for patients who lack capacity to decide: the surrogate in the ICU

Introduction

Around the world, there are various preferred models of medical decision-making. Respect for patient autonomy is emphasized in western countries, and to a much lesser extent, e.g. in Southern or Eastern Europe, South America, and North Africa. In France, the traditional paternalistic model is being replaced through a trend towards more of a shared model.[1] When dealing with serious and life-threatening illness, decision-making requires the most careful attention to patients' preferences, goals, and values because the consequences often include death or diminished quality of life. However, only a small minority of critically ill patients can provide this essential input directly. In the ICU, the health care team deals primarily with surrogate decision-makers, whose role presents a range of complex and challenging issues.

Why is the issue of surrogate decision-making so important?

- Even in countries where 'paternalistic' and unilateral decision-making by physicians has long been the dominant model, the situation is currently in flux and the role of the patient and thus, of the surrogate is expanding.
- For example, in France, the Public Health Code Law of 4 March, 2002 provided for the designation of a '*personne de confiance*', i.e. 'a surrogate', who may be a family member, a close friend, or the person's attending physician and who will be consulted in the event of the person being unable to express his or her wishes or to understand the information required to do so. The designation is made in writing. It can be revoked at any time. When admitted to a medical establishment, the patient is invited to designate a surrogate. When the patient is incapable of expressing his or her wishes, no intervention or investigation may be carried out and no care be curtailed, except in the case of an emergency or unless it is impossible for the act to be performed without prior consultation of the surrogate or family, or in their absence, a close acquaintance of the patient.
- In the UK, independent mental capacity advocates (IMCAs) assist in decision-making in the absence of surrogate/family/confidants. These appointed professionals act in the 'best interest' of patients and allow the introduction of a different perspective that can both balance and extend decision-making considerations in the ICU setting. In addition, the Court of Protection can be approached if surrogates and doctors disagree on decisions to be made. See p196 for more detail on the Mental Capacity Act (2005).
- Published data indicate that over 90% of ICU patients lack decision-making capacity. Even patients who are conscious and seemingly aware often have impaired intellectual function or cannot communicate what they are understanding and thinking because of endotracheal intubation and other impediments.
- Most patients want their families or a close friend to be involved in their care and decision-making.

What is the surrogate's role?

- An ICU patient who has the capacity to make the medical decision at hand, i.e. who understands the relevant information, can weigh benefits, burdens, and alternatives, and communicate the decision clearly, should be the one to make that decision. The ICU team should turn to a surrogate decision-maker only if and when a patient lacks decision-making capacity. In general, an intensive care physician can evaluate capacity without consulting a specialist in psychiatry. There are some tools available to help assess capacity (e.g. the ICU-adjusted confusion assessment method (CAM-ICU) since there is significant evidence that physicians can overestimate capacity in ICU, especially when this fluctuates.[2]
- The strongest basis for a surrogate's decision is clear guidance from the patient in the form of an advance directive (oral or written). In the US, the Patient Self-Determination Act of 1991 mandated that hospitals and other health care institutions and agencies give patients information about their right to participate in and direct their medical decision-making and to accept or refuse medical treatment. France's Public Health Law of April 2005 states that 'any person of age may draw up advance directives in the event of their being unable one day to express their wishes. These advance directives indicate the end-of-life wishes of the person concerning the conditions in which treatment may be curtailed or discontinued. They can be revoked or revised. On condition that the directives were established less than three years before the person lost his or her functional capacity, the physician will take them into consideration concerning any investigation, intervention, or treatment the person may undergo.'
- Unfortunately, many patients have not prepared advance directives and it is difficult for directives to address the full range of circumstances that may arise. Thus, surrogates are typically required to play an interpretive role and may often need to decide without any prior specific input from the patient.
- Many studies have found that concordance between patient preferences and surrogate decisions is poor. A recent systematic review concluded that one third of decisions by surrogates who were specifically designated by patients or were identified as next of kin conflicted with patient preferences.[3]
- Still, there is evidence that patients favour involvement of family or other designated decision-makers, and that 'real-time' decisions by surrogates may be preferred even over patients' directives prepared in advance.[4]

How well do ICU clinicians understand applicable standards for surrogate decision-making?

- In countries where the law is in flux, many clinicians lack clarity and comfort in applying new standards.
  - For example, in France, the 2002 law states that any person admitted to hospital should be invited to designate a 'personne de confiance', but this law is not consistently applied. Few patients are aware of this option and physicians may also be unaware or forget to offer the option to patients.

- On admission to the ICU, most patients cannot make use of the option to designate a surrogate because consciousness is impaired. In France, the medical team can choose a surrogate in consultation with the family, but no study has compared such choices with patients' own designations of a surrogate.
- Even in the US, where authority for surrogate decision-making has long been established, clinicians may lack a clear understanding of the applicable standards, which vary from state to state and can be complex.

How can the ICU team help to optimize surrogate decisions?

- An essential first step is to identify the appropriate surrogate. The patient may have specifically designated a surrogate through appointment of a health care proxy or durable power of attorney. In the absence of a specific designation, applicable law will establish a hierarchy of appropriate decision-makers, beginning usually with a spouse. Laws in this regard vary. In the US, the law is state-specific, both with respect to the extent of decision-making authority of patient-designated surrogates and to the order of various individuals in the decision-making hierarchy.
- The surrogate must be fully informed about the patient's condition, prognosis, and treatments. Existing evidence shows that many families and other surrogate decision-makers are poorly informed, lacking basic information about condition, prognosis, and treatment. As an adjunct to direct physician counselling, the use of printed informational materials for ICU families is increasing and is supported by evidence from randomized, controlled trials. Above all, families and other surrogate decision-makers value the opportunity to meet with an attending physician who can integrate information from various sources and convey it in an understandable way. The meeting also allows for a mutual exchange of information in which the ICU physician listens as well as speaks.
- The surrogate should be encouraged to decide as the surrogate believes the patient would decide, not to substitute the surrogate's own judgement for that of the patient.

What if the surrogate doesn't have capacity?

Decision-making capacity must be evaluated for surrogates as well as for patients.[5] Evidence is accumulating that ICU families are often encumbered by anxiety, depression, and PTSD.[6] These may, at times, challenge the surrogate's capacity to participate appropriately in medical decision-making. A recent study reports that up to 34% of bereaved surrogate decision-makers have features of psychiatric disease,[7] following their involvement in decision-making. Other forms of mental illness or chronic or acute (e.g. inebriation) forms of cognitive impairment could also interfere with the ability of a surrogate to make informed and rational health care decisions.

In addition, involvement in the medical decision-making process can give rise to symptoms of anxiety, depression, PTSD, and guilt in the surrogate. Studies have shown that the presence of these symptoms in the families of ICU patients was proportionate to the extent of their involvement in end-of-life decisions.

An incapacitated surrogate should not be accepted as decision-maker.

If the ICU team has doubt about surrogate capacity, options might include family choice of another competent surrogate, consultation by a specialist in palliative care, and/or presentation of the matter to an institutional ethics committee or to a court-appointed professional (depending on jurisdiction).

What if there is no surrogate for a patient lacking capacity?

- As stated earlier, in the UK, IMCAs assist in decision-making in the absence of surrogate, family, or confidants and act in the 'best interest' of patients. The Court of Protection can be approached if surrogates and doctors disagree on decisions to be made.
- Recent data indicate that in the US, up to 27% of patients dying in ICUs lack decision-making capacity, a surrogate decision-maker, and an advance directive.[8]
- For these patients, state laws, hospital policies, and/or guidelines of professional societies provide procedures for decision-making.
- In practice, however, most life support decisions for these patients appear to be made by physicians without institutional or judicial review, although this practice may not comport with applicable standards.

What are the implications for ICU palliative care practice?

- Clinicians should know the applicable laws and standards, including those for designation of surrogates and for decision-making when an incapacitated patient lacks a surrogate.
- Clinicians should seek to identify an appropriate surrogate (family or other) decision-maker for each patient in the ICU at the time of ICU admission.
- Clinicians should not simply assume, but should explore the decision-making capacity of surrogates as well as patients.
- Ideally, surrogates should be designated before a health crisis such as critical illness. Every hospitalized patient, including all in the ICU who have capacity to do so, should be asked to designate a surrogate.
- The institution may have a formal role in the choice of a surrogate at hospital admission (this is the situation in France), and in the UK, the IMCAs become involved in the absence of surrogate, family, or confidants.
- Surrogates should be included in communications regarding care in the ICU so they can make informed decisions.

Conclusion

The designation of a surrogate is a step towards patient autonomy in the medical decision-making process. The way in which the surrogate is designated and the role assigned to the surrogate differ across societies and time. In all contexts, the main role of the surrogate is to give expression to the patient's values and preferences. For this to be achieved, the surrogate must have decision-making capacity and information relevant to medical decisions, including condition, prognosis, and treatments for the patient. In addition, the ICU must seek a full understanding of the patient's preferences, care goals, and values. Prior discussion between patients and their surrogates may help to clarify these issues when surrogates participate in ICU decision-making.

References

1. Azoulay E, Pochard F, Chevret S, *et al.* (2003). Opinions about surrogate designation: a population survey in France. *Crit Care Med* **31**, 1711–4.
2. Ely EW, Inouye S, Bernard G, *et al.* (2001). Delirium in mechanically ventilated patients: validity and reliability of the confusion assessment method for the intensive care unit (CAM-ICU). *JAMA* **286**, 2703–10.
3. Shalowitz DI, Garrett–Mayer E, Wendler D (2006). The accuracy of surrogate decision-makers: a systematic review. *Arch Intern Med* **166**, 493–7.
4. Sehgal A, Galbraith A, Chesney M, Schoenfeld P, Charles G, Lo B (1992). How strictly do dialysis patients want their advance directives followed? *JAMA* 267, 59–63.
5. Rodriguez RM, Navarrate E, Schwaber J, *et al.* (2008). A prospective study of primary surrogate decision-makers' knowledge of intensive care. *Crit Care Med* **36**, 1633–6.
6. Pochard F, Azoulay E, Chevret S, *et al.* (2001). Symptoms of anxiety and depression in family members of intensive care unit patients: ethical hypothesis regarding decision-making capacity. *Crit Care Med* **29**, 1893–7.
7. Siegel MD, Hayes E, Vanderwerker LC, Loseth DB, Prigerson HG (2008). Psychiatric illness in the next of kin of patients who die in the intensive care unit. *Crit Care Med* **36**, 1722–8.
8. White DB, Curtis JR, Wolf LE, *et al.* (2007). Life support for patients without a surrogate decision maker: who decides? *Ann Intern Med* **147**, 34–40.

Observational studies of families of patients who died in the ICU

Table 4.5 Observational studies of families of patients who died in the ICU

Author	Year	Country	Participants/design
Covinsky (SUPPORT) JAMA (1994).	1994	US.	− 5 centres. − 2,129 families.
Malacrida Crit Care Med (1998).	1998	Switzerland.	− 1 centre. − 123 bereaved families.
Keenan J Palliat Care (2000).	2000	Canada.	− 1 centre. − 33 bereaved families.
Cuthbertson Crit Care Med (2000).	2000	New Zealand.	− 1 centre. − 99 bereaved families.
Abbott Crit Care Med (2001).	2001	US.	− 1 centre. − 48 bereaved families.
Heyland Crit Care Med (2002).	2002	Canada.	− 6 centres. − 624 patients. − 166 bereaved families.
Heyland Chest (2003).	2003	Canada.	− 6 centres. − 256 bereaved families.
Azoulay (FAMIREA) Am J Respir Crit Care Med (2005).	2005	France.	− 21 centres. − 284 patients. − 56 bereaved families.

WH=withholding life support; WD=withdrawing life support; EOL=end-of-life

Measurements	Results
– Adverse caregiving. – Economic burdens.	– Family members assisted patients in one third of cases.
– Family satisfaction.	– Unclear information in 17% of cases. – Lack of information on causes and circumstances of death.
– Family satisfaction.	– Satisfaction with information on the process of WH/WD life-sustaining therapies. – Patient's comfort. – Family ability to voice concerns.
– Family satisfaction. – Family burden.	– Poor communication. – Sleep disturbance. – Financial difficulties.
– Sources of conflict. – Family support.	– Conflicts regarding communication and staff behaviour in 46% of cases. – Need for pastoral care, discussion of patient's preferences. – Conversation with 'doctor in charge' in quiet place.
– Family satisfaction.	– Dissatisfaction: waiting room, frequency of physician communication. – Satisfaction: completeness of information, respect, and compassion.
– Family satisfaction.	– Adequate communication, good decision-making, respect, and compassion were key determinants of family satisfaction.
– Stress-related symptoms. – Symptoms of anxiety/ depression.	– Increased stress-related symptoms in family members who reported poor communication and in those who shared EOL decisions.

Table 4.6 Interventional studies

Author	Year	Country	Participants
Holloran *Surgery* (1995).	1995	US.	− 1 centre. − Surgical Intensive Care Unit patient
SUPPORT *JAMA* (1995).	1995	US.	− 27 centres. − 9,105 patients.
Dowdy *Crit Care Med* (1998).	1998	US.	− 1 centre. − 99 high-risk patients.
Robinson *Lancet* (1998).	1998	UK.	− Witnessed resuscitation.
Lilly *Am J Med* (2000).	2000	US.	− 1 centre. − 530 high-risk patients.
Schneiderman *Crit Care Med* (2000).	2000	US.	− 2 centres. − 70 patients.
Azoulay *Am J Respir Crit Care Med* (2002).	2002	France.	− 34 centres. − 175 patients.
Burns *Crit Care Med* (2003).	2003	US.	− 7 centres. − 873 patients at high risk of conflict.
Campbell *Chest* (2003).	2003	US.	− 1 centre. − 81 patients with MOSF or GCI.
Schneiderman *JAMA* (2003).	2003	US.	− 7 centres. − 476 patients at risk of conflicts.
Lilly *Crit Care Med* (2003).	2003	US.	− 1 centre. − 2,891 patients.
Campbell *Crit Care Med* (2004).	2004	US.	− 1 centre. − 52 patients with terminal dementia.
Moreau *Am J Respir Crit Care Med* (2004).	2004	France.	− 11 centres. − 220 patients.

WH=withholding life support; WD=withdrawing life support; LOS=length of stay;

Intervention	Outcomes	Impact
– A clinical ethics programme with case conference.	– Decrease in LOS. – Earlier WH/WD discussion. – Reduction in costs.	– Decreased LOS.
– Nurse to improve communication on patient's preferences and values.	– Enhancing opportunities for more communication does not change practices.	– Need for proactive measures.
– Proactive ethics. – Consultation.	– Reduction in LOS.	– Improved decision-making. – Decreased LOS
– Grief questionnaire.	– Relatives were satisfied to remain with the patients.	
– Intensive communication with therapeutic goals.	– Decrease in LOS.	– Earlier WH/WD. – Decreased LOS.
– Ethics consultations.	– Family agrees with ethics consultations.	– Decreased LOS and non-beneficial treatment.
– Family information leaflet.	– Increase in comprehension of the diagnosis/treatment.	– Improved effectiveness of information.
– Social workers help identify conflicts and remind physicians about the patient's preferences.	– Increased use of WH/WD and palliative care.	– Improved communication and decision-making.
– Proactive intervention: meeting the family to agree with treatment goals and palliative team support.	– Decrease in LOS. – Earlier palliative care. – Reduction in cost.	– Decreases in the use of non-beneficial resources, LOS and cost.
– Ethics consultation with the centre's consultants.	– Positive views of ethics consultations.	– Decreases in LOS and non-beneficial treatments.
– Intensive communication with therapeutic goals.	– Decreased LOS and ICU mortality.	– Durable reduction in LOS and mortality over four years.
– Proactive palliative care intervention.	– Decrease in LOS and non-beneficial treatment.	– Decreased use of non-beneficial treatments.
– Information provided by junior vs senior physician.	– No difference in terms of comprehension, anxiety, and depression, satisfaction,	– Need to improve communication skills regardless of experience.

MOSF=multiple organ system failure; GCI=global cerebral ischaemia

Table 4.7 Some qualitative studies

Author	Country	Methodology	Purpose	Participants
Cook CMAJ (1999).	Canada.	Ethnography and interviews (same study as Johnson et al. below).	– Understanding the purposes for which life support is withheld, provided, continued, or withdrawn in the ICU.	– 7 intensivists, 5 consultants, 9 ICU nurses, the ICU nutritionist, the hospital ethicist, 3 pastoral services representatives. – 1 ICU.
Johnson Cult Med Psychiatry (2000).	US.	Ethnography and interviews.	– How end-of-life narratives are constructed in ICUs; how withdrawal processes contribute towards perceptions of a good death.	– 7 intensivists, 5 consultants, 9 ICU nurses, the ICU nutritionist, the hospital ethicist, 3 pastoral services representatives. – 1 ICU.
McAdam Intensive Care Med (2008).	US.	Interviews.	– Understanding the contributions to care of family members of patients at high risk of dying in the ICU.	– Family members. – 2 ICUs.
Seymour Soc Sci Med (1999, 2000).	UK.	Ethnography.	– Negotiating a 'natural' death in critical care.	– Observations of nurses, doctors, families, and patients. – 2 ICUs.

Setting	Findings	Conclusions
– 25 ICU rounds and 11 EOL discussions observed.	– Life support technology being used to orchestrate dying. WH or WD can help determine prognosis processes of withdrawal improved methods and timing of death. Decisions are socially negotiated to synchronize understanding expectations for family and clinicians. Life support technology as one discrete support vs general concept.	– Process-oriented as well as outcome-oriented uses of technology.
– 25 ICU rounds and 11 EOL discussions observed.	– Themes: hope dispelled; physiology of dying; WD and WS as a therapeutic act -technology as villain; stepping back; what patient would have wanted; disappearing the patient disappearing as a person.	– What death means and how death is constructed in intensive care.
– N=25 family members of 24 patients.	– Several roles for family members: active presence, patient protector, facilitator, historian, coach, and voluntary caregiver.	– Family members are important to patient care in the ICU. They perform multiple roles that are often not valued or go unrecognized by ICU health care providers.
– 14 case studies.	– Four phases to physician's involvement in decision-making: an initial 'technical' definition of dying informed by results of investigations and monitoring equipment; alignment of technical and bodily dying must have no perceived causative link to death from non-treatment; balancing of medical action with non-action, allowing for diffusion of responsibility for death; and in the fourth phase, the incorporation of the patient's companions and nursing staff into the decision-making process.	– Need to improve on EOL care characterized by rapid cessation of treatment, minimalist palliative care, initiation of a rapid dying process, yet extreme caution to avoid being seen to be instrumental in causing death.

(Continued)

Table 4.7 *(Continued)* Some qualitative studies

Author	Country	Methodology	Purpose	Participants
Swigart *Heart Lung* (1996).	US.	Interviews.	– Assessing families' willingness to forego life-sustaining treatment.	– Families. – 1 ICU.
Tilden *Nurs Res* (2001).	US.	Interviews.	– Stress related to decisions to withdraw life support.	– Bereaved family members. – 4 tertiary centres.
Cassell *Crit Care Med* (2003).	US, New Zealand.	Ethnography.	– Comparing and contrasting EOL care in open, closed, and semi-closed units.	– Patients, staff, relatives. – 3 ICUs.

WH=withholding life support; WD=withdrawing life support; EOL=end-of-life; MV=mechanical ventila

Setting	Findings	Conclusions
– N=30 family members of 16 patients.	– Letting go has three phases: seeking information about critical illness, reviewing the life story— seeking meaning in their life and critical illness, struggling to maintain roles/relationships. When families felt all had been done, then goals of critical care could be relinquished.	– Transitions from cure to comfort only reconciled when families perceived all had been done. Understanding needs (cognitive, emotional, and moral) is essential to effective communication and support to families involved in life support decision-making in the critical care unit.
– 74 family members of 51 decedents, 45 clinicians. – MV withdrawn from 60% of deaths.	– Stress highest in the absence of advance directives. Families, particularly those without an advance directive, were more likely than clinicians to prioritize prolonging the patient's life with all possible aggressive treatments. However, both families and clinicians endorsed the patient's own values and preferences as the most important factor in making the decision.	– The qualities that help patients and families execute advance directives, (good communication skills and closer relationships) may account for lower stress among families of patients with advance directives.
– N=600 (nurses, doctors, Allied Health Professionals, patients, family members, and friends. – 80 EOL care episodes observed.	– Timing different between disciplines of surgery and intensive care for shifts from cure to comfort and extent of family involvement in decision-making. Primary goal of surgeons 'to defeat death' vs resource management by intensivists. Mixed units experienced conflict and miscommunication.	– Administrative models have significant impact on how EOL care is enacted.

Cultural issues, spirituality, and hope

Cultural issues and palliative care in the ICU *128*
Kerry Bowman

Influence of ICU culture on end-of-life care *134*
Peter Dodek

Spiritual care in the ICU *140*
Michele Shields, Denah Joseph

Considering hope in the context of palliative care in the
   ICU *146*
Christy Simpson

The social and financial impact on the families of ICU patients: a
   view from the US *150*
Sandy Swoboda

Cultural issues and palliative care in the ICU

Introduction

In increasingly pluralistic societies, there is a growing demand to integrate end-of-life-care into a broader context that accommodates and respects cultural differences and diversity. We often assume that respect and acceptance of cultural diversity is a given, yet it is important for us to remember that despite our openness to other cultures, our attitudes toward end-of-life care are as much an effect of our cultural beliefs as the many diverse cultures we see in practice. In the face of cultural differences at the end of life, health care providers, patients, and their families may inadvertently not share an understanding of the nature and meaning of death and dying, nor the way it should be approached. Values so ingrained in health care workers as to be unquestioned may be alien to patients from different cultural backgrounds. As a means of understanding our own position, this chapter considers:

- The sociocultural nature of contemporary health care in relation to culture and end-of-life care.
- Areas that may emerge as most potentially problematic at the interface of contemporary health care and cultural differences at the end of life.

To provide an example, a single case of cross-cultural health care at the end of life is explored in depth. Salient areas of cross-cultural differences as well as alternative clinical approaches are provided to better understand and negotiate cultural differences.

Background and significance

Although death is a universal rule, dying is very much a culturally specific experience. Culture refers to learnt patterns of behaviours, beliefs, and values shared by individuals in a particular social group. It provides human beings with a sense of identity, belonging, and a framework for understanding experience. When referring to culture in its broadest sense, the term usually implies a group of people with similar ethnic background, language, religion, familial beliefs, and world view. Culture is a strong determinant of people's views of the very nature and meaning of illness and death:[1]

- How much health or end-of-life decisions can or should be controlled.
- How bad news should be communicated.
- How decisions, including end-of-life decisions, should be made.

As a result of profound demographic changes affecting many western nations, health care workers will increasingly care for patients from cultural backgrounds other than their own. Differences in beliefs, values, and traditional health care practices are of profound relevance at the end of life.[2] Culture shapes the expression and experience of death and dying as patients and families prepare to lose a loved one. With growing awareness that the care of the dying is deficient in relation to many of medicine's accomplishments[3] as well as the multiple initiatives to improve the care of the dying, the burgeoning field of end of life is receiving increased attention. Experts in the field of end-of-life care are being looked towards as a means of improving the care of the dying by clarifying priorities and establishing humane and respectful end-of-life care standards and practices.

The heart of the problem is that health care providers, patients, and their families may not have shared understandings of the meaning of illness or death, and may not agree on the best strategies to plan for the end of life or to alleviate pain and suffering. Good end-of-life care may be complicated by:

• Disagreements between health care workers and patients, miscommunication.
• Decisions or beliefs that are not understood or valued.

Values so ingrained in physicians as to be unquestioned may be alien to patients from different backgrounds. Because of this significant potential for misunderstanding, it is imperative that health care workers be cognizant to potential cultural differences and develop the skills necessary to identify such differences.

An area where we often go wrong in medicine in general and end of life in particular is to see 'cultural differences' as being something rooted solely in our patients' perspectives. We, as health care workers, also represent a 'culture' in which end-of-life perspectives also have a social and cultural history. It is imperative when working with patients new to our society to understand that it represents the interface of two cultures: theirs and ours. It is naive and unrealistic to believe that differences in patients' perspectives can be dealt with without understanding our own perspectives and their genesis. To this end, we must explore contemporary health care's historic and contemporary perspectives on end-of-life care.

The social cultural development of end-of-life care

When considering culture and end of life, it is important to note that despite the broadening of perspectives in the field of end of life, moral agency and individual autonomy remain at the heart of contemporary attitudes towards end-of-life perspective which stands in contrast to many cultures. Many health care workers dealing with people at the end of life recognize the importance of culture, yet argue that despite significant cultural differences, fundamental, inherent, universal, ethical principles exist that can and ought to be applied across cultures, nations, and all forms of human boundaries in the face of death. The argument is frequently forwarded that there are essential ingredients embedded within the world's apparently diverse moral systems such as humaneness, defined as compassion for the pain and suffering of others, and the recognition of the equal worth and basic autonomy of every human being.

If the concepts that stem from the European Enlightenment of the 18th century, (that equal worth and autonomy are applied as universal and our guiding light in the face of death), what then of Asian philosophical traditions grounded in Taoism, Confucianism, or Buddhism in which moral perspective and direction is illuminated by interdependence rather than independence? Such cultures are perplexing to most Westerners because they do not contain references to autonomy or self. We often believe that having an 'open mind' and 'taking our cues from patients' will ameliorate cross-culture misunderstanding. Yet we must first acknowledge that our deepest beliefs related to death and dying are also shaped by culture.

Scenario

The following common procedure illustrates some of these conceptual differences in perspective. A patient comes into an ICU in a cognitively incompetent state. The ICU team meets with the patient's family. They first focus on biomedical explanations of illness and the potential for 'brain death', then make enquiries about the patient's personal wishes about treatment before the incompetent state and encourage an open and direct conversation about the severity of the situation and the potential for death. Hence, the team hopes to arrive at the best plan for this individual's medical care by exploring her perspectives and values through her family.

However, for this family of non-western origin, the focus on individual rights and choices, direct and blunt verbal communication about such a personal and difficult situation, the introduction of the element of choice, and the focus on a purely biomedical explanation of illness and death may be so confusing that it leads to a complete breakdown in communication. Inherent in this relatively standard approach is a belief in a western definition of illness and death, a belief that the timing and circumstances of dying can and should be controlled, and at the heart of each of these paradigms is the fundamental belief in the inherent value of respect for autonomy, even if the patient and her family are unaware of the very concept.

For many people new to scientifically advanced western nations, several factors made death a more frequent, home-based experience that had little to do with choice, including:

- The absence of life-sustaining technology.
- A far shorter life expectancy.
- A higher child mortality rate.
- A closer geographic proximity for many families.

But in western nations, end-of-life decisions abound and the stakes are high. These decisions involve life or death, views about the quality and meaning of life, high costs, moral principles, and legal rights. Not surprisingly, such decisions can generate intense emotions and increase the potential for cross-cultural conflict.

Moreover, substantial differences in culture, combined with social class and education, often exist between health care workers and families. What is known or valued by health care workers may be illusive or irrelevant to families. When differences exist, so too will perspectives on choices, thus creating a greater opportunity for conflict. For families, end-of-life decisions are not abstract philosophical questions or matters of clear-cut clinical judgement. Rather, they are painful emotional experiences, greatly shaped by cultural religious beliefs that can generate profound revelations about mortality and family relationships.

Conclusions

Those working in the domain of end-of-life care must undertake a deeper exploration of social and cultural realities that shape end-of-life experiences. Although end-of-life care increasingly identifies and values interrelationships with others, autonomy and, in turn, the individual, remains at the heart of end-of-life analysis. Our organizational and legal structures assume that the person experiencing the illness is the best person to make health care decisions. This raises the profound question about the adaptability of end-of-life care in a culturally pluralistic society. As many cultures vest in the family or community, the right to receive and disclose information and to organize and make decisions about patient care, we must be constantly cognizant that the application of the concept of autonomy cross-culturally will mean accepting each person's terms of reference for their definition of self. Specifically, we should respect the autonomy of patients and families by incorporating their cultural values and beliefs into the decision-making process. Although this may sound straightforward, it is easy to lose sight of this in our busy practices.

Ultimately, the most effective way to address cultural differences in end-of-life decision-making is through open and balanced communication. The mere acknowledgement of such differences will usually lead to improved communication.

Consider the following questions when working cross-culturally in end of life:

- Do patients value individuality and personal choice or do they focus more on family and collective choices?
- Do they value open communication or do they tend to draw cues from the context of the situation?
- Do they believe a person can and should influence their health or their death?
- Do they believe in a western explanation of illness or do they hold an alternative culturally based view? Is this view blended with western perspectives on illness?

In health care, we often assume that respect and acceptance of cultural diversity is a given, yet it is important for us to remember that despite our openness to other cultures, our attitudes toward end-of-life care are as much an effect of our cultural beliefs as the many diverse cultures we see in practice. We must make a significant effort to raise our awareness and alter our practices in this crucial area.

Table 5.1 is developed from three paradigms from the social sciences. This table represents only trends when dealing with individual patients and families at the end of life.

References

1. Fagan A (2004). Challenging the bioethical application of the autonomy principle within multicultural societies. *J Appl Philos* **21**, 15.
2. Braun KL, Pietsch JH, Blanchette PL (eds.) (2000). *Cultural issues in end-of-life decision-making*. Sage Publications, Thousand Oaks, CA.
3. Clark D (2002). Between hope and acceptance: the medicalization of dying. *BMJ* **324**, 905.

Table 5.1 Considerations in cross cultural end of life care

Perspective	Contemporary medical
Beliefs about causation of death and dying.	• Biologically determined. • Dying occurs when medicine can no longer stave off, treat, or reverse illness. • Death most often occurs in hospitals and the declaration of death is ultimately in the hands of medical personnel.
Social structures.	• Equality. • Independence valued. • Strong acceptance and value given to autonomy.
Communicating about dying to patients and others.	• Information explicitly communicated. • Moral obligation to truth-telling as patient has right to know and must make autonomous decisions. • Information best overtly communicated.
Perception of a religiously/ culturally meaningful death.	• Individual choice. • No direct association to medicine. • Can be an impediment to the acceptance of the futility of further treatment.
Perception of negotiating death (levels of negotiating treatment).	• Patients are largely responsible for defining the 'kind of death' they wish.
Timing of death.	• The timing and circumstances of death can and ought to be controlled as much as possible to respect a patient's autonomous choices.
Non-verbal communication.	• Direct communication, even about difficult matters, is the most ethical approach.

Non-western	Clinical approach
• Death may be seen in a broader and seemingly less tangible manner. • May be viewed as being linked to religious, social, spiritual, and environmental determinants. • Some cultural groups may perceive illness and death as separate entities. • Declaration of death is also socially and culturally determined.	• Anticipate non-medical perspectives on death. • Allow cultural rituals. • Allow flexibility with time spent with the dying or deceased. • Explore perceptions about the causes of the critical illness, its treatment, and death.
• Hierarchy. • Moral value given to interdependence; family decision-making.	• Allow patients/families to make collective decisions (in the absence of coercion).
• Moral duty to protect loved one's from negativity. • Cues taken from the social context. • Frank communication about death often unacceptable. Truth-telling highly problematic.	• Ask patient how much medical info he/she wishes. • Ask how information should be communicated.
• May be the most critical aspect of death. • Greatly shapes the bereavement process.	• Allow rituals. • Flexibility with number and timing of visitors. • Accept non-medical perspectives.
• Suffering and death are largely a matter of fate and may hold profound spiritual meaning.	• Trial of therapy allows patient outcomes to be determined more by 'fate'.
• The timing and circumstances of death and dying are preordained and a matter of fate.	• Allow as natural a process as possible. If life support withdrawn, do gradually.
• Consider body language, respect silences, rituals.	• Listen more than speak. • Consider body language. • Allow and respect silences; consider their meaning..

Influence of ICU culture on end-of-life care

Organizational culture is difficult to define, but may be considered the 'personality' of an organization, a unifying theme that provides meaning in the workplace. Research from industries outside health care has demonstrated the profound impact that organizational culture can have on individuals' perceptions, attitudes, and behaviours. Cultures help members of an organization deal with uncertainty, on both an individual and collective basis, by defining what is important in a given situation, providing guidance on how individuals should perceive situations and interact with each other, and providing members with accepted ways of expressing and affirming beliefs, values, and norms. Hence, organizational culture provides its members with direction, purpose, and perspective. Furthermore, there are demonstrated associations between improvements in organizational culture and improvements in outcomes in other industries.

Within the context of the ICU, and especially related to end-of-life care, family members may be more satisfied with the treatment of the patient as well as their own treatment in high procedural justice cultures. This is because family members are more likely to have been the recipient of helping behaviours from the staff, but more importantly, they would have observed positive values amongst the staff which signal that individuals are valued and can expect to be treated with dignity. The purpose of this chapter is to highlight what we know and what we need to know regarding the role of organizational culture in addressing the needs of patients near the end of life and their families.

Some problems with end-of-life care

Before addressing the role of organizational culture, it is important to understand gaps between patients' and families' preferences and providers' actions in end-of-life care:

- Despite preferences for comfort care, many patients die after receiving high-technology treatments.
- About half of physicians are unaware of their patients' preferences regarding resuscitation, and about half of DNR orders are written within two days of death.
- About a third of patients who die spend at least ten days in an ICU.

Needs and perceptions of family members of adult ICU patients

Basic needs of family members include information and knowledge, hope and reassurance, preservation of relationships (including those with the patient and with other family members and friends), and assistance (comfort in the waiting room and at the bedside, flexible visiting hours, and financial help). Perceptions of family members during an ICU encounter often follow this pattern:

- They experience acute stress just after admission, decreasing by discharge.
- They are least satisfied with the lack of information.
- Attending physicians are viewed as more controlling than nurses.

- Bedside nurses are viewed as more affiliative.
- Family members develop a sense of optimism related to meeting needs and to perception of affiliation from physicians.

ICU staff may underestimate satisfaction and overestimate stress scores of family members.

Components of a 'good death'

Studies of patients, family members, and providers have revealed common themes about what constitutes a 'good death':
- Pain and symptom management.
- No prolongation of the dying process.
- Sense of control.
- Clear decision-making.
- Relieving burden.
- Strengthening relationships.
- Preparation for death and completion.

Recommendations to improve end-of-life care

To achieve the elements listed above, family members have called for the following improvements in care:
- Better communication.
- Greater access to physicians' time.
- Better pain management.

Family satisfaction with end-of-life care in ICUs[1]

Perspectives on the quality of end-of-life care from family members may vary depending on the geographic location of the patient. From the family members of patients in six Canadian ICUs:
- 96% felt that the patient was mostly to totally comfortable in final hours.
- 88% felt supported to very supported by the health care team.
- Overall satisfaction was associated with:
  - Completeness of information received.
  - Respect and compassion shown.
  - Amount and level of care received.

Perspectives from family members in four American ICUs were notable for:
- Poor symptom control (pain, dyspnoea).
- More favourable perspectives associated with:
  - Control of pain.
  - Control of events.
  - Preparation for death.
  - Concern for dignity and self-respect.

Withdrawal of life support

The final active intervention in end-of-life care for critically ill patients is the withdrawal of life support. From one Canadian ICU, family members had the following perspectives:
- 83% strongly agreed that the patient's death was compassionate and dignified.

- Satisfaction with care was associated with:
  - Discussion initiated by the appropriate person.
  - Explanation of the process.
  - Opportunity to voice concerns.
  - Preparation of family and friends.
  - Privacy during the withdrawal of life support.
  - Withdrawal proceeding as expected.
  - Patient appearing comfortable.

What is most important to dying patients and their families?

Satisfaction carries most weight if the specific items being assessed are also important to the family members. From a multicentre study, the following items were most commonly rated as very important by patients and their family members:

- Trust and confidence in physicians.
- Avoidance of unnecessary life support.
- Effective communication.
- Continuity of care.
- Closure and life completion.

Opportunities to improve care of dying patients and their families

Areas that are both important and have gaps in level of satisfaction include:

- Plan of care after hospital discharge.*
- Symptom relief.*
- No burden on family.
- Trust and confidence in physician.
- Adequate provision of information.*

What is organizational culture?

- ' ... how things are around here.'[2]
- ' ... the invisible force behind the tangibles and observables in any organization, a social energy that moves people to act. Culture is to an organization what personality is to the individual—a hidden, yet unifying theme that provides meaning, direction, and mobilization.'[3]

Organizational culture is reflected by:[2]

- What is valued.
- Dominant leadership styles.
- Language and symbols.
- Procedures and routines.
- Definitions of success.

* Also according to family members

Cultures that convey beliefs, values, and norms suggesting that members of the group are respected and fairly treated have been known to impact specific attitudes and behaviours of those members, including increasing helping behaviours, performance, and lowering absenteeism.

Is organizational culture linked to outcomes of critical care?

• Caregiver interaction, including culture, leadership, coordination, communication, and conflict management, are associated with a lower length of stay, lower nurse turnover, higher technical quality of care, and better provider's perception of the ability to meet family needs.[4]

Furthermore, improvements in safety culture, a subset of organizational culture in ICUs, have been associated with improvements in safety outcomes such as the incidence of ventilator-associated pneumonia and central venous catheter-related bloodstream infections, and a reduction in ICU costs.

Organizational culture and end-of-life care

There are few studies about the role of organizational culture and end-of-life care, but a qualitative study of different models of ICU service delivery revealed the following about two different models:

• In semi-closed ICUs, surgeons and intensivists were more often in conflict and surgeons were reluctant to accept death.
• In a closed, intensivist-run ICU, there was more consideration of quality of life and withdrawal of life support.[5,6]

Furthermore, power relationships with physicians may inhibit nurses from giving information to families.

Discrepancies between physicians and nurses

Culture is not an objective measure, but is assessed from the perspective of the worker. It is not surprising that perspectives of physicians and nurses may be different:

• Decision-making regarding end-of-life care is perceived as satisfactory by more than two thirds of physicians, but by only one third of nurses.
• Quality of death and dying are perceived better by attending physicians (and family members) than by nurses and residents.
• Moral distress is greater in nurses than in physicians; this difference is related to conflict about level of care.

What can we do now? Promote an ethical practice environment

In the absence of clinical trials of interventions aimed at improving organizational culture, action can be based on what we have learnt from observational studies:

• Clarify personal and professional values.
  • 'If I were dying, what would I consider a good death?'
• Clarify organizational values.
  • 'What are the key elements of care that every dying person should expect from each professional at this institution?'
• Monitor ethical performance.
  • Accountability for upholding norms, specific measures, morbidity/mortality reviews.

What else can we do now?

Other opportunities for improvement in organizational culture that may influence end-of-life care are drawn from assessments of organizational culture and from assessments of knowledge, skills, and attitudes regarding end-of-life care:

- Improve collaboration.
  - Conflict resolution/communication.
  - Recognition of different roles and values.
  - Share control of information.
- Improve medical education in end-of-life care.

What do we need to know?

Although it is important to act now, it is also important to develop a research agenda to inform future practice in this area. Examples of some research questions to be answered are:

- Is there an independent relationship between organizational culture and patient/family perceptions of end-of-life care?
- Which domains/types of organizational culture are most strongly associated with perceptions of end-of-life care?
- How can we change organizational culture to improve perceptions of end-of-life care?

References

1. Heyland DK, Rocker GM, O'Callaghan CJ, Dodek PM, Cook DJ (2003). Dying in the ICU: perspectives of family members. *Chest* **124**, 392–7.
2. Cameron KS, Quinn RE (1999). *Diagnosing and changing organizational culture based on the competing values framework*. Addison–Wesley, Reading, Mass.
3. Kilman RH (1986). *Gaining control of the corporate culture*. Jossey–Bass, San Francisco, CA.
4. Shortell SM, Zimmerman JE, Rousseau DM, *et al.* (1994). The performance of intensive care units: does good management make a difference? *Med Care* **32**, 508–25.
5. Cassell J, Buchman TG, Streat S, Stewart RM (2003). Surgeons, intensivists, and the covenant of care: administrative models and values affecting care at the end of life—updated. *Crit Care Med* **31**, 1551–7.
6. Baggs JG, Norton SA, Schmitt MH, Dombeck MT, Sellers CR, Quinn FR (2007). Intensive care unit cultures and end-of-life decision-making. *J Crit Care* **22**, 159–68.

Spiritual care in the ICU

The meaning and practice of spiritual care

By taking a holistic approach to health care, spiritual caregivers respect and respond to the values and beliefs of patients and their families. For many people who face health crises, spirituality is a resource for coping with and healing from illness and injury. Some patients and families express spirituality in religious communities with traditional religious practices, rituals, and beliefs. Others focus their spirituality outside traditional faith communities and practices. In general, many people who do not describe themselves as 'religious' still see themselves as 'spiritual.' The uncertainty and upheaval experienced as a part of health concerns or crises often raise 'spiritual' issues.

Chaplains play an essential role in supporting patients and families of diverse traditions and backgrounds and in collaborating with the health care team in the development of comprehensive care plans. In an age of increasingly patient- and family-centred care, spiritual care is no longer an optional service for hospitals to provide, but an essential one.

A general screening question can be helpful in determining a patient's or family's spiritual perspective. 'Do you have any spiritual beliefs or practices which are important to you? As your physician/nurse/caregiver, I'd like to be supportive of these.' This question can elicit patient preferences and provide the treatment team with opportunities for an improved plan of care.

Whether they consider themselves to be 'religious' or not, people tend to share some basic core spiritual needs. To attend to these needs in the chaotic environment of the ICU, a spiritual caregiver endeavours to be a calm, non-anxious, embodied presence and to establish a trusting relationship with the patient and family.

Assessing core spiritual needs and making spiritual interventions

Concerns related to the human need for self-worth and belonging to the community may be indicated by a patient's self-blaming as well as a deep appreciation for the presence of visitors, family, and other social support. The patient minimizes his/her needs and fears burdening others in circles of community, of which the patient may not feel worthy.

Mrs T, a 62-year old married, Filipina, Roman Catholic with six children, suffered multiple medical problems, including renal failure. Although she felt weary and no longer wanted aggressive treatment, her family exhorted her to 'keep trying.'

The spiritual caregiver embodies or incarnates valuing and community

Intervention

The health care team offered to facilitate a family meeting to discuss goals of care. The patient expressly did not want to be present for this, but was relieved that others on the team were willing to speak for her wishes. In providing this voice, the team affirmed that they had listened to her story, understood her needs, and valued her perspective. In the family meeting, the team reframed the family's wish for her to continue treatment as evidence of their great love for her and suggested than an even greater act of love might be to support her wishes to go home, stop dialysis, and have as much time as possible with her loved ones. The family grieved openly and shifted their opinion about how best to support and affirm the patient in the days ahead.

The need to make meaning and find direction may be indicated by a patient's difficulty in making decisions, expressing concerns related to the larger meaning of his/her life and/or questioning why this is happening in order to make sense of this stage of life.

Mr C, a 41-year old father of two teenage daughters, received a heart transplant 20 years ago. He spent three months in the ICU for intractable infections, eventually facing the last chance prospect of one more surgery. He despaired over his inability to find any meaning in his suffering, his diminishing treatment options, and the prospect of another major surgery, and agonized about what to do. Previously, he had been an avid hiker, and found solace and nurturance in nature. He had lost this connection in the barren technological wilderness of the ICU.

The spiritual caregiver embodies or incarnates a guide

Intervention

The chaplain suggested guided visualizations and meditation, which he welcomed. This was a powerful support to reconnect him with a deep sense of his inner resources. In creatively imagining other times and environments, he accessed a sense of trust, guidance, and knowing what was enduring and meaningful in his life. This enabled him to regain his equilibrium and go forward with the surgery.

Concerns related to the need to love and be loved in reconciled/completed relationships may be indicated by a tendency to blame others, evidence of broken or estranged relationships, expression of a need to forgive and/or be forgiven, an inability to grieve losses and/or an unwillingness or inability to say goodbye.

Ms O, a married, 38-year old mother of a toddler, was intubated and sent to the ICU after collapsing at home. Although she had end-stage ovarian cancer with brain metastases, she was 'for resuscitation' and wanted everything done to prolong her life. During previous hospitalizations, she and her husband expressed great anger at the staff for failing to cure her disease, at pollution for causing her cancer, and at another hospital's physicians for 'abandoning' her. She and her husband insisted on limiting her pain medication, out of fear that this would hasten her death and mean that 'everyone had given up' on her.

The spiritual caregiver embodies or incarnates a truth teller

Intervention
The chaplain compassionately and directly addressed the patient's and husband's blaming of others, and fracturing of relationships as indicative of their need for reconciliation. She suggested that they reflect on their own contributions to the breakdown of relationships and alternatives. Unfortunately, the intervention was unsuccessful. The couple dismissed the caregivers as much as they could. The patient died intubated in the ICU, with the husband so embittered that he failed to connect, even with his wife as she lay dying.

Spiritual issues in the transition from curative to comfort measures
The decision to limit life-prolonging interventions is most often fraught with difficult emotions and distress for patients, families, and often, clinicians. Attention to the spiritual needs of patients and families during this process can greatly facilitate this transition and alleviate some of the suffering and dissatisfaction with care associated with accepting that the end of curative treatment has arrived.

During discussions about the transition to comfort measures, it is essential to encourage patients and families to express their views and seek to understand the hopes and fears they have regarding death, including worries about being a burden to others, losing control, uncertainty, the impact of the death on those left behind, and potential pain and suffering.

Culture can impact patient and family views concerning the use of advance directives and decisions about end-of-life care, such as the use or discontinuation of feeding tubes, levels of pain medication, palliative sedation, and the degree of openness and transparency in any treatment-related communication.

Often, patients and families experience goals of care conversations at the end of life as a form of abandonment; this can be ameliorated by clearly communicating that during the transition, the focus continues to be the well-being of the patient through optimal symptom and pain management as well as greater attention to the relief of spiritual distress and suffering.

Often, death in an ICU follows the decision to withhold or withdraw life-sustaining treatments. Such decisions can raise intense feelings of guilt, confusion, and ambivalence, especially for family members or other substitute decision-makers called upon to make the decisions when patients are not capable of doing so. Staff can help families cope with these difficult emotions and clarify the ethical basis of their decision-making process.

There are occasions when a family's religious belief may lead to the sense that allowing the team to stop treatment amounts to giving up on God or a loss of faith in God's love and healing power. In some faith traditions, the withdrawal of life-sustaining treatment is never sanctioned. Identifying and understanding these views can help the team work within the family's frame of reference and forestall painful emotional conflicts.

Ritual and sacrament in end-of-life care in the ICU

Spiritual caregivers in the ICU may design and lead rituals, ceremonies, sacraments, and other interventions such as:

- Prayer, meditation, and reading of sacred texts.
- Worship services.
- Blessings.
- Religion-specific sacraments and holy objects.
- Weddings and sacred unions.
- Observances of holy days.
- Guided meditation for pain reduction and relaxation.
- Music, sacred or familiar to the patient/family.
- Life review and creation of a legacy document or DVD.
- Guided meditation for inner guidance or connection to God or a Higher Power.
- Times of remembrance for staff to recall and commemorate a beloved patient.

At the end of life, most faith traditions have specific rituals and prayers that may be very important to families to observe with the dying patient. In addition, there may be significant post-mortem practices related to care of the body in preparation for burial. The beliefs and values of patients and families need to be identified and respected in as much as the health care team can ethically and reasonably accommodate them. Spiritual care professionals can help to negotiate and provide appropriate observances meaningful to the family members involved.

Other spiritual tasks of patients at the end of life

Creating an optimal environment for accomplishing 'tasks' of dying is much more difficult to achieve in an ICU setting. The noise, dominance of technology, constant monitoring, lack of privacy, and sense of urgency that pervade most ICUs may preclude the quiet and calm that support the 'work' of the dying described below. It is of utmost importance that ICU staff seek to create as much as possible both an outer and inner environment in which such work can be pursued and sustained. Recognizing that spiritual well-being is a core component of quality of life at the end of life can motivate staff to facilitate the provision of this kind of care.

- Patients and families need quiet private time when they are not interrupted or hovered over by well-meaning staff, where the tasks of saying goodbye, repairing relationships, and/or expressing gratitude can proceed without the added strain of feeling that these intimate moments are on public display.

- Caregivers need to acknowledge that sometimes, there may be aspects of patients' and families' suffering that are beyond medicine to 'solve.' At such times their simple presence and compassionate witness are still gifts they can offer.
- Patients and families are often unprepared for the crisis that precipitates an ICU admission and are often worried by unfinished financial or legal matters. Facilitating the resolution of such concerns can greatly alleviate distress.
- Even when a patient cannot participate in the tasks of dying outlined above, doing this work with the family around the patient's bedside may also be of great value to both patients and those who will be grieving later on.
- Grieving can promote a sense of completion and peace as well as a sense of the possibility of experience of the transcendent inherent in the dying experience.
- Help in facing fears and finding sources of comfort, hope, and healing in the face of impending death is of critical concern to most patients and families facing dying. Acknowledging the universality of all forms of spiritual distress can itself be helpful.

Considering hope in the context of palliative care in the ICU

Introduction

In the ICU setting, there is much intensity and focus on saving patients. Making a shift (sometimes very quickly) in the goals of care towards palliative care—recognizing and accepting that a patient is dying—can be difficult for patients, families, and health care providers alike.

Hope is frequently understood to be a vital aspect of health care. Patients and families ask about and seek hope from their health care providers. In likewise fashion, many health care providers believe that they have a responsibility to foster, instill, or enhance hope in patients and families.

While there may be many different things to hope for in the ICU, the hopes intertwined with issues of living and dying often take centre stage.

Accordingly, considering the role of hope in the context of death and dying in the ICU in more depth becomes relevant.

What is hope?

- Hope means something different to each person. There is no one agreed upon definition, and yet there are some key, common features that recur in many of these definitions. Hope:[1]
  - *Is related to our desires and wants as well as our values and/or goals.* Hope is influenced by who we are and what is important to us. As our goals and values change or are ranked differently, especially when faced with life-limiting illness or injury, so will our hopes typically change.
  - *Is influenced by what we imagine to be realizable possibilities.* Hope is also shaped by the situations we are faced with and experience. Each of us, whether patients, families, or health care providers, may see the same situation differently or relate more to certain aspects of what is happening. This may then influence what we see as possible, as something to hope for, in the near or distant future.
  - *Involves action.* When people hope for something, they often act in ways that will help to bring about hope. People may also do things that will help support their hope such as by turning to those they love and trust, including, e.g. their families and faith communities.
- Overall, it can be said that hope as well as what is hoped for is person-relative and context-dependent.
- For many people, hope is based in their spiritual or religious beliefs. For others, hope is primarily found in their relationships with family and friends. Still, others discover hope in nature or through meaningful activities.
  - As the sources of hope are quite broad, this gives health care providers a number of ways to engage with and discuss the possibility of hope with patients and family members.

Examining assumptions about hope at the end of life, especially in the ICU

- Some have suggested that there is no hope at the end of life or that, when the goals of care are no longer curative, a particular case is hopeless. These statements are predicated on the assumption that the 'only' hope that health care providers can offer to patients is found in curative approaches.
- When stated like this, most appreciate that what can be offered to patients who are dying and/or family members goes well beyond treatments alone. Having hope is possible in the context of impending death.
- Some have assumed that hope is not part of dying as hope is future-focused. During the dying process, the timeline envisioned for hope may be shortened. Hopes may become more focused on what will happen in the next hour, day, or week rather than months or years down the road. This shift in future focus can facilitate the identification of a number of shorter term hopes.
  - Still, patients may maintain hopes about distant goals, hopes for after they are dead (i.e. hopes for family members), and hopes that pertain to an afterlife, if this is part of their belief system. These hopes are ways of expressing what is important to the patient.
  - Many patients state that having hope, regardless of what it is for, is what is most important to them. The experience of being hopeful or having hope in the present adds to their quality of life.
  - This does not mean that health care providers cannot question or discuss specific hopes with patients. What it means is that health care providers should not become so focused on what a particular hope is for that they ignore what hope itself represents for patients.
- Others have suggested that it is not possible to maintain hope and be honest with patients (and family members), especially about terminal illness or injury. It is true that telling patients that they are dying is a direct challenge to the possibility of hope. It is only natural for patients to lose some specific hope(s) when hearing this information. The question is whether the possibility of finding something (new) to hope for is left open for patients.
  - This may be done, not through promising unachievable goals for patients (such as a cure is 'just around the corner'), but by supporting patients and allowing them the opportunity to ask questions, seek support, express their anger, fear, or sadness.
  - In other words, how information is shared makes a fundamental difference to whether dying patients are able to find something to hope for.

Hope for a good death?

- One of the key aims of palliative care is to facilitate a good death. Finding ways to (help) realize the hope for a good death often becomes the focus for health care providers and family members.
- However, it needs to be acknowledged that the hope for a good death represents an ideal, something that we strive for with good palliative care. Some deaths get closer to this ideal than others.

In the ICU context, some very real challenges exist for achieving a good death. These include, concerns about privacy, potentially intractable symptoms, the ability for family members to be present, and the presence of medical technology.

• Further, what the hope for a good death may mean in practice can vary from person to person. Being clear about what is important to the patient and, secondarily, for family members can help ensure that it is their hope(s) that are central rather than what the hope for a good death means to health care providers themselves.

Magnifying hope and shrinking hopelessness[2]

There is a focus in health care on magnifying hope and on trying to foster hope for patients and family members. While this is valuable, it may sometimes be just as important to consider the ways in which the despair or fear—the opposites of hope—that patients and family members experience can be addressed. By attempting to shrink hopelessness, health care providers can acknowledge where patients and family members are at emotionally.

There are some common sources of hopelessness. These include:[3]

• The 'skidding effect': a loss of control can exacerbate hopelessness, especially when people are used to being in charge of what happens. Dying or witnessing someone dying is often experienced as an ultimate loss of control.
  • Finding ways to offer some control back, even with small choices, can be helpful. Naming this experience can also be helpful as it provides an opportunity to identify what is being experienced.
• The 'alien effect': feeling isolated and separate (alienated) from others contributes to hopelessness. This can include not being given an opportunity to talk, ask questions, or share one's feelings as well as feeling that others are not understanding what is being said.
  • Providing opportunities for conversation—opening up the topic of death and dying—will help to lessen the sense of isolation. Patients have indicated that they do want to talk about death and dying, but that they will often wait for signals from their health care providers to indicate that their condition is serious and/or that 'now' is the time to talk about dying.[4]
• The 'bruising effect': repeated trauma can make it difficult to find hope. Trauma can be experienced physically, emotionally, and/or spiritually. In the ICU context, there may be much to process in a relatively short period of time which can add to the sense of being bruised and tender. People often respond to the feeling of 'being bruised' with anger or by withdrawing.
  • Acknowledging this experience and finding ways to help people feel supported (or that the 'bruise' is protected) can help address hopelessness.
• Hope also fluctuates. On a day-to-day basis, people's hopes or level of hopefulness naturally go up and down. Recognizing this gives an opportunity to share with others that just as hope can go down, it can also come back up.

- Sensitively sharing difficult information, addressing questions and concerns, and honestly talking about what is happening can help to address expectations, and thereby, temper unnecessary fluctuations in levels of hopefulness.

Considering the hope(s) of health care providers

Much of the discussion about the role of hope in health care, in dying, and in the ICU context focuses primarily on the hope(s) of patients and family members. It is equally important to consider and not overlook the hope(s) of health care providers.

- Some starter questions to stimulate reflection and conversation about the hope(s) or lack thereof of health care providers include:
  - Does what a health care provider hopes for make a difference to how he/she cares for a dying patient and family members?
  - Is it possible, as a health care provider, to convey hope if he/she does not have it?
  - How do health care providers cope when their hope is lost or challenged?
- Finding ways to talk about and support the hope(s) of health care providers may have an impact on their sense of burnout, moral distress, and defeat, especially when patients die.

References

1. Simpson C (2004). When hope makes us vulnerable: a discussion of patient-health care provider interactions in the context of hope. *Bioethics* **18**, 428–47.
2. Wendy Edey, counsellor at the Hope Foundation of Alberta, who coined phrase. Available from: http://www.ualberta.ca/hope.
3. Edey W, Jevne R, Westra K (1998). Key elements of hope-focused counselling: the art of making hope visible. The Hope Foundation of Alberta, Edmonton, Alberta http://www.ualberta.ca/hope.
4. Davison SN, Simpson C (2006). Hope and advance care planning in patients with end-stage renal disease: qualitative interview study. *BMJ* **333**, 886.

The social and financial impact on the families of ICU patients: a view from the US

Introduction

The unit of care for the ICU generally, and for palliative clinicians in particular, includes the family as well as the patient. An ICU stay radically affects this entire unit, family as well as patient, from the moment of admission. Among the many burdens for families are social and financial disruptions, which can be especially overwhelming when the period of treatment is prolonged. These burdens may not be immediately apparent to ICU clinicians, but deserve consideration as part of the comprehensive plan of care, particularly in settings outside of the UK without similar welfare support services.

Realities

The Study to Understand the Prognosis and Preferences for Outcomes and Risks of Treatment (SUPPORT) in the US found that:
- More than half of the families reported at least one severe caregiving or financial burden.
- Approximately 20% of family members had to make a major life change in order to provide care to a patient.
- Up to 31% of families lose most or all of their family savings as a result of caregiving, despite the fact that approximately 96% of the patients had hospitalization insurance.
- 24% of patients required considerable caregiving from a family member after discharge and many patients require home care and incur disability costs.

In a study examining the impact of a prolonged, surgical ICU stay of greater than six days:
- Most patients were still in the hospital one month later.
- As the illness continued, more family members needed to leave work to meet the care needs of the patient.
- Family members withdrew from other social activities due to the illness of the patient.

These changes occurred during all phases of the illness, beginning early in the ICU stay and continuing for several months, even after discharge from the hospital.

Initial Impact of the ICU

Difficult challenges face families from the moment the patient enters the critical care unit. The outside world moves forward, but the family is now in a state of 'suspended animation.' Normal routine become impossible. Costs and consequences start accumulating very rapidly. For example, a family's frequent visits to the ICU and hospital entail costs associated with:
- Travel, parking, meals.
- Rearranging schedules, day care.

- Car pooling.
- Perhaps most importantly, the inability to meet work responsibilities.

If a patient is admitted to a facility beyond driving distance to the home, the family member may have no place to stay. Many families in this situation have to 'relocate' to the ICU waiting room, where sleep and personal hygiene are difficult or impossible to maintain. Appointments and deadlines are missed. Self-care by families is swallowed by the crisis of the critical illness.

More time in the ICU, more problems
As critical illness continues over a prolonged time, social and financial problems continue and accumulate concerning:
- General household maintenance, food shopping, and bill paying.
- Strained relationships between those at home.

In the US, the Family Medical Leave Act guarantees leave to care for a seriously ill family member. But this leave is unpaid and there is a limit to the number of days allowed.

The impact is not generally short-lived; it carries on throughout the hospitalization and rehabilitation phases, well into the first year after the initial ICU stay.

Specific needs of different individuals
Needs are not uniform. Consider:
- The needs of the spouse are different from the needs of a parent which are different from the needs of the child assuming care responsibilities for a parent.
- Female caregivers will often put the needs of others in front of their own, minimizing the severity of their own health issues or the level of exhaustion or fatigue.
- Ethnic differences should also be considered. For example, African Americans and Hispanic caregivers are more likely to experience economic burden compared to Caucasians.

Changing roles
During a critical illness, the patient is cared for by the multidisciplinary ICU team who manage the day-to-day, hour-to-hour changes in the patients. The family takes on a supportive role at the hospital and dynamics at home can change. If the patient is the primary breadwinner or household manager, then the family may need to intervene and step into these roles.
- While caregiving can take as little as several hours a week, it can be the equivalent of a full-time job and the sense of responsibility of the caregiver can be overwhelming.

What can the ICU team do?
The goals of palliative care include the attempt to improve the quality of life of not only the patient, but also of the family members. Many families are unprepared to cope with the impact a prolonged ICU stay and the health care teams' efforts should include interventions to address these issues proactively. These issues arise for almost all patients and families,

whether or not patients survive or succumb to the critical illness. The following interventions should help:

- Social work referral should be almost universal.
  - Assessment of the insurance status, financial status, and emotional state of the family members. A concerted effort should be made to address these issues early on in the patients' illness in order to identify the proper resources to help family members during this critical time.
- Provide a list of nearby hotels or facilities that can accommodate visiting families.
- Provide a list of places to eat. Tell them where they can shower, etc.
- Explore their personal needs and coping skills related to the current illness.
  - Discover relationships between family members and the patient before making assumptions of the roles of family members by 'family title'.
  - Assess the impact of visitation on daily routines and schedules.
  - Assess the burden the illness may have on the family to include financial, emotional, and spiritual needs.
  - Provide access to resources to assist with stated needs as appropriate and to help families navigate through the health care system.
- Referrals to support services early on such as spiritual counselling.
- Reassessment of the needs of the family on a routine basis. This can be accomplished on daily rounds with staff members and/or with family members if they are present during rounds.

Patients who recover

- Resource and support services should not end with the discharge from the ICU, but should continue to assist the family until discharge from the hospital.
- The financial and social impact of any prolonged illness is not short-lived, and is sometimes delayed as bills and insurance coverage changes and disability payments are slowly processed.
- Sometimes there can be delays in realizing the full impact of the illness until several months after the initial prolonged hospitalization.

Beyond the ICU, other social work teams will need to continue the supports mentioned above. This will ensure the best possible social outcomes for patients and families during this critical phase.

The uninsured in the US

Many patients without medical insurance or who have little insurance may need to sell their home or relocate due to cost savings and inability to make ends meet. In the above mentioned study of family impact, six families filed for bankruptcy; all patients were less than 65 years old and lacked private insurance. Reasons for bankruptcy filing included lost income, loss of savings, and inability of the patients or family member to return to gainful employment. None of the families expected or planned for a catastrophic illness and many of the expenses related to care outside the hospital were not covered by insurance. As a baseline, hospital costs in

1996 that exceeded $100,000 were predictive of some degree of financial loss at 1 year post-ICU discharge.

Families of younger patients (<65 years old) often have more economic burden associated with a prolonged illness in the ICU, which could be explained by less time to accrue savings and non-eligibility for social support services which may be limited to the older population.

The social impact of dying in the ICU

The social impact of dying in the ICU is an important consideration. Having space and time to grieve with the patient and loved ones is important to many family members, which is sometimes difficult to arrange in the ICU environment. Being cognizant of individual religious or cultural beliefs surrounding a dying patient is essential.

As the patient's condition deteriorates, resuscitation status, limitation of life support, and the death experience should be discussed compassionately with the patient and their families as soon as possible.

• Discuss death in terms understandable to the patient and family and how to be prepared for death in the ICU.
• Determine the religious and/or cultural needs that are important during this time.
• Assess the emotional impact this type of death experience may have on the family surrounded by hospital equipment, in a sterile 'hospital' environment.
• Assess desire with transfer to a floor bed after withdrawal of care for a more nurturing environment and whether this is supportive for the family.
• Provide access to resources to assist with funeral services and post-death care.
• Possible follow-up with the family after the ICU death experience in an effort to debrief from the death experience and discuss findings of autopsy or the ICU experience.

Each dying experience is unique to the patient and family as they experience it in the ICU. There is no specific 'protocol' to follow. However, certain aspects of this experience can be addressed early on to assist the family during this emotional time. Members of the multidisciplinary team can be instrumental in assuring this process is as sacred and comforting as possible.

The price of death

For families of patients dying in the ICU, particularly in the US, additional expenses arise, often with fewer available resources to meeting them.
• Funeral costs.
• Loss of income (self).
• Lack of access to funds due to the death of the patient.

When a patient dies, all sources of income stop and the 'last pay cheque' may have to be returned and reissued due to the patients' date of death. For a patient with a prolonged hospitalization and ICU stay, insurance coverage may abruptly end or 'run out', which could put a strain on personal finances due to excess expenditures.

Further reading

1. Covinsky KR, Goldman L, Cook EF, et al. (1994). The impact of serious illness on patients' families. SUPPORT investigators. Study to understand prognosis and preferences for outcomes and risks of treatment. *JAMA* **272**, 1839–44.
2. Swoboda S, Lipsett P (2002). Impact of a prolonged surgical critical illness on patients' families. *Am J Crit Care* **11**, 459–66.
3. Hanratty B, Holland P, Jacoby A, et al. (2007). Financial stress and strain associated with terminal cancer—a review of the evidence. *Palliat Med* **21**, 595–607.
4. Cuthbertson SJ, Margetts MA, Streat SJ (2000). Bereavement follow-up after critical illness. *Crit Care Med* **28**, 1196–201.

Teamwork, relationships, and moral distress

The role of teams in palliative ICU care *156*
Vicki Spuhler

Collaboration as an essential element of palliative ICU care *160*
Vicki Spuhler

Relationships and iatrogenic suffering: part 2 *162*
David Kuhl

Educating trainees in the ICU: the value of death rounds *168*
Martha E Billings, Catherine L Hough, J Randall Curtis

Moral distress in critical care health care workers *174*
Freda DeKeyser Ganz

Burnout syndrome in ICU nurses and physicians *180*
Bara Ricou, Paolo Merlani

The rapid response system: a role in risk reduction *186*
F Rubulotta, P Calzavacca, M DeVita

The role of teams in palliative ICU care

Introduction
As we strive to balance curing with caring in the ICU, we need a level of commitment by all health care providers to work together in true collaboration in highly effective teams. At no time is this more important than when planning and providing palliative care.

Team purpose
In a general sense, critical care practice aspires to create a health care system that responds to the needs of patients and families and seeks to improve the care for patients who suffer from critical illness. These values are espoused in the mission and vision statements of respective nursing and medicine professional societies around the world.

Teamwork and teams are an essential part of ICU care delivery, but even the most effective team can promote fragmentation of care if left to perform their roles in isolation of other teams of care providers. As the complexity of care delivery increases, it seems improbable that any one group of professionals could have all the skills necessary to adequately support patients as they prepare for end-of-life care in the ICU. The purpose of teams providing palliative care is to offer the most skilled, compassionate care in a collaborative manner in order to assure the best outcomes for the dying patient and the patient's family. However, not all groups are teams. Four essential elements that differentiate a team from a group[1] are depicted in Table 6.1.

Table 6.1 Essential elements of a team

Essential element	Palliative care examples
Shared goals: a reason for working together	Provide consistent communication to families of dying patients.
Interdependence: recognition that team members need one another's experience, ability, and judgement in order to arrive at mutual goals.	Nurse conducts symptom assessment; physician confers with pharmacist; physician prescribes medication; nurse repeats symptom assessment.
Commitment: working together, which leads to more effective decisions than working in isolation.	Physician and patient's nurse confer with social worker to determine options for family support.
Accountability: being accountable as a functioning unit within a larger organizational unit.	ICU team members develop guidelines for withdrawal of life-sustaining therapies when the goal is a comfortable death.

Transferring the four elements of a team into an effective and cohesive unit requires a shared expectation for accomplishment, trust, and respect.[2] The Society of Critical Care Medicine in the US has identified multidisciplinary critical care teams as one of its core values (available from: http://www.sccm.org/about/mission.html). This implies a shared value for the work that can be accomplished by effective teams.

Palliative care team roles

The core goals of integrative palliative care include the optimization of comfort and emotional and practical support for families, beginning with the diagnosis and without regard to prognosis. Palliative care teams consist of specially trained and supported physicians, nurses, social workers, chaplains, and others who provide consultation for patients and their families with life-threatening or terminal disease.[3]

Palliative care (that includes, but is not limited to, end-of-life care) should be delivered as part of comprehensive critical care. Billings *et al.*[4] described a successful process of merging the culture of ICU and palliative care through a programme which promoted a palliative care nurse champion and incorporated a palliative care specialist on rounds. Specialized training, mentoring, and role modelling were part of the implementation plan. This process led to an increase in palliative care consultations and to a process for conducting family meetings. Nurses on the unit reported considerable improvement in job satisfaction and comfort with end-of-life care. This kind of collaboration between palliative and critical care should underpin initiatives to ensure ongoing improvement to the quality of care for all our critically ill, dying patients. (See a more detailed discussion of quality evaluation in 📖 Ch. 2).

Characteristics of good ICU teams providing palliative care

Good teams do not spring up by magic. There are three basic elements to a team providing palliative care. Consideration of each element provides opportunities for improvement in the manner in which palliative care is provided.

Team size

The size of the palliative care team may expand and contract, depending on the patient's and family's needs. The team may include the ICU physician, patient's nurse, social worker, chaplain, patient's primary physician, and others. Questions to ask about a core team for a particular palliative care patient include the following:

- Can the team convene easily and frequently?
- Can communication occur easily and frequently?
- Are discussions open and interactive for all members?
- Does each member understand the other's skills and role on the team?
- Do you need more people to achieve your goals?
- Are sub-teams possible or necessary?

Complementary skills on teams providing palliative care

- Are there adequate levels of complementary skills? The complexity today in critical care demands many skill sets and clinicians whose education and training reflect an area of specificity and expertise. This training may not yet have included palliative care skills. Making sure that the bedside team has access to and utilizes those with the right skills and expertise is essential to team success.[2] Evaluate whether the three categories of skills noted in Table 6.2 are either actually or potentially represented across the membership. Consider whether any skill areas that are critical to team performance are missing or under-represented and whether members, individually and collectively, are willing to spend the time to help themselves and others learn and develop skills.

Table 6.2 Complementary skills

Skill category	Skill examples
Functional/technological	Physician prescribes medications for complex patient symptoms.
Problem-solving	Social worker works with the family to bring others together for a family conference.
Interpersonal	Nurse works with the patient's family to understand goals of care.

Accountability

Team accountability is about the sincere promises we make to ourselves and others, promises that underpin two critical aspects of teams: commitment and trust.[2]

- Is there individual and joint accountability for the team's purpose, goals, approach, and outcomes?
- Can progress against specific goals be measured?
- Do all members feel responsible to accomplish all measures?
- Are the members clear on what they are individually and jointly responsible for?
- Is there a sense that 'only the team can fail'?

Answering the preceding questions can establish the degree to which the team functions as a real team in providing palliative care.

Patient and family as members of the team

Clear and effective communication with the patient, the patient's family, and significant others is of paramount importance in the provision of optimal end-of-life care. Communication with patients and their loved ones is as integral a part of the care as symptom control. Generally, discussions which include the patient and family do not take away hope. In fact, if handled with sensitivity and support, these discussions tend to bring the reassurance and increased ability to cope that is associated with diminished uncertainty.[5]

- The identification of the patient's needs that are central to their care must be understood within the context of the relationships that are important to them; those needs are often identified by their families.
- Indeed, caring for the patient must include caring for the family.
- It is important for the clinicians within the team to appreciate the patient and their family as the ones that define the goals that drive the care delivery process.
- The establishment of an ethical environment based on respect and dignity will support this reality.
- It is also important for the clinical team to remember that the stress and fatigue that accompany serious life-threatening illness often makes it necessary that families and patients hear the same information several times so that it can be absorbed and they can feel reassured.[5]
- Respect means we attend to the whole person, to his or her physical health, emotional, psychosocial, spiritual, and culturally bound needs.[6]

When the team includes the patient and family as team members, the patient and their families will feel 'heard' and supported. By involving the patient, whenever possible, and the family in decision-making, we show respect[6] for them and their palliative needs. The team that provides family-centred care, bearing witness to the crisis and grieving that they are experiencing, demonstrates a shared value for the importance of teamwork and patient/family palliation.

References

1. Reilly AJ, Jones JE (1974). Team-building. In: Pfeiffer JW, Jones JE (eds). *The 1974 annual handbook for group facilitators*, pp 227–37. University Associates, San Diego.
2. Katzenbach JR, Smith DK (2006). *The wisdom of teams: creating the high performance organization. First Collins Business Essentials.* Harper Collins Publishers, New York.
3. Hawryluck LA, Espin SL, Garwood KC, *et al.* (2002). Pulling together and pushing apart: tides of tension in the ICU team. *Acad Med* **77**(10 Suppl), S73–6.
4. Billings JA, Keeley A, Bauman J, *et al.* (2006). Merging cultures: Palliative care specialists in the medical intensive care unit. *Crit Care Med* **34**(11Suppl), S388–93.
5. Mcdonald N, Oneschuk D, Hagen N, Doyle D (eds) (2006). *Palliative medicine; a case-based manual*, p11. Oxford University Press, New York.
6. Rushton CH (2007). Respect in critical care: a foundational ethical principle. *AACN Adv Crit Care* **18**, 149–56.

Collaboration as an essential element of palliative ICU care

Collaborative interprofessional teamwork should be the basis upon which quality end-of-life care is provided to patients and their families.[1] Collaboration occurs through relationships and trust is the foundation for building effective relationships.[2] Teams providing palliative care in ICUs must be able to identify the problems they face in offering options to patients and families for moving forward in planning goals of care, and then make the necessary adjustments and decisions about how to proceed. To do this requires excellent interpersonal and communications skills and trust within the team.

Interpersonal skills

Establishing a common purpose and understanding cannot occur without good interpersonal skills.[3] These skills include risk-taking when team members discuss with each other their perhaps differing views of the patient's prognosis. The skill of recognizing the interests and accomplishments of others promotes collaboration by relying on the expertise of colleagues such as social workers and chaplains to assist with grieving families.

Communication skills

Developing effective communication skills is essential for effective team-work.[3] Failure to communicate is one of the primary causes of dissatisfaction for ICU family members. Skilled communication is more than a one-way delivery of information; it is a two-way dialogue in which people think and decide together.[4] Badger has identified effective communication leading to team consensus as a primary factor allowing nurses (and others) to move from cure to comfort care for their patients.[5]

There are four basic elements of effective communication:[6]

- Simplify the message. The key to effective communication is simplicity. Be clear about the message you are sending, and remember, it is not just what you say, but how you say it (see 📖 in 'Relationships and iatrogenic suffering: part 1' p94 and 📖 in 'Relationships and iatrogenic suffering: part 2' p162). This is especially important when team members discuss with family members the patient's prognosis and the option of comfort care.
- See the person. Effective communicators focus on the people with whom they are communicating. Be present. Attend to not only the words of the communication, but the body language.
- Show the truth. Credibility precedes good communication. Believe in what you say and act in accordance with what you believe. Nurse-physician relationships only become true partnerships if both can demonstrate their unique contribution to care and are positioned as intellectual peers. In a healthy work environment, good communication skills are as important as good clinical skills.[2]
- Seek a response. Don't just talk 'at' people. Seek their input. Show sensitivity.

The importance of trust

Trust is a foundational element for good collaboration. Without trust, the heart and soul of relationships are shattered, team collaboration compromised, and patient care becomes undermined.[2] True collaboration is ongoing and built over time, eventually resulting in a culture that supports shared decision-making.[4] When we practice the behaviours that build trust, we invite collaboration.[2] The following eight behaviours build trust and lay the groundwork for true collaboration to occur:[2]

- Act with mutually serving intentions.
- Keep agreements.
- Be consistent in word and deed.
- Seek open, unrestricted access to information.
- Use effective communication skills.
- Speak with good intent.
- Provide timely and honest feedback.
- Develop clinical competence.

Successful teams strive to practice the behaviours that will build trusting relationships. When high team trust exists, individuals involve each other and make decisions collaboratively. 'When communication is clear and constructive and practice is truly collaborative, the end-of-life care provided to ICU patients and families by satisfied and engaged professionals will improve markedly.'[1]

References

1. Puntillo KA, McAdam JL (2006). Communication between physicians and nurses as a target for improving end-of-life care in the intensive care unit: challenges and opportunities for moving forward. *Crit Care Med* **34**(11 Suppl), S332–40.
2. Reina ML, Reina DS, Rushton CH (2007). Trust: the foundation for team collaboration and healthy work environments. *AACN Adv Crit Care* **18**, 103–7.
3. Katzenbach JR, Smith DK (2006). *The wisdom of teams: creating the high performance organization*. First Collins Business Essentials. Harper Collins Publishers, New York.
4. AACN (2005). Standards for establishing and sustaining health work environments: a journey to excellence by the American Association of Critical Care Nurses. *Am J Crit Care* **14**, 187–97.
5. Badger J (2005). Factors that enable or complicate end-of-life transitions in critical care. *Am J Crit Care* **14**, 6.
6. Maxwell JC (2002). *The 17 essential qualities of a team player: becoming the kind of person every team wants*. Thomas Nelson Inc., Nashville Tennessee.

Relationships and iatrogenic suffering: part 2

Questions for self-reflection

With a high incidence of death and dying in a modern day adult ICU, we need to know ourselves if we are to be less likely to cause iatrogenic suffering through the way we communicate with others in such a setting.

Effect and influence of past experiences and important relationships

Dying and death[1]

- What did you feel about death prior to studying medicine (during your childhood, adolescence, and early adulthood)? What do you feel about death now?
- How was death talked about and treated in your family of origin?
- How were family funerals and memorial services held?
- When did you go to your first funeral/memorial?
- What did you think about it and how did you react?
- What do you think about that event now?
- Do any people who have died, such as a parent, spouse, or friend, continue to have an effect on your life?
- Does the patient you are about to see or whom you will be speaking to about code status or a life-altering diagnosis remind you of a family member or a friend?
- Have you had any close calls with death such as an illness or an accident?
- Have you been closely involved with anyone's death?
  - Have you grieved that death? (Grief might be regarded as wanting more of what one will never get again. It is a complex emotion that may include sadness, anger, fatigue, isolation. Grief stays with us until all the sense of loss belonging to the death has been experienced.)
  - What was your life like with the person in it?
  - What did you gain from the relationship?
  - What did the other person gain from the relationship?
  - What would your life be like if the person was still part of your life?
  - What did the person give to you in relationship that as stayed with you following the person's death?
  - How do you feel about it—guilty, resentful, angry, or peaceful?
- What was the most significant death you experienced? Did it change your life? If so, how?
- How have your ideas about death evolved (especially since you entered/completed your medical training)? What kind of death would you like to have? Is death or could death be a friend for you or is to be fought, dreaded, or yet to be accepted?
- Have you previously had conversations with patients regarding a serious or terminal illness? What was that like for you? What might you have done differently?

Family[1]

- How do you define your family? Who is your family? Who is in your family of origin (grandparents, parents, siblings, aunts, uncles, other people you experienced as 'family')? Who is in your family of adulthood (spouse/partner, children, grandchildren, friends you have chosen as family)?
- Has anyone in your family ever been seriously ill? Has anyone in your family died? (See the section on 'dying and death' above.)
- Which family members played a significant role in shaping your life as a child and young adult—in positive ways, in negative ways? What are the features of those individuals that remind you of the role they played in your life? Is there someone in the family that you are about to speak with that reminds you of anyone in your own family? Who in your adult family has been important in how your life has unfolded to this point in time? What would another person have to know about your family to understand you and how you have come to be the person you are?
- How were emotions (anger, sadness, pleasure, pride) expressed in your family? How do you respond to loud expressions of anger? How do you respond to people being silent when they are angry? How do you experience anger? Frustration? Anxiety? Ambiguity?
- How were decisions made in your family? Who held the power and/or the control in your family? Who made the decisions? What were the rules in your family, the 'shoulds' and 'oughts'? How was conflict addressed and resolved?
- What were (are) the strengths and weaknesses in your family? What are some of your favourite memories? Some of your painful memories? Was there anyone in your family that you were afraid of or fearful for? What experiences have torn your family apart or made you closer?
- How do relationships in your family of adulthood reflect or contrast with those in your family or origin? Which familiar patterns (e.g. attitudes, values, strategies, behaviours, world views) have you chosen to carry forward or pass on? Which have you wanted to change?

Reflecting on the effect of your work

Burnout[2] (see also 📖 in 'Burnout syndrome in ICU nurses and physicians' p180)

- Burnout is a work-related syndrome that is characterized by emotional exhaustion, depersonalization, and feelings of a reduced sense of personal accomplishment and commitment to one's profession.
- Most likely to happen in professions that involve an extensive care of other people.
- Assessed using the 22 item Maslach burnout inventory–human services survey (MBI–HSS).
- May affect patient care.
- Some examples of questions pertaining to burnout:
  • Do you feel run down and drained of emotional energy?
  • Do you find that you are prone to negative thinking about your job?
  • Do you find yourself getting easily irritated by small problems or your co-workers and team?
  • Do you feel misunderstood or unappreciated by your co-workers?

- Do you feel that you have no one to talk to?
- Do you feel that you are not getting what you want out of your job?
- Do you feel that you do not have time to do the many things that are important to doing a good quality job?
- Do you feel that you are in the wrong organization of the wrong profession?

Moral distress[3] (see also 📖 *in 'Moral distress in critical care heath care workers' p174)*

- Feelings resulting from a situation in which moral choices cannot be translated into moral action.
  - Anger.
  - Frustration.
  - Guilt.
  - Powerlessness.
- Occurs when one acts in a way that is contrary to personal and professional values, thereby undermining authenticity and integrity.
- People working in an environment in which moral distress exists may experience:
  - More communication.
  - Lack of trust.
  - High turnover rates.
  - Defensiveness.
  - Lack of collaboration across disciplines.
- Ask:[4] am I feeling distressed or experiencing signs of suffering? Is the source of my distress work-related? Is it affecting the other members of the team? If so, how?
- Affirm: affirm distress and commitment to take care of yourself. Validate feelings and perceptions of others.
- Assess: identify source(s) of your distress. When does it happen? How do you experience the distress? Do others that you work with experience the same? Examples:
  - A particular patient care setting: you are asked to provide care (by other team members, physicians, family members) that you feel is not wanted by the patient or you feel that it is unnecessary.
  - A unit policy or practice.
  - Lack of collaboration.
  - Questions to ask: how important is it to you to try to change the situation? How important would it be for your colleagues/unit to have the situation changed? How important would a change be to the patients/families on the unit? How strongly do you feel about trying to change the situation? How confident are you in your ability to make changes occur? How determined are you toward making this change?
- Act: determine risks and benefits to maintaining the status quo, to making changes that will diminish or eliminate moral distress. Develop a plan of action.

Vicarious trauma[5] (often used interchangeably with compassion fatigue and secondary trauma)

- A stress reaction experienced by therapists and researchers who are exposed to disclosures of traumatic images and materials by clients and research participants, in which therapists or researchers experience enduring changes in the manner in which they view self, others, and the world.
- Occurs over time.
- Process of accumulation (sedimentary layers of horrible stories building until one cannot distinguish one from another).
- Long-term, inevitable, expectable consequence of working with suffering people, causing:
  - A transformation of the system of meaning in the sufferer.
  - A darkening of one's world view, spirituality, and relationships.
- Impaired domains:
  - Safety.
  - Trust.
  - Esteem.
  - Control.
  - Sensory intrusion.
- Most common signs:
  - Increased rates of illness.
  - Cynicism.
  - Sadness.
  - Intolerance of emotion.
  - Addictive responses.
  - Exhaustion.
  - Depression.
  - Loss of efficiency.
  - Judgement errors.
- Sample questions (from ProQOL, a measurement of compassion fatigue, burnout, and compassion satisfaction).[6] To be scored between 1 and 5 (0=never; 1=rarely; 2=a few times; 3=somewhat often; 4=often; 5=very often). As this is only a sample of the questions, your score cannot determine the degree of compassion fatigue, burnout, or compassion satisfaction you are experiencing.
  - I am happy.
  - I am preoccupied with more than one person I help.
  - I get satisfaction from being able to help people.
  - I feel connected to others.
  - I jump or am startled by unexpected sounds.
  - I feel invigorated after working with those I help.
  - I find it difficult to separate my personal life from my life as a helper.
  - I am losing sleep over traumatic experiences of a person I help.
  - I think that I might have been 'infected' by the traumatic stress of those I help.
  - I feel trapped by my work as a helper.

Trauma: a sense of helplessness in the face of unfixable suffering[7]

- What effect does incurable, irreversible disease have on you?
- What effect does failed resuscitation have on you?

- Which patients keep you awake or wake you up in the middle of the night?
- Which patients do you avoid in your conversations with other health care professionals who also cared for those patients or which patients do you not forget?

Working to prevent iatrogenic suffering, the suffering that characterizes health care providers and patients

- Maintain balance in your life with time spent in physical, social, psychological, and spiritual activities. Keep in contact with close friends and family.
- Improve and enhance your communication skills.
- Make certain that you have a family physician.
- Ask people who know you well if and how you have changed or are changing as you continue working in health care. Are you empathic, cynical, angry, compassionate?
- Be aware of your own emotional responses to patients, their family members, your family members, and friends. Do you feel indifferent, apathetic, disinterested in the stories people are telling you?
- Do you feel that no one understands you or the 'important' work you do?
- Ask for professional help with people who are skilled in assessing your psychological, emotional, mental, and spiritual well-being. Work against the stigma of asking for help in these domains. Asking for help does not mean you are pathological.
- Spend time outdoors and in nature.
- Develop and maintain interests outside of health care.
  - Music.
  - Art.
  - Dance.
  - Sports.
  - Literature.
  - Recreation.
- Know yourself.
- Spend time in self-reflection.
- Be still.
- Be silent.
- Suspend judgement of yourself and of others.
- Pay attention.
- Listen.

References

1. Birren JE, Deutchman DE (1991). *Guiding autobiography groups for older adults exploring the fabric of life.* The Johns Hopkins University Press, Baltimore.
2. Leiter MP, Maslach C (2001). Burnout and quality in a sped-up world. *Journal for Quality and Participation* **24**, 48–51.
3. Rodney P, Starzomski R (1993). Constraints on the moral agency of nurses. *Can Nurse,* **89**, 23–6.
4. Rushton CH (2006). Defining and addressing moral distress: tools for critical care nursing leaders. *AACN Adv Crit Care* **17**, 161–8.
5. Pearlman LA, Saakvitne KW (2005). Treating therapists with vicarious traumatization and secondary traumatic stress disorders. In: Figley CR (ed), *Compassion fatigue: coping with secondary traumatic stress disorder in those who treat the traumatized,* pp 150–77. Brunner/MazelPearlman, Levittown PA.
6. Stamm BH (2005). The professional quality of life scale: compassion satisfaction, burnout, and compassion fatigue/secondary trauma scales (the ProQOL Manual) Sidran Press, Baltimore.
7. Hermann J (1997). *Trauma and recovery.* Basic Books, New York.

Educating trainees in the ICU: the value of death rounds

Preparing physicians for coping with death in the ICU

Despite efforts to improve on palliative care education during both medical school and postgraduate training, most trainees still feel unprepared to care for dying patients, and many report not being well prepared to manage their feelings about death. The ICU is a setting where many deaths occur, some of which are the most disturbing and dramatic to physicians-in-training. It is also a setting that is frequently overlooked for palliative-care education despite the high prevalence of dying and end-of-life care.

The impact of a death

The death of a patient can have a strong emotional impact on physicians.

• In one study, a quarter of resident and attending physicians surveyed reported a patient's death as very disturbing, including physicians who had completed training.[1]

• Trainees are more likely to view deaths as shocking and disturbing compared to attending/consultant physicians.

• Among the unexpected and shocking deaths, trainees felt a lack of emotional and intellectual closure, and felt more responsible for the patient's suffering.

Physicians-in-training are also more likely to interpret the death as a personal failure related to a sense of their own incompetence.

• Trainees often have difficulties with managing their own reactions to death and coping with grief.

• Trainees have described feeling that displaying emotions would imply unprofessionalism or guilt.

• Medical students have similar reactions to deaths, finding them very disturbing or causing feelings of shock and worries of fault.

Learning how to cope with these feelings is a critical step in the development of physicians and there is clearly a need for a time to process the emotional reactions to a patient's death for physicians-in-training.

Insufficient support and guidance

Studies also reveal a lack of support and guidance from the medical teams after a death and a focus on the medical aspects. Teams would not only fail to acknowledge the death, but also make insensitive comments such as 'we can cross [the patient] off the list'. Trainees, interviewed about an emotionally powerful death, also noted a lack of discussion with the team or with consultants, and as a result, feeling emotionally isolated. Trainees also describe intense feelings such as frustration, anger, and guilt about patient suffering 'over-treated' deaths or deaths where conflict occurred with either the family or within the team. Trainees struggle with how to voice their opinions about end-of-life care when they conflict with either their own superiors' or family choices. Trainees need an opportunity to process reactions and reflect on a patient and their death for the team. Death rounds—a focused time for discussion devoted solely to patient deaths on the service—is one way to serve this need.

A recent publication described one approach to formalizing such an opportunity to discuss and address emotional reactions to death during an ICU rotation for trainees.[2] This opportunity, called 'death rounds', has been implemented in the ICUs at several institutions, including the University of Washington and University of Utah. We are not aware of similar initiatives outside of the US. We will describe some of the key features that we have found important for the implementation of death rounds. Box 6.1 provides an overview of the goals and potential benefits of death rounds.

- All members of the team should be invited to attend death rounds, including interns, trainees, fellows, and attendings (consultant physicians). Other non-physician members of the team who provided care for the deceased patients can be included such as nurses, spiritual care providers, pharmacists, and nutritionists. However, members of the team should not be required to attend if they choose not to do so. Other physician services closely involved in the deceased patient's care may be included, such as palliative care or key consultants.
- Death rounds can be structured to occur monthly or every two weeks, depending on the typical volume of the service and number of deaths. Box 6.2 provides a summary of important aspects for structuring death rounds. It should be scheduled for a time usually dedicated to teaching or rounding when all members of the team are available to attend. Each session could last between 30 to 60 minutes. The sessions should occur in an ICU team room around a table, where all participants can see each other and privacy is ensured to allow open discussion.
- Sessions can by facilitated by a chief medical resident or equvalent, a palliative care specialist, spiritual services, fellow or attending or consultant in critical care. No specific training in facilitation is required. The facilitator should provide the names of all patients who died on the ICU service during the prior two-week or one-month period.
- Death rounds are meant to be informal and non-didactic discussions, yielding spontaneous responses and reflections about the patients who died. Each death can be discussed in depth and length as needed by the team. For each patient, a resident can give a brief medical history and relevant hospital course. The team interactions with the patient and family and challenging dynamics should be part of the discourse. The discussion should also focus on the details and quality of the death. All clinicians involved in the case should be invited to contribute to the discussion and identify issues.
- The facilitator need not prompt any specific questions; often, the best discussions are generated from the trainees. The facilitator could ask the trainees open-ended questions such as: 'Did you have any concerns about how care was provided?' or 'How did this make you feel?' Box 6.3 provides some examples of the types of questions the facilitator can ask.
- In reflecting on the death, medical issues are often raised. However, the purpose of the rounds should not be to replace morbidity and mortality conferences or search for error. Discussion of other medical issues such as pain control may use be useful.
- Facilitators should resist the urge to use these sessions for didactic teaching or to lecture participants in how they 'should feel' about caring for patients or their families.

- Writing bereavement cards to the families of the deceased patients may also be incorporated into the death rounds format and can be of benefit to family members as well as to clinicians.
- The informal and conversational approach is an important component and allows trainees to begin with the comfortable medical, social, and situational aspects of providing end-of-life care and naturally delve into ethical and emotional issues as they process their reactions. Team and interdisciplinary unity builds as difficult revelations generate empathy and support.
- The rounds provide an opportunity to review aspects of providing end-of-life care. Trainees are free to ask basic questions about dealing with patients' death which are not typically addressed on morning rounds such as the awkwardness of pronouncing death and dealing with issues of organ donation.
- Discussions often touch on common themes such as dealing with deaths of young patients, trainees' concerns that they had not done everything possible to prevent the death of a patient, the frustration of working with families who have unrealistic expectations, and the difficulty of guiding families in end-of-life decision-making in the setting of medical uncertainty.

Reflecting on death

Death rounds can be an effective way to reflect on the deaths of patients in the ICU, process emotional responses, learn palliative care, and foster team development. A survey of trainees at the Universities of Utah and Washington, performed after death rounds were implemented, found that most trainees felt death rounds were worthwhile. The vast majority of trainees thought that death rounds should be incorporated into ICU rotations.[1] Those trainees attending more than three sessions felt that death rounds improved their ability to cope with death and provide end-of-life care. Given restrictions on resident work hours and limits on teaching time, trainees valued death rounds over attending other rounds or other conferences.

Implementing death rounds beyond the ICU

After implementation at our institution, death rounds were adopted into the training culture. Medical trainees were eager to share the difficult personal and professional aspects of dealing with dying patients. Death rounds have subsequently been implemented in:

- Inpatient neurology service.
- Surgical critical care.
- Neurosurgical critical care services.
- Additional medical ICU within the larger institution.

Death rounds have become a key aspect of palliative care education as well as resident support during various critical care rotations at this institution.

Death rounds normalize death as a natural part of critical care medicine and therefore, enables the discussion of a subject formerly considered taboo. The focused conference brings attention to the fact that death needs to be discussed overtly and not hidden. Trainees, fellows, attendings, and clinicians from other disciplines learn how to cope with death. Death rounds can provide trainees an opportunity to validate their intense emotions and feelings of insecurity and guilt, and provide closure. Our hope is that our positive experiences of death rounds can be emulated in ICUs outside of the US.

Box 6.1 Goals and potential benefits of death rounds

- Reflect on the deaths of patients, open acknowledgement, provide closure.
- Process emotional responses: feelings of guilt, fault, suffering, frustrations.
- Discussion of ethical issues raised with dying, conflicts with the family or within the clinical team.
- Learn palliative care, end-of-life decision-making.
- Foster team development, build unity, empathy, and support.
- Improve ability to cope with death, prevent isolation.

Box 6.2 Structure of death rounds

Mechanics of setting up death rounds

- For all physician members of the team: interns/house staff, trainees, fellow and attending.
- Other members of the team: nursing, spiritual care, pharmacy, and nutrition.
- Occur monthly or every two weeks for 30 to 60 minute sessions.
- Time when all members of the team are available to attend.
- Informal and non-didactic; spontaneous conversation.
- Around a table and in a private location, where all participants can see each other.
- Facilitator should provide the names of those who died to initiate discussions.

Discussions during death rounds

- Deaths discussed in depth and length as needed by the team.
- Discussion of ethical issues raised during care.
- Talk about interactions with the patient and family and challenging dynamics.
- Discussion of the details and quality of the death.
- The focus should **not** be a search for medical error.

Box 6.3 Potential questions for the death rounds facilitator to ask

- 'What went well in caring for this patient and family?'
- 'What could we have done better in caring for this patient and family?'
- 'Do you have any concerns about how the care was provided?'
- 'How did this make you feel?'

References

1. Redinbaugh EM, Sullivan AM, Block SD, *et al.* (2003). Doctors' emotional reactions to recent death of a patient: cross-sectional study of hospital doctors. *BMJ* **327**, 185.
2. Hough CL, Hudson LD, Salud A, Lahey T, Curtis JR (2005). Death rounds: end-of-life discussions among medical residents in the intensive care unit. *J Crit Care* **20**, 20–5.

Further reading

1. Jackson VA, Sullivan AM, Gadmer NM, *et al.* (2005). 'It was haunting … ': physicians' descriptions of emotionally powerful patient deaths. *Acad Med* **80**, 648–56.
2. Ferris TG, Hallward JA, Ronan L, Billings JA (1998). When the patient dies: a survey of medical house staff about care after death. *J Palliat Med* **1**, 231–9.

Moral distress in critical care health care workers

Introduction

The term 'moral distress' was originally coined by Jameton in 1984 and refers to the painful feelings and psychological disequilibrium experienced when a person knows the appropriate or right thing to do in a given situation, but cannot carry out that action because of various obstacles or constraints. Feelings of moral distress have been reported among several types of health care workers, including physicians, nurses, pharmacists, and respiratory therapists. The ICU is a setting where risks of moral distress are high, particularly in regard to end-of-life decision-making and provision of palliative care or the lack of it. The following discussion will further define moral distress, its prevalence among health care workers, factors which are associated with its development as well as outcomes of moral distress and recommendations aimed at decreasing it.

What is moral distress?

The care patients receive in the ICU is not only a function of the knowledge and skills of those who deliver health care, but is also related to the institutional environment, administrators, policies, resources, and legal limitations. These seemingly external factors can create obstacles which prevent health care workers from delivering the level of care they feel their patients deserve. Often, situations arise which create a moral problem such as:

- Unsafe staffing levels.
- Disagreement between staff members and family members related to end-of-life decisions. These are situations in which staff members often must act against their own beliefs and values.

Such actions may lead to uncomfortable feelings or distress. These feelings have been coined moral distress.

Within the current medical literature, the focus is often on the distress of nurses, and to a lesser extent, on physicians within adult critical care who, in the current medical system, must take the greatest responsibility for making treatment decisions.[1] However, other health care workers must live with these decisions, even if they don't agree with them and may feel that they are victims of moral choices made for them by more powerful agents in the health system, causing them to suffer moral distress.

Moral distress and moral dilemmas

Several authors have differentiated between moral dilemmas and moral distress.

- Moral dilemma: a situation in which there is a choice between two or more conflicting courses of action which are equally desirable or are equally unsatisfactory alternatives to a problem that does not have one satisfactory solution. In this case, more than one right action is correct. However, only one action is possible and there is no obvious reason to choose one alternative over another.

- Moral distress: a failure to carry out an action that is thought to be right because of an error in judgement, personal failing, or circumstances beyond one's control. Here, there is an inconsistency between one's beliefs and one's actions.

Levels of moral distress among critical care nurses are moderately high, with the highest scores occurring when:
- The number of staff is so low that the care is considered inadequate.
- Providing intensive care to those not expected to benefit from it.
- There are no end-of-life decisions.
- There are communication and hierarchical problems.

Nurses often report higher levels of moral distress than physicians,[1] but respiratory therapists also are reported to suffer from moral distress with their greatest concerns related to unsafe staffing and not acting in the patient's best interest.[2]

Stages of development of moral distress
- Initially, the health care worker finds himself/herself in a specific situation in which internal factors (such as the belief system or the personality of the worker) and external factors (such as the organizational culture or environmental context) impact on the worker causing him/her to determine that there is a moral problem involved in this situation.
- After assessing the situation and appraising it, the worker comes to a moral judgement about what action to take or not to take.
- If there are no obstacles to this decision, the worker then feels that he/she has 'done the right thing' and will feel no moral distress.
- However, if some type of barrier prevents the worker from doing what is thought to be right, then emotional distress is the result.
- The worker must decide whether to do nothing or to do the wrong thing, according to his/her own moral judgement.
- This leads to initial distress followed by outcomes such as feelings of frustration, anger, and anxiety.
- If these feelings continue and are not resolved, feelings of reactive distress occur, leading to further outcomes such as decreased job satisfaction and burnout (see Fig. 6.1).

Factors associated with the development of moral distress
As shown in Fig. 6.1, there are two major factors associated with the development of moral distress:
- Internal factors associated with the health care worker.
- External factors associated with the health care environment.

Internal factors may include fear, doubt, or feelings of powerlessness on the part of the worker, especially among medical students, nurses, and respiratory therapists.
External factors have been categorized into four basic categories:
- Lack of resources, including:
  - Low staffing level.
  - Lack of staff time.
  - Economic considerations such as cost containment.
  - Inadequately trained or inexperienced staff.

- Rules vs praxis: this category refers to differences between written policies and procedures and what workers actually do in practice.
- Conflict of interest. This includes:
  - Conflicting goals between physicians, nurses, families, and patients.
  - Unclear definitions of responsibilities.
  - Medical prolongation of dying or aggressive treatment without letting patients or families know of such choices.
- Lack of support from colleagues and administrators showing a lack of an ethical work environment.

Outcomes of moral distress

Outcomes of moral distress are short-term as well as long-term. Uncomfortable early feelings such as unease, fear, frustration, guilt, or anger can be reinforced by physical responses such as sweating, shaking, headaches, diarrhoea, and crying. If not resolved, moral distress may affect the health care worker's psychological health, leading to:

- Decreased self-esteem.
- Sense of loss of integrity and self-worth.
- Depression, shame, and grief.

Long-term consequences include:

- Decreased job performance, leading to decreased quality of patient care.
- Avoidance or withdrawal.
- Decreased job satisfaction.
- Burnout.
- High staff turnover.
- Leaving the profession.

All moral distress outcomes do not have to necessarily be negative. Moral distress, if addressed, can lead to personal growth and more compassionate patient care. When action is taken to decrease moral distress, feelings of accomplishment and attainment of professional goals can occur.

Recommendations to decrease moral distress

With the relative high incidence of moral distress and its devastating consequences as described above, measures to decrease and possibly avoid moral distress are highly recommended. One model introduced by the American Association of Critical Care Nurses, called 'AACN's model to rise above moral distress', was developed to help nurses as individuals when personally confronted with moral distress. The model is based on four major actions (ask, affirm, assess, and act).

- ASK: when experiencing feelings of distress such as anger or frustration, the health care worker should ask questions of himself/herself in order to understand the distress. Some of the relevant questions to ask are 'what are these feelings?', 'what are the dimensions of the situation?', 'who are the relevant stakeholders?', 'what is the extent of my responsibility in this situation?', 'what risks am I willing to take to advocate for what I believe is right?', and 'are others also experiencing such feelings?'

- AFFIRM: affirm the distress and make a commitment to take care of oneself. This includes validating your feelings with others and gaining support from colleagues and friends. Role models may be very beneficial in such circumstances.
- ASSESS: this includes identifying the source of the distress and its severity as well as one's readiness to act while weighing the risks and benefits of such actions.
- ACT: when taking action, one must be ready for setbacks and have strategies for coping with them. Action could include communication with the relevant parties, developing educational strategies for future situations, and even leaving the present place of employment. By choosing to act, the health care worker can decrease the negative impact of moral distress and use the feelings as a motivation for change.

Several sources on moral distress have recommended actions on a unit or organizational level.

- Create an ethical work environment: described as a unit where trust, respect, and open communication are used to create a sense of equality and shared decision-making among members, thereby removing a sense of imbalance of power. Unit managers are recommended to create a positive care environment or culture where ethical practice is considered standard practice.
- Develop a shared governance model: where the management structure of the unit should become more open, thereby increasing feelings of health care worker's autonomy and empowerment.
- Revise policies and procedures in accordance with current practice. This creates a standardization of practice and a situation in which formal policies and procedures are in accordance with actual practice.
- Encourage open communication about moral concerns with peers and with other members of the health care team.
- Support communication and collaboration between the patient, family, and all members of the health care team, including management, which can improve decision-making processes and provide support. This might include the development of support groups where members can share their feelings and experiences. Such discussions may also include the recognition of different sets of values between various members of the health care team and patients and families.
- Use review processes, multidisciplinary rounds, ethics rounds, ethics consultations, or continuing education where previous situations are discussed and evaluated.

Summary

Moral distress has been found among health care workers in the ICU. It has been shown to lead to negative, short- and long-term consequences. However, there are actions that can decrease such feelings. It is hoped that increased knowledge about moral distress and its identification in practice will allow health care workers to become more aware of their personal values and beliefs, strengthen their resolve to learn from their previous negative experiences, and initiate the process of healing, eventually leading to improved quality of patient care.

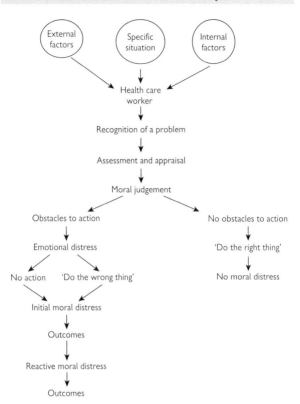

Fig. 6.1 Model of moral distress. Adapted from: Fry ST, Harvey RM, Hurley AC, Foley BJ (2002). Development of a model of moral distress in military nursing. *Nurs Ethics* **9**, 373–87; Tiedje LB (2000). Moral distress in perinatal nursing. *J Perinat Neonatal Nurs* **14**, 36–43.

References

1. Hamric AB, Blackhall LJ (2007). Nurse-physician perspective on the care of dying patients in intensive care units: collaboration, moral distress, and ethical climate. *Crit Care Med* **35**, 422–9.
2. Schwenzer KJ, Wang L (2006). Assessing moral distress in respiratory care practitioners. *Crit Care Med* **34**, 2967–73.

Further reading

1. Elpern EH, Covert B, Kleinpell R (2005). Moral distress of staff nurses in a medical intensive care unit. *Am J Crit Care* **14**, 523–30.
2. Fry ST, Harvey RM, Hurley AC, Foley BJ (2002). Development of a model of moral distress in military nursing. *Nurs Ethics* **9**, 373–87.
3. Corely MC (2002). Nurse moral distress: a proposed theory and research agenda. *Nurs Ethics* **9**, 636–50.
4. Rushton CH (2006). Defining and addressing moral distress. *AACN Adv Crit Care* **17**, 161–8.

Burnout syndrome in ICU nurses and physicians

Introduction

This chapter will help the readers to understand the burnout syndrome (BOS), its causes, and effects among ICU nurses and physicians around the world. The contributing factors leading to this syndrome as well as the important impact on caregivers and the health system are described. Some key solutions are suggested, especially for ICU managers.

Definition of BOS

BOS is a psychological syndrome in response to chronic emotional and interpersonal, professional stressors. The syndrome can be measured by a self-administered questionnaire. The most commonly used is the Maslach burnout inventory (MBI).[1]

BOS is composed of three dimensions:
- Emotional exhaustion, characterized by:
  - Emotional instability.
  - Avoidance of commitment.

The clinician affected by BOS is overwhelmed by small events, reacts aggressively, or bursts into tears easily. He/she may become unable to participate in normal activities of the service. Emotional exhaustion can lead to a feeling of extreme professional exhaustion. Ultimately, the clinician with BOS will want to change jobs.

- Depersonalization, characterized by:
  - Excessive detachment.
  - Cynicism.
  - Lack of empathy.

The clinician affected by BOS does not feel concerned by others' problems, including the patient's suffering. He/she may surprise those around him or her by cynical jokes, especially when confronted with difficult situations. Communication with patients or their family members has tones of indifference. This depersonalization can lead to a feeling of culpability and to social withdrawal, leading to more and more isolation.

- Lack of personal accomplishment, characterized by
  - A sense of lack of recognition by others.
  - Doubt about his/her own capacities.

The person thinks that he/she is not recognized enough in his/her job despite all he/she did. This feeling leads to frustration, increasing doubts about his/her capacity or expertise, insecurity, and lack of self-confidence. In extreme examples, the sense of lack of personal accomplishment can lead to a feeling of failure and a decision to quit.

Epidemiology of BOS

- The syndrome is not specific to developed countries, and has been described among ICU nurses and physicians in Europe, the US as well as in Asian countries.

- The syndrome is more frequent among ICU caregivers than on general wards.
- The prevalence of BOS among ICU caregivers is high, affecting as many as 28 to 47%, according to differing definitions.[2–4]
- Stress and BOS: recent data suggest that stress and burnout are related.
- Nurses: compared to general workers, ICU nurses feel more stressed. Reported causes of stress include:
  - Greater pressures at work and at home.
  - Difficulties with living fully at work and at home.
  - Nurses find their work more psychologically burdensome than general workers.
  - More frequent important professional and private conflicts.
- ICU physicians endure high degrees of stress too. Important factors include:
  - The effects of work on personal and family life.
  - The lack of recognition of one's contribution by others.
  - A sense of loneliness in making the right decision.
  - Keeping up to date with knowledge.
  - Too much responsibility at times.
- Although BOS is more commonly described among nurses, the syndrome affects physicians equally.

Factors contributing to the development of BOS

Factors that favour the occurrence of BOS are similar for nurses and physicians and are detailed below.

Organizational aspects
- The workload.
  - Nurse/patient ratio.
  - Number of admissions/discharges.
  - Severity of disease of patients.
  - Shortage of personnel/absenteeism.
  - Insufficient equipment.
  - Administrative work.
  - Time pressure.
- The stressful ICU environment.
- Evening or night shifts.
- Relentless demands from:
  - Patients and families.
  - Hierarchy.
  - Colleagues.
  - Other units.
- Requirement to keep up with knowledge.

Emotional aspects
- The patient's poor condition.
  - Pain and suffering for patients.
  - Critical illness in young people.
  - Uncertainty of prognosis.
- Proximity of death, end-of-life care.

- Participation in the limitation of treatment discussions.
- Conflicts with other nurses or physicians.
  - Poor communication.
  - Lack of humour.
  - Lack of respect.
  - Individualism.
  - Lack of common objectives.
  - Lack of mutual support.
  - Aggressiveness.
- Conflicts with patients or relatives.
- Difficulties reconciling private life and professional life.
- Fear of committing errors.

Factors that seem to decrease the risk of BOS
- Good relationships within the team.
- Good relationship within the hierarchy.
- Increasing number of years of professional experience.

Factors with less certain impact
- Age.
- Gender.
- Professional category (physicians vs nurses).
- Parenthood.
- Geographical vs cultural factors.

Medical practitioners in ICUs are naturally prone to BOS. They are confronted daily with dramas, including death, disablement, or life-altering diseases. These circumstances can all lead to anxiety, harassment, frustration and disillusionment, and a high-risk of dehumanization where the individual patient can disappear. In the past, 'clinical detachment' was considered mandatory for doctors' efficacy. Nowadays, the need for empathy requires emotional commitment from caregivers.

Impact of BOS
Clinical impact of burnout on nurses
- Psychological symptoms are more frequent in caregivers with BOS and are described in as many as 65% of ICU caregivers. These factors interfere unfavourably in everyday life (in decreasing order of frequency):
  - Sleep disruption.
  - Insomnia.
  - Irritability.
  - Thinking about changing job.
  - Eating problems.
  - Spending too much money.
  - Memory troubles.
  - Libido disorders.
  - Depressive symptoms.
  - Difficulties with concentration.

PTSD

PTSD has been described in 24% of British ICU nurses. The list of traumatic events related to work and associated to the occurrence of PTSD includes:

- Post-mortem care, seeing patients die, combative patients, involvement with end-of-life care.
- Verbal abuse from family members, physicians, other nurses.
- Open surgical wounds, massive bleeding, trauma-related injuries.
- Feelings of providing 'futile' care to patients.
- Performing CPR.
- Stress related to feeling overextended due to inadequate nurse/patient ratio.
- Stress related to not being able to save a specific patient.

In summary, these situations are mostly related to deaths in the ICU, to difficulties in communication and occasions where there is aggressive behaviour at work.

- Physical symptoms are more frequent in caregivers with BOS (in decreasing order of frequency):
  - Back pain.
  - Pain in shoulder, neck, legs, or feet.
  - Stomach pain, gastrointestinal difficulties.
  - Head aches, migraine.
  - Cold extremities.
  - Visual troubles, fatigue.
  - Heart troubles.

Secondary effects of BOS in nurses

- Many nurses take some type of medication against pain and self-medication is frequent (analgesics, antacids, and hypnotics). Drug abuse, smoking and/or alcohol abuse are also mentioned. Many nurses take care of themselves through non-medical means to relax such as sophrology, osteopathy, homeopathy, or massages.
- The impact of BOS on nurses' health is a real problem since the number of vacant positions of ICU nurses is rising at the same time as the demand for ICU beds is increasing. In Europe as in the US, ICU nurse numbers are falling. There is an exodus of nurses towards less stressful positions. Absenteeism or days off due to health problems compounds this problem.

Clinical impact of burnout on physicians

Data reporting the emotional reactions of physicians are limited. However, there are often clues to indicate that physicians also suffer from impact on their well-being.

- Grief symptoms.
  - Physicians do not easily admit to be touched by death. However, when questioned about their feelings when confronted to death, many express their disappointment. In a study outside the ICU, in internal medicine, residents have reported being disturbed by death, emotionally affected, and experiencing grief.
  - Very few expressed their need for support, the majority relied on talking each other and with other residents as a source of support.

The striking finding of this work was that more than a third of the interns thought that their needs for support were unmet.

- Depression.
  - The rate of depression is high among French ICU physicians. A total of 81% of doctors who present with a high BOS score are depressed and 51% among them want to leave their job.[3]
  - In the UK, a third of ICU physicians confess to being distressed. More importantly, 12% show signs of depression and 3% have indicated suicidal thoughts.[5]

Secondary effects of BOS in physicians

In surveys of medical residents, a majority met criteria for burnout. Among them, half reported that they were providing suboptimal care to patients, and this feeling was strongly associated with burnout.

- These residents said that, among other things:
  - They ordered medical or physical constraints to agitated patients without evaluating them.
  - They paid little attention to the social or personal impact of the disease on the patient.
  - They had little emotional reaction to the death of their patients.
  - They felt guilty about how they treated their patients from a humanitarian point of view.
- Burnt out physicians in US make more frequent medical errors, essentially due to sleep deprivation. In addition, they report difficulties in sleeping and in concentrating at work, rate their health as poor, work despite illness or work when impaired, and fear being regarded as depressed.
- Car crashes and needlestick injuries are more frequent among overworked residents.

Impact on patients or families

ICU caregivers who have BOS may adversely affect the quality of patient care.

Solutions to reduce BOS

Time restriction for physicians—when residents had shorter working days, the consequences were:

- A significant reduction of the number of medical errors, especially regarding diagnostic and treatment procedures.
- Fewer car crashes.
- A slight decrease of the degree of BOS, especially in the emotional exhaustion dimension.
- An overall increase in resident satisfaction.

Some potential solutions:

- Organizational
  - Regulate admissions and discharges to minimize patients rapid turnover.
  - Adjust nursing staff and medical rotation schedules to maximize continuity of care.
  - Establish a staff support group (facilitators).

- Enlist palliative care experts, pastoral care representatives (teach and model end-of-life care).
- Facilitate rituals for the staff to mark patient's death.
- Personal management.
  - Support caregivers to better balance their private life and work.
  - Support colleagues caring for dying patients.
  - Communicate regularly with interdisciplinary team regarding goals of care.
  - Better manage tensions and conflicts.
  - Improve the image of the profession.

Conclusions

- Burnout syndrome is common and affects both ICU nurses and physicians.
- Burnout impacts not only caregivers, but also the care of patients and families.
- Heads of ICUs should be aware of this problem and lead investigations to assess the most important contributing factors in their respective units.
- Projects aiming at reducing extent of BOS among caregivers are needed.
- The available data suggest that the BOS is not intrinsic to the type of clinician, but is related to the job and its environment. Therefore, managerial efforts should focus not on the persons, not on changing personal, but on the conditions of work and the work environment.

References

1. Maslach C, Schaufeli WB, Leiter MP (2001). Job burnout. *Ann Rev Psychol* **52**, 397–422.
2. Poncet MC, Toullic P, Papazian L, *et al.* (2007). Burnout syndrome in critical care nursing staff. *Am J Resp Crit Care Med* **175**, 698–704.
3. Embriaco N, Azoulay E, Barrau K, *et al.* (2007). High level of burnout in intensivists: prevalence and associated factors. *Am J Resp Crit Care Med* **175**, 686–92.
4. Verdon M, Merlani P, Perneger T, Ricou B (2008). Burnout in a surgical ICU team. *Intensive Care Med* **34**, 152–6.
5. Coomber S, Todd C, Park G, *et al.* (2002). Stress in UK intensive care unit doctors. *Br J Anaesth* **89**, 873–81.

The rapid response system: a role in risk reduction

Assessing patient's preferences and values before ICU admission

- Early identification of patients at risk for life-threatening illness makes it easier to manage them appropriately and prevent further deterioration.
- Many clinical problems, if recognized early, can be managed with simple measures such as oxygen, respiratory therapy interventions, intravenous fluid resuscitation, or effective analgesia. At this stage, physicians should ask patients about preferences and needs.
- Rapid response systems (RRS) could be the tool to start end-of-life decision-making discussions outside ICUs. 'How sick is this patient?' is one of the most important questions a clinician must answer. However, 'what does this patient expect from me or from the treatment I am doing' is one the most important question often unasked or unanswered.

RRS

There are four components[1] (see Fig. 6.2):
- Event recognition and response trigger (afferent arm).
- Provision of personnel and equipment resources (efferent arm).
- Process improvement activities post hoc.
- Administration infrastructure to support the entire system.

Several studies have demonstrated that physiological deterioration precedes cardiopulmonary arrests by hours, suggesting that early intervention could prevent the need for resuscitation, admission to the ICU, and other sentinel events. An RRS requires and creates a new culture within the hospital. Within an existing and a changing culture, a timely approach to end-of-life discussions is a skill that needs to be learnt.

Medical emergency team (MET)

- A RRS is an organized structure, composed of several elements and, in particular, the response or efferent arm is called MET or rapid response team (RRT).[2]
- A MET is composed of a trained group of health care practitioners who respond to crises outside the emergency room (ER) or the ICU. The purpose of the MET is to improve patients' outcome. The longer the interval between the onset of an acute illness and the appropriate intervention, the more likely it is that the patient's condition will deteriorate, even to the point of cardiopulmonary arrest.
- Similarly, METs should be able to assess critically ill patients' preferences, and to make end-of-life decisions over the 24 hours preceding ICU admission, although sick patients may present with confusion, irritability, impaired consciousness, or a sense of impending doom. This challenges communication.
- However, a call for the MET helps the team to identify patients at risk. The MET can follow up these patients and be part of a process to clarify preferences and values or eventually to hold an end-of-life

discussion with their relatives. These patients might have experienced rescue efforts and can more easily know whether they wish to receive resuscitative efforts again. They might know the burden and benefits of CPR, having had it. MET can become one possible way to assess whether CPR is needed or required.

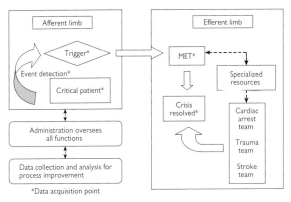

Fig. 6.2 Structure of the afferent arm and efferent arm in rapid response system.[1]

Criteria for calling the MET

There are five syndromes:
• Hypotension.
• Rhythm disturbances.
• Respiratory distress.
• Neurological derangements.
• Oliguria.

More recently, a sixth syndrome has also been described, characterized by a worry of the nurse ward staff as the trigger for the call. Together, these syndromes allow for faster recognition and treatment of MET-called patients and are useful also for descriptive purposes/evaluation.

Decision-making/setting goals

Hospitals that have implemented a RRS show an increase in DNR orders of 10–25%.[3] Several hospitals in the UK and US, Denmark, and Australia have recorded staff satisfaction after RRS introduction and implementation. No conflicts were recorded in making a DNR decision on the ward, triggered by a MET review. Ward staff confirmed that the interaction with the MET brought them a higher quality of care. It has to be highlighted once more that in all those centres where the surveys were performed, continuous education programmes were available for both MET components and ward staff. Continuous interaction between MET and ward staff is a fundamental element to facilitate the improvement of a RRS. An Australian study conducted at the Austin Hospital (personal communication) showed that a delay in MET activation increases mortality. Similarly, the mortality rate decreases with the rise in the number of MET calls. This is a powerful example showing the importance of the continuing MET/ward staff members interaction.

Anticipating/avoiding cardiac arrests

The primary goal of a RRS is to decrease the rate of unexpected in-hospital cardiac arrest. When a patient deteriorates, the RRS brings resources to the patients' bedside to meet immediate medical needs. For most patients, this enables a rapid implementation of critical care. For some patients, palliative care is more appropriate and can be delivered after discussion with the patient and family. Because the system is activated before a cardiac arrest, there can be more time available to deliberate regarding the appropriate goals of care.

Conclusions

The early recognition and assessment of a critically ill patient is difficult, but essential for minimizing critical illness and preventing deaths/cardiac arrests. The manifestations of impending critical illness are often non-specific. RRS can contribute to improved knowledge of patient's preferences and values through the opportunity to discuss with conscious patients and their families treatment that can be started before ICU admission. RRS could provide a good opportunity to teach end-of-life care outside of ICUs and contribute to a systematic and timely recording of patients' preferences.

References

1. Devita MA, Bellomo R, Hillman K, et al. (2006). Findings of the first consensus conference on medical emergency teams. *Crit Care Med* Sep; **34**(9): 2463–78.
2. Galhotra S, DeVita MA, Simmons RL, et al.; members of the Medical Emergency Response Improvement Team (MERIT) Committee (2006). Impact of patient monitoring on the diurnal pattern of medical emergency team activation. *Crit Care Med* **34**, 1700–6.
3. Jones D, Duke G, Green J, et al. (2006). Medical emergency team syndromes and an approach to their management. *Crit Care* **10**, R30.

Legal issues and conflict resolution

Palliative care in the ICU through a legal lens *190*
Jocelyn Downie

The Mental Capacity Act (UK) *196*
Graeme Rocker

Difficult cases *200*
Malcolm Fisher

Conflicts, negotiations, and resolution: a primer *202*
Thomas J Prendergast

The ethics consultant and clinical ethics committees *208*
Jean-Claude Chevrolet, Philippe Jolliet

Euthanasia: the Belgian experience *214*
Ruth Piers, Nele Van Den Noortgate, Wim Schrauwen,
Dominique Benoit

Palliative care in the ICU through a legal lens

Scenarios

An elderly man with amyotrophic lateral sclerosis (ALS) that has predominantly affected his glottic structures is dying of progressive respiratory failure secondary to pneumonia. He has a tracheostomy. One day he turns to you and writes, 'I really can't go on like this. I don't want to go on like this. Can't you help me to die? I've had a good life and I'm ready to go now.'

A 28-year old man is brought into the emergency department following a severe motorcycle accident. He is stabilized and, still unconscious, taken to the ICU. His mother arrives at the ICU. She says, 'I have his living will and his donor card. He made it very clear that he did not want treatment if he would end up a quadriplegic. He made me promise not to let him be kept alive if that was going to be the outcome. And he made me promise to make sure something good came of his death by making sure that his organs were donated to people who could use them.' It was very clear that while he would survive, the man was not going to recover the use of his body and would, in fact, face a life with quadriplegia. His mother, having this explained to her, refused all treatment, including artificial hydration and nutrition. She also mentioned that she had read in the newspaper recently about non-heart-beating donors and she asked whether her son could be a candidate for that.

A 14-year old girl is in the ICU with hypotension secondary to blood loss following resection of a large intra-abdominal mass. She is able to tell you that she is a Jehovah's Witness and so refuses all blood products.

A 70-year old woman is admitted to the ICU. She has advanced Alzheimer's disease and septic shock secondary to bowel perforation in a setting of colon cancer. You believe that a DNR order would be in her best interests. Her son disagrees and refuses to consent to the DNR order being placed on his mother's chart.

These scenarios highlight the range of legal issues that can arise in the context of palliative care in the ICU. The following should help you to be able to identify the issues and know what to do and where to turn for help when confronted by any of them.

Definitions*

- Advance directives are legal instruments through which an individual, while competent, lays out what decisions are to be made (also known as advance decisions, instruction directives, living wills) or who should make decisions on their behalf (also known as lasting powers of attorney, proxy directives, durable powers of attorney for health care) should they become incompetent
- Withdrawal and withholding of treatment means stopping or not starting treatment.
- Mature minors are individuals under the age of majority (the specific age depends on the jurisdiction) who have the capacity to understand and appreciate the nature and consequences of the decision before them.
- Unilateral withdrawal and withholding of treatment means stopping or not starting treatment against the wishes or without the knowledge of the patient or his substitute decision-maker.
- Total sedation means sedation given in amounts intended to induce complete unconsciousness.
- Potentially life-shortening symptom relief means medication given to relieve symptoms (e.g. pain) in amounts that may, but are not certain to, shorten life.
- Assisted suicide means killing oneself with the assistance of another.
- Euthanasia means one person killing another with the intention of alleviating that person's suffering.

Sources of legal obligations

Legal obligations come from a variety of sources. It is important to be aware of them all so that you can determine what your legal obligations are in any particular situation.

Legislation

Many jurisdictions have legislation dealing directly with health matters (e.g. consent legislation such as the Mental Capacity Act 2005 in the UK). Many jurisdictions also have legislation dealing indirectly with health matters (e.g. child protection legislation, the criminal law, Human Rights Acts, and constitutional law). The legislation may take the form of statutes and regulations, and comes about as a result of action taken by the legislative branch of government (e.g. Parliament or Congress).

---

* Many of these definitions are based on those provided in: J Downie (2004). *Dying justice: a case for decriminalizing euthanasia and assisted suicide in Canada*. University of Toronto Press, Toronto.

Case law

This is law found in cases that have been taken to court and in which the judges have interpreted legislation. Case law provides guidance as to the meaning and application of specific pieces of legislation.

Common law

This is judge-made law based on precedent (prior cases) and traditional core legal principles rather than statute. Of particular importance in this context is tort law. This is common law that explores whether you have any obligations to the patient and if so, whether you breached them through your acts or omissions. If you are found to have had a duty of care, breached the standard of care, and damages resulted from the breach, you may be found liable for damages to the patient. It is in tort law that you will find much of the law that relates to informed consent.

Civil law

Some jurisdictions (e.g. Quebec, Louisiana, and France) use civil law, either alone or in conjunction with common law. Civil law is a legal system in which the laws and legal principles are codified and not left to judges to create through the common law. If one lives in a civil law or hybrid civil and common law jurisdiction, then one must also be aware of legal obligations set out in the Civil Code.

Legal questions

As the law varies across jurisdictions, it is not possible to provide a single description of the legal status of the various activities in end-of-life care in the ICU that could raise legal issues. Health law varies between countries and in federal systems, can even vary between the various components of the system (e.g provinces and territories such as in Canada, states such as in the US, and states and territories such as in Australia). What can be provided is a set of questions that you should be sure you can answer before proceeding with any of the activities set out above.

Advance directives

- Is there any advance directives legislation in your jurisdiction? Is there any common law on advance directives in your jurisdiction? If so, does it establish advance decisions or instruction directives and/or proxy directives or lasting powers of attorney?
- If there is advance directives legislation and/or common law, does the patient have a valid advance directive? If so, what are the rules with respect to following a valid advance directive?

Withholding and withdrawal

- Who has decision-making authority for the patient in cases of refusals of treatment? If the patient is a competent adult, it will be the patient. If the patient is a child, it will usually be the parents. If the patient is a mature minor or an incompetent adult, decision-making may vary by jurisdiction so you must ask whether there is mature minor legislation or relevant common law or whether there is incompetent persons or mental capacity legislation or relevant common law.

- Who has decision-making authority for the patient in cases of requests for treatment? Is there legislation or common law on the issue of unilateral withholding or withdrawal of treatment?
- Are there any legal limits on what the patient or substitute decision-maker can refuse? For example, is artificial hydration or nutrition treated differently in the law from other forms of treatment?
- Are there any legal limits on what the patient or substitute decision-maker can demand? For example, can substitute decision-makers demand that resuscitation be attempted or that a patient be admitted to the ICU?

Pain and suffering control
- Is there any legislation or common law on total sedation?
- Is there any legislation or common law on the provision of potentially life-shortening symptom relief?

Assisted suicide
- Is it legal to provide assistance with suicide? Check the criminal law in your jurisdiction for an answer to this question. As of May 2008, it was explicitly legal only in the Netherlands, Oregon (US), Switzerland, and Luxembourg.

Euthanasia
- Is it legal to provide euthanasia? Check the criminal law in your jurisdiction for an answer to this question. As of May 2008, it was explicitly legal only in the Netherlands, Belgium, and Luxembourg.

Determination of death
- Is there any legislation or common law on the definition of death? Is there any legislation or common law on whether death is to be determined by neurological and/or cardiological criteria and tests? These questions are of particular importance in circumstances in which the patient is a prospective organ donor. The issues raised by these questions are particularly complex legally in the context of 'donation after cardiac death' (also known as donation by non-heart-beating donors), especially in relation to how much time must pass between cessation of cardiac function and organ procurement.

Framework for analysis
The following steps may provide a useful guide for working through a case that appears to raise legal issues.
- Gather all of the relevant facts.
- Discover what the relevant legal rules and principles are.
- Consider the underlying philosophy and spirit of the legal rules and principles.
- Ascertain the patient's interests, wishes, and rights.
- Consider the interests, wishes, and rights of other affected parties.
- Consider your duties to your patient, your patient's family, others affected by any action or inaction, your colleagues, your institution, your profession, society.
- Identify your own personal values.
- Identify the choices available to you.

- Calculate the possible consequences of each of the choices.
- Identify the scope of your discretion.
- Discuss the situation with others (within the constraints of respect for confidentiality and privacy).
- Engage in self-reflection.
- Identify the priorities as between any competing consequences.
- Choose/implement a course of action/inaction.
- After the fact, review the choice(s) you made and make any necessary adjustments (personal, professional, institutional).**

Best practices

Talk, talk, talk.
It is important to promote good communication across the team and between the team and the patient or her substitute decision-maker. Decision-makers (whether the patient herself or her substitute decision-maker) have the right to information about their diagnosis, prognosis, and the potential consequences of any treatment/non-treatment decisions. The need for the involvement of lawyers and courts in conflicts over end-of-life decision-making can often be prevented through careful, thorough, and respectful communication.

When in doubt, consult.
You may feel uncertain or conflicted about a variety of legal issues. When confronted with a legal issue in end-of-life care, you may need more medical facts, help facilitating communication, or more information about law or ethics. Therefore, consultation with the following may be very helpful:

- Physicians, nurses, respiratory therapists, or other health professionals.
- Social workers.
- Ethicists.
- Lawyers.

As a last resort, go to court.
There may be times when the best communication and careful consultation cannot resolve a conflict about end-of-life care. For example, when a young child's substitute decision-maker is refusing treatment that you believe to be in the child's best interests. In such circumstances, you may need to go to court to advocate for the child's interests and to seek an order to treat.

Further reading

Canada

1. Downie J, Caulfield T, Flood CM (2007). *Canadian health law and policy*, 3rd edn. LexisNexis Canada, Markham.
2. Picard EI, Robertson GB (2007). *Legal liability of doctors and hospitals in Canada*, 4th edn. Carswell, Toronto.

** This framework is based on related frameworks for analysis developed by Jocelyn Downie, Françoise Baylis, and Richard Devlin.

United States
1. Furrow BR, Greaney TL, Johnson SH, Josh TS, Schwartz RL (2000). *Hornbook on health law*, 2nd edn. West Publishing Co.
2. Horn C, Caldwell DH Jr, Osborne DC (2000), *Law for physicians: an overview of medical legal issues*. American Medical Association Press.

United Kingdom
1. Grubb A (ed) (2002). *Principles of medical law*, 2nd edn. Oxford University Press, Oxford.
2. Montgomery J (2002). *Health care law*, 2nd edn. Oxford University Press, Oxford.

Australia
1. MacFarlane P (ed) (2002). *Health law: commentary and materials*, 3rd edn. Federation Press, Australia.
2. McIlwraith J, Madden B (2006). *Health care and the law*, 4th edn. LawBook Co., Australia.

New Zealand
1. Skegg P, Paterson R (2004). *Medical law in New Zealand*. Thomson/Brookers, New Zealand.
2. Johnson S (ed) (2004). *Health care and the law*, 3rd edn. Thomson/Brookers, New Zealand.

The Mental Capacity Act (UK)

While it is beyond the scope of this handbook to consider in detail legislation relating to professional issues within the ICU in differing jurisdictions, the trend towards a more patient-centred approach in health care has resulted in changes to statute law in many countries. The Mental Capacity Act (MCA) in the UK is one such example. While the MCA is much broader in scope than a focus on end-of-life/palliative care, some components relevant to the UK ICU practice are summarized below. These are based on more detailed descriptions of the MCA in government documents and in the Oxford Handbook of Palliative Care, 2nd edition, 2009. For more details, please see 'Further reading.'

The Mental Capacity Act

The MCA, introduced in 2007, provides the UK with a legal framework to:
- Define and govern clinical decision-making process for people who lack mental capacity.
- Protect and promote patients' rights (particularly autonomy).
- Involve and guide relatives/representatives.
- Protect and guide professionals (with a binding 'Code of Practice').

The MCA has five key principles.
- Presumption of capacity: capacity is assumed unless established otherwise.
- Supported decision-making: the right to receive all practical support to enhance capacity and hence, optimize self-determination.
- Acceptability of unwise decisions: the right to what might appear to be eccentric or unwise treatment decisions.
- The requirement of best interests: any action or decision made for people without capacity must be in their best interests.
- Least restrictive interventions: any action or decision made for people without capacity should be the least restrictive of their basic rights and freedoms.

Capacity

A person lacks capacity on an issue if, because of their brain or mind dysfunction, they cannot understand, retain, and use the relevant information to reach and then communicate their decision on that specific task at that time. To demonstrate capacity, a person must satisfy five required domains:
- Brain or mind dysfunction/impairment that is not sufficient to impair decision-making on a specific issue at a specific time.
- Understand the relevant information: information must be tailored to individual needs (use of simple language or visual aids). 'Relevant information' includes: the nature and need for a decision, the likely consequences of accepting/refusing a treatment and of any alternative options or of not deciding.
- Retain that information: for sufficient time to reach a decision, i.e. not necessarily any longer.
- Use or weigh the relevant information: to reach a balanced decision.
- Communicate their decision: this can be by any means.

Decisions about treatment
- Respect for patients' autonomy is a fundamental aspect of medical professionalism; it is a prerequisite of the doctor-patient relationship and is enshrined in UK law.
- A patient with capacity can refuse any treatment for any or no reason, rational or not, even if their life may be shortened.
- Medical treatment in the ICU (e.g. mechanical ventilation, technically assisted hydration/nutrition, renal dialysis, and CPR) may potentially prolong life, but in advanced disease, such interventions may offer relatively little meaningful survival or symptomatic benefit and doctors may be unsure of their true value. Many patients may not desire a prolongation of life that is only possible through what they see as 'intolerable' means.
- An open discussion and agreement with patients prevents the pursuit of inappropriate and undesirable medical interventions.
- In general, a health care professional is not even allowed to touch a patient without consent (otherwise, it is a battery, even if an intervention has proved helpful).
- However, there are exceptions. Consent has not been needed in common law if there is necessity or in an emergency:
  - Doctrine of necessity: acting in the best interests of a patient who is not competent to give valid consent (now reflected in the MCA).
  - Emergency: to prevent an immediate serious harm to a patient or to others or to prevent a crime.
- In the UK, doctors are not, as a rule, legally obliged to follow requests for a specific treatment that is against their best judgement, i.e. if it appears:
  - Clinically unnecessary.
  - Futile or inappropriate.
  - Lacks any reasonable expectation of cost-effectiveness.
- However, a demand for artificial nutrition and hydration to be kept alive from a patient with capacity must be followed at risk of legal proceedings.
- Of note, once capacity is lost, patients no longer have the same absolute right to artificial nutrition and hydration to keep them alive.

MCA 2005: deciding best interests
Central to the MCA is that any decisions made for people without capacity must be in their best interests. In deciding best interests:
- Confirm the person lacks the capacity for that decision at that time.
- Weigh the relative medical benefits of the treatment.
- Clarify current wishes and feelings of the person who lacks capacity.
- Clarify past wishes, feelings, beliefs, and values, i.e. what that person wants from a review of:
  - Any written statements from the person (formal and informal).
  - Views of legally designated decision-makers and all other relevant sources, including carers and family as well as professionals.

When deciding best interests around life-sustaining treatment, there is a strong presumption in favour of continuing treatment to prolong life:

- Unless the prolonged quality of life would be 'intolerable' for the patient (thus not be in their best interests).
- And any determination to stop treatment must not be motivated by any desire to bring about death.

Ultimately, if there is uncertainty or disagreement after appropriate consultation, it is a judge (not a doctor) who makes the determination of 'best interests' for a patient lacking capacity.

MCA 2005 and advance decisions to refuse treatment (previously advance directives or living wills)

According to the MCA, an 'advance decision' describes the formal provision of clear instructions to cover any future loss of capacity, so a person can specify which treatment(s) should be then stopped or not started and under which circumstances.

Advance decisions to refuse treatment are outcomes of, and not a substitute for, ongoing communication and careful deliberation. Advance decisions:

- Can only be made by informed, adult patients with the specific capacity.
- Must stipulate the relevant treatments and circumstances.
- Only cover refusal of treatment.
- Can be oral or written, unless authorizing refusal of life-sustaining treatment when they must:
  - Be written.
  - Be signed.
  - Be witnessed.
  - State 'even if life is at risk'.

Health care professionals, advance decisions and liabilities

- Health care professionals are liable to follow an advance decision to refuse treatment if it appears valid and applicable to the prevailing circumstances, as if the person had made a contemporaneous decision with capacity (failure to comply could risk a claim of battery).
- Health care professionals carry no liability for the consequences of providing or not providing a treatment according to an advance decision that they have sufficient grounds to reasonably believe to be valid and applicable.
- Advance decisions to refuse life-sustaining treatment are not valid unless they satisfy criteria stated above.

MCA 2005 and lasting power of attorney

A 'power of attorney' is a legal document that enables a person to choose someone else to act on their behalf. The MCA has updated and extended the scope of the previous UK statute on '(enduring) power of attorney', replacing it with 'lasting power of attorney' (LPA) which can, in addition to covering finances, cover decisions on health and welfare. The new documents allow a person, the donor, to choose one or more representative(s), the 'donee(s)', to officially act on their behalf. The scope of legal authority passed within an LPA can cover any or all aspects within either or both types of LPA:

- Property and affairs:
  - Replaces the previous enduring power of attorney.
  - Can be activated either before or after capacity is lost, as specified
- Personal welfare:
  - A new option to appoint someone to 'consent' on health.
  - Other welfare matters can only be activated once the donor has lost capacity.

Further reading

Books

1. British Medical Association (1995). *Advance statements about medical treatment: code of practice with explanatory notes.* BMJ Publishing Group, London.
2. British Medical Association (2001). *Withholding and withdrawing life-prolonging medical treatment: guidance for decision-making*, 2nd edn (3rd edn now available). BMJ Publishing Group, London.

Articles

1. Jacoby R, Steer P (2007). How to assess capacity to make a will. *BMJ* **335**, 155–7.
2. Johnston C (2007). The Mental Capacity Act 2005 and advance decisions. *Clin Ethics* **2**, 80–4.
3. Samanta A, Samanta J (2006). Advance directives, best interests, and clinical judgement; shiftingsands at the end of life. *Clin Med* **6**, 274–8.
4. Sheather J (2006). The Mental Capacity Act 2005. *Clin Ethics* **1**, 33–6.
5. Travis S, Mason J, Mallett J, Laverty D (2001). Guidelines in respect of advance directives: the position in England. *Int J Palliat Nurs* **7**, 493–500.

Official documents

1. Department for Constitutional Affairs (2007). The Mental Capacity Act 2005: code of practice. The Stationery Office, London. Available from: http://www.opsi.gov.uk/acts/en2005/ukpgaen_20050009_en_cop.pdf (accessed Dec 2008).
2. Department of Health (2007). Background to the IMCA Service. Available from: http://www.dh.gov.uk/en/Policyandguidance/Healthandsocialcaretopics/Socialcare/IMCA/DH_4134876 (accessed July 2007).
3. Department of Health (2007). Mental Health Bill, www.dh.gov.uk/en/Publicationsandstatistics/DH_063423
4. Her Majesty's Stationary Office (2005). Mental Capacity Act 2005. Queen's Printer of Acts of Parliament, London. Available from: http://www.opsi.gov.uk/acts/acts2005/20050009.htm.
5. Re B (Consent to treatment: capacity) [2002] All ER 449.

Difficult cases

Introduction

Patients, relatives, and medical staff usually accept the inevitability of the dying process, but situations arise when disagreement occurs between clinicians and patients/families about the appropriate level of treatment. Five main areas of conflict may occur.

The patient who requests treatment be withdrawn inappropriately

Under most circumstances, identifiable and remedial problems such as inadequate explanation, depression, or uncontrolled pain play a major role in such demands. Nevertheless, it is essential to explore the basis of the request. In our experience, most patients who request their treatment be terminated leave hospital alive. Usually, an understanding can be reached in which the patient agrees to a temporary extension of treatment in which successful efforts to improve the patient's circumstances lead to withdrawal of the request.

A patient demands that relatives should not be informed that the patient is going to die

Our experience with this problem is not sufficient to be confident in dealing with it appropriately, but again as a broad principle, it appears to us important to explore issues and listen in efforts to understand impaired caregiver adjustment during early phases of bereavement. This is probably the best way to lead to a change in the patient's or relative's demand. A death which is unexpected by any particular group is more likely, in our experience, to lead to complaints and anger from relatives.

Relatives request inappropriate withdrawal of treatment

In most circumstances, an explanation that the providers of care also have rights and at present, do not feel they have adequate data to make a decision with a promise of review in a few days is accepted. Such requests from relatives are usually based on concerns for the suffering of their loved ones, but may be related to personal and vested interests related to their relatives own suffering or, rarely, the necessity of financial gain. These requests are unusual and respond to negotiation.

Relatives request inappropriate continuation of treatment

This is one of the most difficult problems. In most circumstances, we prefer to acquiesce and renegotiate later, although at the time of acquiescence, our reluctance to engage in further intervention is stressed. Usually, explanations over time that continued supportive treatment is without benefit and also burdensome enables a consensus to be reached. Religious leaders or community elders may be invaluable in assisting families and other providers with expertise such as palliative care specialists. The family doctor may also help with the negotiations. In Sydney, our practice is to involve additional experienced colleagues with ongoing discussions. Elsewhere in the world, interventions through an ethics committee may also prove helpful. This is discussed in detail in Ch. 7 in 'The ethics consultant and clinical ethics committees'. On occasion, treatment may be limited or even withdrawn without consensus if this cannot be achieved and if the medical situation is hopeless. Fortunately, such instances are rare.

In these situations in New South Wales (Australia), the family's rights to a court appeal are explained and a date set for the withdrawal of artificial forms of life support. Recently, we have observed behaviour patterns that suggest achieving consensus is not possible and complaints to the media and our Health Care Complaints Commission are virtually inevitable. The difficulty arises usually when a family are from a small ethnic or religious group and have a medical or nurse family member. Often, there is disagreement among the family members. Repeated consultation occurs and treatment (and often suffering) is continued as the health care team believes/hopes the family will become reasonable with time. Over this period, the family's demands become more unrealistic, the staff is accused of negativity, demands for only particular doctors or nurses to be involved occur, conferences are not attended, and there may be physical assaults and other inappropriate behaviour. In this situation, detailed documentation is vital and the possibility of outside help should be considered prior to offering time to consult a lawyer and setting a date for the removal of artificial forms of life support. When physicians believe protracted life support cannot be justified and all other avenues of conflict resolution have been explored, they should not be afraid to approach the courts for an order to limit life support.

Conclusion

- It is our belief that if a humane environment is created in the ICU, the problems regarding withdrawal of treatment may be dealt with by health care providers, patients, and families in a sensible and beneficial manner without recourse to committees or courts.
- The major principles in establishing such an environment are the generation of trust between the consumer and clinician, and early frank, open, and realistic discussions between the consumer and someone who has established credibility by being seen as heavily involved in trying to save the patient.

Further reading

1. Fisher M, Raper RF (2000). Delay in stopping treatment can become unreasonable and unfair. *BMJ* **320**, 1266–8.
2. Cook D, Rocker GM, Heyland D (2004). Dying in the ICU: strategies that may improve end-of-life care. *Can J Anaesth* **1**, 266–72.

Conflicts, negotiations, and resolution: a primer

The patient was a 75-year old woman admitted for elective surgical repair of aortic stenosis. Three days post-operatively, she developed atrial fibrillation with a rapid ventricular response, causing hypotension. Her ventricular rate was controlled after several hours and she converted to sinus rhythm. However, the prolonged hypotension caused both a hypoxic-ischaemic encephalopathy and an ischaemic insult to her kidneys, resulting in acute renal failure. She was heavily sedated for 'agitation', intubated for respiratory support, and treated with haemodialysis three times a week. On post-operative day 12, the surgical service performed a tracheotomy. It proved impossible to wean her from the ventilator.

On post-operative day 50, a new attending intensivist (Dr F) came on service to assume care of the patient. At that point, the patient was ventilator- and dialysis-dependent and had only a withdrawal response to pain. Dr F was told that there was no advance directive. Further, he was advised that the patient's daughter was 'very difficult' and that both nursing and medical staff had been completely cut off in any discussion of limiting life-sustaining therapies.

How can we work our way out of this impasse? Mediation, negotiation, and conflict resolution are areas of active research in schools of business, law, and international relations. The model below comes from outside a medical context. It is the model of principled negotiation, developed at Harvard Law School and popularized in a series of books by Roger Fisher and colleagues. The best known of these is 'Getting to yes'. Fisher and colleagues identify four simple principles for effective, principled negotiation:

• Separate the people from the problem.
• Focus on interests, not positions.
• Invent options for mutual gain.
• Insist on using objective criteria.

To make it clearer how these principles apply to the medical context, we will describe and simultaneously walk through a process of negotiation that requires the parties to respect divergent opinions and to work together towards a consensus, while avoiding the very similar power-based strategies of autonomy and futility.

The negotiation model rests upon a specific understanding of the three main types of relationship between physician and patient.

• Under the model of paternalism, the physician is assumed to know the best answer for the patient and to act on that knowledge.
• Under the model of autonomy and informed consent, the physician is assumed to have access to the correct information which he/she provides to the patient.
• Under the negotiation model, the physician accepts the patient as an equal partner in a discussion in which the physician has a fiduciary interest in the patient's decision.

When I say they are equal partners, of course, I do not mean that they have equal information. They do not. They are equal in that each brings to the discussion something essential:

- The physician brings his or her knowledge, experience, and genuine interest in the patient's welfare.
- The patient brings his or her set of values and goals, need to know, and willingness to accept uncertainty or risk.

These are the raw materials of decision-making in a negotiation model which does not assume that either party can make the correct decision without the input of the other.

Although communication between two people has informational aspects and emotional aspects, medical education systematically emphasizes informational content over emotional content. Furthermore, medical training conditions one to dissociate emotional responses from cognitive assessments. In some contexts, particularly in emergency situations, it may be important for effective practice to respond automatically. However, it is one thing to be aware of and to block out emotional responses that threaten good clinical decision-making and quite another to ignore those responses altogether. If physicians have a tendency to emphasize information in communications and a predisposition to block the emotional side of interpersonal interactions, then they may enter into family conversations with a bias that these interactions are about truth in some objective sense and not about perceptions, emotions, and the interplay of communication.

Fisher's four principles

Separate the people from the problem

This principle opposes the natural tendency of many physicians to iden-tify the patient as the problem, just as it is natural to many patients and families to personify problems with their physician. How often have you heard a physician referred to as impossible to talk to or a family member described as someone you cannot deal with? Those allegations may be true, but more often, they reflect disagreements on the issues.

We need to remind ourselves that when you interact with people, you interact with:

- Perceptions (theirs and yours).
- Emotions (theirs and yours).
- PLUS all the inherent difficulties of communications such as transference, counter-transference, inattention.
- AND the tendency to talk at someone and not to them, and to risk misunderstandings that can arise when technical language is interpreted in a non-technical context.

Define the problem

The first step in analyzing the patient's situation above is to separate the surrogate decision-maker from the problem. To do so, it is essential to define the problem clearly: the patient is elderly, she had poor functional status preoperatively, and now has been in the ICU for seven weeks, where she remains ventilator- and dialysis-dependent. She is unlikely to recover cognitive function and we do not know what her wishes for care would have been in this circumstance.

We need to do more than to identify the surrogate decision-maker. We must attempt to see the interaction from her point of view, to understand how emotions enter into and affect decision-making. The patient was widowed. She had three children, two of whom lived on the opposite coast. The daughter who lived locally was her mother's primary caregiver and, by all accounts, looked after her very conscientiously. The patient initially had not wanted to have aortic valve surgery, but the daughter saw how severely limiting her progressive aortic stenosis was and, sincerely believing it was in her mother's best interests, persuaded the patient to go ahead with surgery that was recommended by her internist and consultant CT surgeon. After all the post-operative complications, the daughter worried whether she had done the right thing, felt responsible and guilty, and doubted her judgement. That was the surrogate decision-maker coming to the discussion. She had been framed as a 'difficult' person, but an equally valid and more productive framing would present her as a loving daughter troubled by her mother's illness and her own role in it.

Focus on interests and avoid staking out positions

This sounds easier than it is. Physicians are taught to identify the correct answer, i.e. to find a right way to do things. If we have made a considered decision that, on reflection, we believe to be correct, then the tendency when faced with disagreement is to focus on the factual basis for our conclusion and to ignore the interests that may lead someone to arrive at a different position. We may wind up arguing over positions—in this case, the daughter's position that her mother should continue to be treated in the ICU and the ICU staff's position that continued critical care was no longer appropriate—with the resultant stalemate, i.e. she had been in the ICU for more than seven weeks with essentially no clinical change for the past five weeks. Why was there no movement? Each party had staked out its position and neither had the skills to bridge the gap.

Identify interests

How can we identify interests? Do not guess. Ask. Specifically, ask why someone holds the position that they do, not to demand justification, but to understand the needs, hopes, and fears that the position serves for them.

What are the interests here? For the intensivist, interests are:
- Practical.
- Theoretical.

Practically, the patient is occupying a scarce resource, but is not going to improve to her prior baseline and, from an administrative perspective, her presence in the ICU is leading to bickering and morale problems among the staff who feel that her continued treatment is inappropriate. Just as important, the intensivist has an ethical interest, namely, a clear responsibility to make sure that the treatment the patient is receiving is in accordance with her wishes.

What are the daughter's interests in continuing medical therapy? She was confident that her mother was receiving excellent care. However, the daughter was uncertain how much cognitive function the patient would recover, she was concerned about criticism that she might receive from her brother and sister (who left decisions about their mother's care to her) about a decision to limit their mother's life support. Finally, she questioned her own judgement since she perceived that she had gotten her mother into this mess in the first place.

Once these interests are identified, the 7-week stalemate becomes a very different situation, leading to discussions of:

- Excellent care: we will reassure the patient's daughter that the patient will continue to receive excellent care.
- Uncertainty over recovery of function: we will act to reduce uncertainty by reconsulting services that may be able to help define specific prognostic questions.
- Criticism from family: we will acknowledge how difficult it is to be carrying the burden of the decision alone, but we will shift that burden in two ways.
  - First, we will make it absolutely clear that the person guiding us in what to do is the patient herself. If we elect to discontinue life support, we do so not because we have grown weary ('given up'), but because we respect the patient's wishes ('letting go').
  - Second, as physicians, we avoid the Chinese menu approach to informed consent, i.e. here are the data, make up your mind, it is not my decision. We have an interest in the decision, namely, that it be bearable for the surrogate decision-maker, maintain the integrity of the family unit, and respect the patient's wishes. If we need to talk with the siblings, fine. We are involved, not detached.
- Question her judgement: we will reassure the daughter that both the patient and the surgeon agreed with the decision to proceed to surgery, and we work to have the CT surgeon reinforce that message.

Invent options for mutual gain

The most common interim practical measure is to establish a time-limited trial of therapy, e.g. dialysis, mechanical ventilation, antibiotic therapy, etc. In this case, therapy had been continued, but there had been no attempt to establish an outcome or point at which therapy would be reassessed. However, there was a point about which both the daughter and the clinicians were in complete agreement, namely, that we both wanted to respect the patient's wishes for care.

Critical insight

The decision on how to proceed is not about:

- Intensive care resource allocation.
- The ICU staff's frustration.
- What the patient's daughter wants.

The decision is about what the patient would have wanted in this situation, and our only access to that information is through the patient's daughter.

Insist on using objective criteria

Although prediction is imperfect, there is often a lot that can be said about the medical facts. In this case, we reconsulted nephrology who confirmed that renal failure was permanent. We repeated the patient's magnetic resonance imaging (MRI) scan and asked neurology to revisit the consult, pushing them to commit to a likelihood of recovery. They were unable to say exactly what the final outcome would be, but were able to narrow the range of possibilities: the best case outcome would be a limited ability to recognize her family, perhaps to enjoy visiting with them, but that higher function, including communication was extremely unlikely and self-care was out of the question. With that information, we were able to shift the frame of the discussion from withdrawal of life support to what the patient would have wanted in the event of this sort of calamity.

Getting to yes

Dr F came on service on a Monday. The patient's daughter lived about an hour away and was still working full-time, so she visited every other day. He met with the daughter and her husband several times, with the discussions being informed by curiosity and a desire to understand the daughter's perspective. Dr F initially told the daughter that:

• He needed time to make sense of a long and complex hospital course.
• He wanted more information about the patient's prospects for recovery.
• AND once he felt comfortable with the patient's course and had gathered the best information he could, then he would meet formally with the daughter to talk about long-term goals.

Dr F was doing the groundwork of breaking bad news: finding out what the person knows, sharing information (aligning and educating), responding to the person's feelings, and establishing follow-up.

Dr F, Dr M (the CT surgeon), the daughter, and her husband met together in the ICU conference room. Dr F had requested that the cardiothoracic surgeon who had performed the valve replacement attend because the daughter needed to hear directly from him that the surgery was the right decision, regardless of the post-operative complications. Dr F explained the neurologist's findings and asked the daughter if she thought their prognosis was surprising. The daughter stated that she knew that her mother would never be the person she once was.

Shared understandings

Having established a shared understanding of that outcome in a non-threatening way, Dr F then asked the daughter, in light of her current condition, what her mother would have wanted:

Dr F:
'What would your mother have wanted?'
Patient's daughter:
'Oh, she'd never have wanted any of this!!'
[Pause]
Dr F [quietly]:
'What do you think we should do now?'
Patient's daughter [sobbing]:
'We should stop!'

And the patient's daughter started to cry. The team withdrew life support the following day.

This scenario will be familiar to those who have worked in modern intensive care in western Society. Why? What caused this woman to be treated for two months in an ICU with no realistic hope of recovery and— apparently—against her wishes? Were her physicians 'unable to face death'? No, her physicians were trying to do the best they could and believed they were being stymied. Was her daughter completely unrealistic or difficult? No, her daughter was trying to be the best daughter she could be.

The best way to explain what happened is that each side had forgotten how to talk to one another. Fisher and colleagues' genius is to remind us that we can develop the skills to communicate, even in difficult conversations, if we stop to reflect systematically on the process of talking to each other.

Further reading

1. Fisher R, Ury W, Patton B (1991). *Getting to yes*, 2nd edn. Penguin Books USA, Inc., New York.
2. Prendergast TJ, Puntillo KA (2002). Withdrawal of life support: intensive caring at the end of life. *JAMA* **288**, 2732–40.
3. Stone D, Patton B, Heen S (1999). *Difficult conversations: how to discuss what matters most.* Penguin Books USA, Inc., New York.

The ethics consultant and clinical ethics committees

Introduction
Modern ICU practice often involves difficult decision-making, particularly in a setting of end-of-life issues. When conflicts arise within or between members of the ICU team and families, many institutions and ICUs make use of an ethics consultation service. Clinicians within an ICU may often be asked to participate in the deliberations of an ethics committee and should understand the roles and constitution of such a service.

Background
Ethics consultations in hospitals are largely a product of the 1970s in the US. Their development was encouraged by the US administration, particularly when the influential 1983 report of the President's Commission for the study of ethical problems in medicine and biomedical and behavioural research entitled 'Deciding to forgo life-sustaining treatment' gave significant support to the role of ethics committees. By the mid 1990s, the majority of the large US hospitals had created such committees. These committees also proliferated to variable extents in Europe and in different countries in different ways with respect to their roles and functions.

Over many years, concerns have arisen about their proper role and mode of operation. For example, some of the concerns below are related to theoretical issues concerning:
- The physician's 'authority' or loss of it, a concern more often expressed among surgeons than among non-surgeons and in southern Europe.
- The practical functioning of these committees.
- The additional bureaucracy they may introduce in medicine.
- Amateurism that might become evident in the proposed advice of these committees.
- Role confusion between ethics consultants responsible for individual patient counselling when an ethical question is raised and clinical ethics committees as administrative bodies whose task is advising on institutional policies.

We feel that these committees should have a large and influential role in our health care institutions. In our view, these committees should be of help both in a direct way to patients and caregivers when a moral dilemma arises (and these are common in an ICU setting), and they should guide hospital authorities by encouraging appropriate consideration of ethical dimensions as part of health care decision-making.

Contemporary hospital activity is often characterized by the need to consider complex issues; decision-making related to end of life or scarce resource allocation in an ICU is particularly difficult.

Recent research suggests that ethics consultations can:
- Benefit patients, especially in the critical care setting, leading to reductions in the use of non-beneficial therapies, thereby decreasing suffering and costs.
- Help resolve conflicts involving caregivers, patients and family members, and/or other hospital personnel.

- Provide assistance that is useful to nurses and doctors.
- Provide assistance that is somewhat useful to families and patients.
- Be accessed more frequently when nurses and doctors are more trained and competent in ethical matters.
- Be perceived and valued differently across various European countries, explaining the evolution of different modalities of ethics support services across the European continent.

Characteristics of clinical ethics committees

Composition and members

Membership of the clinical ethics committee properly reflects the following groups:
- Physicians.
- Nurses.
- Social workers.
- Representative of the legal profession.
- Administrator.
- A pastoral care provider and/or an ethicist.
- Lay community members.

Lay members act as representatives of the non-institutional culture. These members are selected on the basis of expertise, prudence, and concern for others. There are often concerns related to whether or not a lawyer, a professional ethicist, or a pastoral care representative should be members of a clinical ethics committee. The fear expressed by some relates to the concern that such 'specialists' could potentially bias discussions because of their perceived expertise in the area. Concern about possible conflict of interest also occurs, e.g. in the case of a lawyer who is also an employee of the institution. While these concerns are not without merit, they may be equally applicable to physicians and nurses on the committee. In our view, a strong education programme and clearly stated regulations for the functioning of the committee can help to prevent these problems. Finally, the person chosen to chair the committee should be someone well respected within the hospital. Often selecting an experienced clinician to be the chair can enhance the acceptability and credibility of the committee, at least during the early stages of its functioning.

Position in the hospital and role

- The committee should have strong institutional support. The freedom of action of the committee should not be questioned or influenced by the hospital authorities.
- Clinical ethics committees do not make explicit decisions about patient care within the ICU or elsewhere. Rather, they are specifically designed to be a consultative and advisory body for patients, families, clinical and other hospital staff. The committee's scope of practice is limited to considering and offering recommendations related solely to ethical issues impinging on patient care.
- The committee uses a facilitative and collaborative approach to discussion and decision-making. This is achieved by ensuring all key stakeholders are identified, invited to participate, and given equal opportunity to speak during the process. An authoritarian approach to

ethics consultations would wrongly place the emphasis on consultants as the primary, moral decision-makers, excluding other legitimate and relevant parties (patient, family, eventual surrogate decision-makers, and/or caregivers) from participating in moral decision-making.

- An 'ethical facilitation approach' recognizes that societal values, law, and institutional policy have implications for a morally acceptable consensus, which should be the final goal of the ethics consultation.
- An ethics committee is especially helpful when the members are able to identify and analyze the nature of the uncertainties and value conflicts underlying the request for consultation. This will be particularly relevant in an ICU setting where the prognosis is imprecise and the potential for conflict is greater than in many settings.
- The purpose of such discussions is not simply to negotiate a consensus on a particular moral question, but also to enhance capacity for considering and reflecting on moral rules and principles in a given institution, opening the way to broader moral expertise.

Law, clinical ethics committees, and ethics consultants: responsibility and immunity

Legal status of ethics committees and consultants varies according to local legislation, and in each institution, it is important to know about the extent of protection of the individual members of these committees, and/or whether broad legal protection or 'immunity' exists.

Such an immunity provision shields people who act in good faith from liability. However, civil and criminal immunity can be conferred only by legislation through specific laws.

Difficulties and concerns

Clinical ethics committees had been in existence for about thirty years in the US before the American Society for Bioethics and Humanities reported on 'Core competencies for health care ethics consultation'. Four problematic issues were identified:

- Debate concerning the value of the hospital ethics committee vs a specialized consultant such as a professional ethicist. The difference between achieving a quorum of clinical ethics committee members in less than 72 hours vs a single ethics consultant for rapid decision-making in the case of emergency consultations is evident. However, the committee consultation with its diverse perspectives should be the goal.
- Committee membership:
  - Basis for selecting/appointing members: interest, expertise, or experience in ethics?
  - Power concerns: potential for one or several individual(s) with strong personalities dominating the discussion and decision-making.
  - Emotion vs reason: personal perspectives, expectations and opinions of those individuals most interested in the issue may preclude or limit deeper analysis, i.e. the medical staff, the patients, and the family facing difficult situations.

For these reasons, an alternative model has been proposed in which an individual ethics consultant would discuss first-hand with the consultation requestor(s) and then refer the case to the ethics committee as a quality control body. Each ethics consultant at the facility could be a member of the ethics committee, but not every member needs to function as a consultant.

- Certification/education for professional bioethicists and hospital ethics committees.
  - Bioethics implies contributions from law, medicine, philosophy, and sometimes, theology, sociology, cultural anthropology, heath care economics, and/or politics.
  - As well, questions pertaining to a difficult ethical dilemma concerning a patient necessitate specialized and very often sophisticated knowledge of medical and nursing skills.

It is very unlikely that one person would embody this broad expertise. One could argue that this concern is of such paramount importance that every hospital, or at least every major centre, supports specific career advancement/additional training for nurses and physicians to develop appropriate expertise related to the effective functioning of the clinical ethics committee. However, it is clear that committee membership must represent more than nurses and physicians. Therefore, the committee has to be opened to the wider public and should include some non-institutional members. The committee should reflect the norms and values of professional health care, the institution, and larger society, and therefore, must be broad-based and multidisciplinary.

Education is the *sine qua non* of any functioning clinical ethics committee. Each institution has to find its own way to provide sufficient and appropriate ongoing education to the members of the committee. A budget has to be allocated to this task. Such education initiatives may include, but are not limited to:

- Lectures given by experts.
- Seminars.
- Reviews of opinions of recognized ethicists, etc.

The main point is that clinical ethics is a specific activity requiring a particular expertise. Continual self-education of the committee is the only way to work towards excellence in its process and output. Periodic evaluation is essential in areas of:

- Activities of the committee and/or of the consultants.
- Competencies of the members.
- Consequences and outcomes of their recommendations.
  - Source of 'moral expertise: who is a 'moral expert'? In a general sense, the ethics consultant is a 'facilitator of moral inquiry'. This formulation has several important implications. Because moral questions are so clearly linked with political, social, and psychological issues, the ethics consultant should be well informed about medicine, law, and philosophy, and recognize her/his own personal position on moral questions. In addition, the ethics consultant needs to be seen as a recognized and respected part of the fabric of a health care community. This is essential to ensure credibility when expressing advice related to difficult ethical dilemmas that arise in health care contexts.

Conclusion
- Clinical ethics committees are often perceived as helpful, although the nature of evidence of such a claim is not always clear-cut.
- These committees, when created, function best when built according to principles of multidisciplinarity, competence, and professionalism.
- The role and work of these committees should be regularly evaluated.
- We think that the development of ethics committees, ethics consultations, and other modalities of ethics in our hospitals is not so much related to a lack of perception or lack of caregiver expertise for resolving ethically problematic situations, but rather reflects an increasing moral sensitivity to these issues by contemporary nurses and doctors.

It is encouraging that doctors and nurses requesting ethics input have understood the high value of dialogue, diverse perspectives, and the sharing of expertise to help their patients.

Further reading
1. Paris JJ, Reardon FE (1986). Ethics committees in critical care. *Crit Care Clin* **2**, 111–21.
2. Kelly D, Hoyt J (1996). Ethics consultation. *Crit Care Clin* **12**, 49–70.
3. Orlowski J, Hein S, Christensen J, Meinke R, Sincich T (2006). Why doctors use or do not use ethics consultation. *J Med Ethics* **32**, 499–502.
4. Hurst S, Perrier A, Pegoraro R, et al. (2007). Ethical difficulties in clinical practice: experiences of European doctors. *J Med Ethics* **33**, 51–7.
5. Schneiderman LJ, Gilmer T, Teetzel HD (2000). Impact of ethics consultations in the intensive care setting: a randomized, controlled trial. *Crit Care Med* **28**, 3920–4.
6. Pochard F, Azoulay E, Chevret S, Zittoun R (2001). Toward an ethical consultation in intensive care? *Crit Care Med* **29**, 1489–90.
7. Aulisio MP, Arnold RM, Youngner SJ (2000). Health care ethics consultation: nature, goals, and competencies. A position paper from the Society for Health and Human Values–Society for Bioethics Consultation Task Force on Standards for Bioethics Consultation. *Ann Intern Med* **133**, 59–69.

Euthanasia: the Belgian experience

Introduction
- Euthanasia is illegal in most countries (see 📖 Palliative care in the ICU through a legal lens, p190 and 📖 The Mental Capacity Act, p196).
- In Europe, Belgium is the second country after the Netherlands to approve a law on euthanasia. The law came into force in 2002, together with the law on patient's rights and the law on palliative care.

These three laws have emerged from the growing support for respect of the patient's autonomy.
- The palliative care movement in Belgium has arisen as a reaction to a medical culture where more emphasis is placed on medical technology than on empathy and human dignity. One of the primary goals of the palliative movement in Belgium was to reduce 'futile' interventions at the end of life and to give to patients the right to die in dignity. Viewed from the perspective of the patient, who must be offered the chance to choose the manner in which he/she wishes to die, euthanasia is considered within the spectrum of other end-of-life decisions. As a consequence, euthanasia is considered to be an extension of good palliative care in Belgium (Federation of Palliative Care Flanders).[1]

Definitions
- Euthanasia: the administration of lethal drugs with the explicit intention of ending the patient's life, at the patient's explicit request.
- Physician-assisted suicide: the prescription or supply of drugs with the explicit intention of enabling the patient to end his or her own life.
- Palliative sedation: the intentional administration of sedative drugs in dosages and combinations required to reduce the consciousness of a terminal patient as much as necessary to adequately relieve one or more refractory symptoms. This is not considered to be euthanasia since the primary or main intention is not to terminate life.

Belgian Act on euthanasia
- Physician-assisted suicide is not (yet) legal (in contrast with the Netherlands).
- Belgian law places ultimate responsibility for the act of euthanasia solely on the physician.
- No physician can be compelled to perform euthanasia. However, physicians should communicate their moral objections to perform euthanasia at the beginning of the patient-doctor relationship in order to enable the patient or his/her relatives to search for another physician.
- The physician who has performed euthanasia is required to send a registration form to the Federal Control and Evaluation Committee.
- There is central registration of advance directives concerning euthanasia.

The law allows euthanasia under strict conditions:
- Request for euthanasia.
  - The patient is a major and is/was competent at the time of the request for euthanasia.
  - Request is voluntary, well-considered, and repeated, and does not result from any external pressure.
  - The patient has an incurable condition with constant and unbearable **physical or mental** suffering that cannot be alleviated.
  - The physician must discuss the possible therapeutic and palliative courses of action and their consequences with the patient.
  - A second (independent) physician must confirm the incurable nature of the disease and the fact of unbearable suffering.
  - The physician must discuss the request with the nursing team.
  - The physician must discuss the request with the relatives of the patient (only after patient's consent).
  - The request for euthanasia must be written down and signed by the patient.
  - Additionally, in a competent, but not terminally ill patient (the patient will not die within a short-time period, according to a physician's appraisal):
    - A third physician (expert or psychiatrist) must confirm that there is unbearable suffering and that the request is voluntary, well-considered, and repeated.
    - A period of at least one month must pass between the time of the written request and the act of euthanasia.
- Advance directive concerning euthanasia.
  - Only applicable when the patient is in an irreversible coma.
  - A second physician (expert) must confirm the irreversibility of the coma.
  - The directive must be discussed with the nursing team.
  - The directive must be discussed with the surrogate decision-maker.
  - The directive must be renewed every five years.

Incidence of euthanasia in Belgium
- In comparison to other end-of-life decisions such as withdrawing or withholding life-sustaining therapies, euthanasia is rare.
- In the EURELD 1 study, important variation among six European countries concerning end-of-life decisions was observed (Table 7.1).[2]
- The Federal Control and Evaluation Committee publishes data concerning reported euthanasia cases in Belgium. (The numbers presented here are data from 2005.)
  - A total of 393 cases of euthanasia were reported, representing 0.36% of all deaths.
  - In 98%, it reflected a request from a competent patient; in 2%, it was in accordance with an advance directive.
  - Terminal illness in 93%, non-terminal illness in 7%.
  - A total of 85% malignancy (solid tumour or haematological malignancy), 4% neuromuscular disease.
  - In 52%, the euthanasia was performed in a hospital, 41% at home, 5% in a nursing home.
  - In most cases, thiopental for induction of deep coma (alone or in combination with a muscle relaxant) was given intravenously.

Table 7.1 Three ways to measure quality of care: the structure-process- outcome model*

	Country					
	Belgium	Denmark	Italy	Netherlands	Sweden	Switzerland
Number of studied deaths	2950	2939	2604	5384	3248	3355
Sudden and unexpected death*	34(32–35)	33(32–35)	29(27–31)	33(32–34)	30(29–32)	32(30–34)
Non-sudden death, no end-of-life decision	27(26–29)	26(24–28)	48(46–50)	23(22–25)	34(32–36)	17(16–19)
Total end-of-life decisions	38(37–40)	41(39–42)	23(22–25)	44(42–45)	36(34–37)	51(49–53)
Doctor-assisted dying	1.82 (1.40–2.36)	0.79 (0.53–1.18)	0.10 (0.03–0.34)	3.40 (2.95–3.92)	0.23 (0.11–0.47)	1.04 (0.75–1.45)
Euthanasia	0.30 (0.16–0.58)	0.06 (0.01–0.26)	0.04 (0.00–0.27)	2.59 (2.19–3.04)	..	0.27 (0.14–0.51)
Doctor-assisted suicide	0.01 (0.00–0.28)	0.06 (0.01–0.26)	0.00 (")	0.21 (0.12–0.38)	..	0.36 (0.20–0.63)
Ending of life without the patient's explicit request	1.50 (1.12–2.01)	0.67 (0.44–1.04)	0.06 (0.01–0.29)	0.60 (0.43–0.84)	0.23 (0.11–0.47)	0.42 (0.25–0.70)
Alleviation of pain and symptoms with possible life-shortening effect	22(21–24)	26(24–28)	19(17–20)	20(19–21)	21(20–22)	22(21–23)
Non-treatment decisions	15(13–16)	14(13–15)	4(3–5)	20(19–21)	14(13–16)	28(26–29)

Data are weighted % (95% CI). *Including all people for whom the reporting doctor had his or her first contact with the patient after he or she had died.
Source: Reprinted from: van der Heide A, Deliens L, Faisst K, et al.; EURELD consortium (2003). End-of-life decision-making in six European countries: descriptive study. Lancet **2**, 345–50. Copyright 2003, with permission from Elsevier

What to consider when confronted with a request for euthanasia?

- Practical stepwise recommendations are given in Fig. 7.1.

Professional roles

Nurses and euthanasia

- In a hospital setting, nurses are at the bedside of the patient 24 hours a day. As a consequence, they are more often confronted with the patient's anxieties and questions regarding prognosis or end-of-life issues than physicans. Nurses are sometimes the first to sense a wish to die.
- Nurses (can) have a significant and meaningful contribution in finding a solution for thc patient's request.
- Nurses (can) provide assistance in administering lethal medication by supporting the patient.
- The aftercare for the family members of the deceased patient is most often given by nurses.

Consultants

- In Belgium, 'LEIF' physicians ('LEIF' stands for 'LevensEinde InformatieForum', meaning 'End of life Information Forum') are trained in end-of-life care and can be called upon to be the second physician in the process of providing euthanasia. They also give advice to colleagues on other end of life issues.

Communication

- Physicians and other health care providers need to be sensitive to signals indicating a desire to talk about end-of-life issues.
- The exploration of end-of-life preferences should be the priority in these discussions in order to provide insight into the patient's thoughts and feelings.
- An important aspect is the clarification of the euthanasia request:
  - Why is the situation unbearable for this individual patient?
  - What exactly does the patient expect from the physician and other health care providers?
- Euthanasia requires an emotional involvement from patient, family, and caregivers; an open communication among all parties involved is required in order to go through a qualitative process and to minimize feelings of guilt afterwards.
- Remark: although not included in the Act on euthanasia, caregivers also have a guiding task towards family members. Families should be involved in the whole process as much as possible.

Euthanasia and the ICU?

- Currently, euthanasia is very rarely performed in the ICU. The main reason is that withholding and withdrawal of life-sustaining treatments in the ICU most often precede death and as a consequence, there is less need for shortening life by active administration of medication with the intention to hasten death.
- Moreover, only about 5% of the patients admitted in the ICU are capable of participating in end-of-life decisions. In order to give the

other 95% a voice, Belgian law has made it possible to write down preferences regarding end of life in an advance directive. As in most other countries, living wills contain wishes regarding all life-sustaining treatments. The Act on euthanasia in Belgium has also made it possible to write an advance directive explicitly concerning euthanasia (only applicable in cases of irreversible coma).

• In the future, we expect that the use of these advance directives in ICU will increase. However, good communication between surrogate decision-makers and ICU caregivers will be necessary, even in cases where there are advance directives, as the interpretation of these advance directives in specific situations is not always clear-cut.

Changes in daily clinical practice since euthanasia became legal

• Physicians are more often confronted with conflicts between their own norms and values and the preferences of their patients.

• Since the law on euthanasia has appeared, people talk more easily about end-of-life issues. However, a lot of misunderstanding remains, not only among patients and families, but also among health care providers. As an example, withdrawing life-sustaining therapy is often wrongly interpreted as euthanasia.

• Among physicians, the impression exists that since the legalization of euthanasia, a natural death is less often tolerated by patients and families.

Conclusions: 'euthanasia in Belgium'

• The legalization of euthanasia has emerged from the growing respect for autonomy of the patient.

• Euthanasia is considered to be an extension of good palliative care.

• Euthanasia is rare in comparison to other end-of-life decisions.

• A physician who performs euthanasia commits no criminal offence when he/she has respected the conditions and procedures as provided in the Act on euthanasia.

• Euthanasia should only be performed after good communication and clarification of the patient's request.

• Euthanasia should be the result of interdisciplinary communication and decision-making.

• Since euthanasia has become legal, patients and families talk more easily about end-of-life issues. However, there remains a lot of misunderstanding among the public and also among health care providers.

1. Exploration of the request

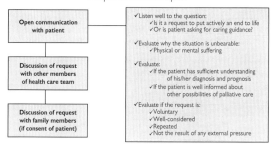

2. Decision-making

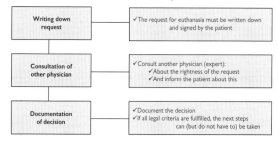

3. Accomplishment

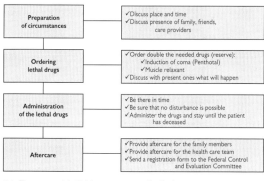

Fig. 7.1 The approach in Belgium to requests for Euthanasia.

References

1. Bernheim JL, Deschepper R, Distelmans W, Mullie A, Bilsen J, Deliens L (2008). Development of palliative care and legalization of euthanasia: antagonism or synergy? *BMJ* **336**, 864–7.
2. Van der Heide A, Deliens L, Faisst K, *et al.* (2003). End-of-life decision-making in six European countries. *Lancet* **362**, 345–50.

Cardiopulmonary resuscitation

Discussing cardiopulmonary resuscitation: a personal
   (semi-structured) approach *222*
Stephen Workman

Cardiopulmonary resuscitation: an overview of outcomes *230*
Peter G Brindley, Gurmeet Singh

A decision aid for communication with hospitalized patients
   about cardiopulmonary resuscitation preference *234*
Christopher Frank, Jeannette Suurdt, Daren Heyland

Cardiopulmonary resuscitation: a decision aid for patients in
   hospital and their families *236*

Discussing cardiopulmonary resuscitation: a personal (semi-structured) approach

Overview

- Where there is no explicit advance directive, discussions about the utility and meaning of cardiopulmonary resuscitation (CPR) have many implications. These implications, including the potential death of the patient, mean that important symbolic meaning often arises. However, in many circumstances, CPR has a very low success rate and significant medical consequences (including the initiation of life support and admission to an ICU). This paradox requires a compassionate approach to opening discussions and making decisions with patients if they are able to participate, and with their family members if patients agree. Both patients and families frequently struggle to understand or accept outcomes that they may not fully understand or appreciate.

- It is the responsibility of the treating physician, in conjunction with his/her team, to determine the likelihood that CPR could be effective. Once this determination has been made, and ideally, team consensus on this point has been reached, determinations of efficacy can structure decision-making and the presentation of treatment options that may include palliation.

- A comprehensive understanding of the medical and psychosocial factors involved is needed. This comprehensive understanding is best achieved within an interdisciplinary team meeting with patients or more often, their family members. Such meetings must be deliberately planned and carried out in an attentive and respectful way. Listening to the concerns of family members is key.

- Complex discussions will be best achieved and decisions respected within a relationship of trust between the health care team and the patient and family.

Prognostic assessment is central

- Prior to addressing CPR, consider prognosis, both long- and short-term, the natural history of the underlying disease and other comorbidities (if present), overall patient performance, frailty measures on pre-admission, patient competence, and potentially effective treatments. Ideally, a patient's prognosis should be assessed and compassionately communicated at admission and whenever it changes significantly. The possibility or probability of death, even with optimal treatment, should be assessed and explained.

Consider the utility of CPR

- Is CPR a realistically effective option or would it only be expected to prolong the dying process? Consider the underlying diagnosis, natural history, illness severity, and functional status.

- Recognize potential sources of bias that have the potential to make CPR less desirable to medical personnel, but not necessarily less effective or desirable such as resource pressures or pre-existing disability.

- Recognize that families may have cultural, religious, or strongly held personal beliefs that will affect discussions and that must be taken into consideration. Determine who will need to work with you to perform a family assessment and provide emotional and instrumental support to the family—clinical nurse specialist, social worker, or pastoral care services.

Determine if you wish to offer CPR

- Determine if it is medically advisable to offer CPR. Consider whether your clinical colleagues would support your medical assessment as reasonable.
- Recognize that it is impossible to seek explicit permission to withhold CPR without demonstrating that CPR will be provided upon demand— recognize when preparing to meet with families that it will be important to help them to understand that CPR is approached as any other specific treatment decision. In some cases, it will be appropriate and in others it will not.

Is the patient clearly dying—is palliative care the only treatment option?

(For example, a patient with advanced cancer develops fluid-refractory hypotension.)

Goal: prepare patients and family members for the death of the patient and provide emotional support:

- Focus on efficacy of treatments and prognosis. Tell patients that they are dying and explain this to their family members. This should be done in the most compassionate way possible. Attentive listening is likely the cornerstone of such compassionate care. Provide reassurance that further treatments cannot change the fact that the patient is dying. Use words such as 'die' or 'dying'. Do not say the patient is critically ill or has an uncertain prognosis or is failing to respond to treatment. Involve palliative care services and offer pastoral care or other forms of emotional and spiritual care. Do not focus upon treatment options, even non-viable ones, until some measure of acceptance has been reached. State clearly that you are not abandoning the patient and family and will continue your support. Families should also be clear about unrestricted visiting and the importance of their continued involvement in care.
- Describe the importance of taking steps to ensure patient comfort and emotional and spiritual support for patients and their families. Be concrete—talk about symptoms that may appear and how they will be dealt with. Do not ask about preferences for CPR or previous advance care plans or living wills after establishing that the patient is dying and that CPR cannot alter this fact.
- Consider describing to patients or their family members the need to write a 'no code' order on the chart in order to meet institutional policies. Take steps to 'normalize' the idea of discussing and making shared decisions about end-of-life care. Explain such assessments and decisions are an important part of care, and are done to help ensure that patients do not receive treatments they do not or would not want.

- Patients and/or family members should be encouraged and given the opportunity to ask questions. Generally, the more time they have to talk and express their concerns, the more satisfied they will be with a family conference and the care in general.

CPR clearly not effective, but survival remains possible

(For example, an elderly patient with dementia, renal failure, pneumonia, and some evidence of sepsis.)

Goals: prepare family members and patients for the possibility of death and convey the bad news that CPR would not be effective if the patient's heart were to stop. Be careful to explain your reasoning in a language that the family will understand.

- Establish rapport, determine expectations, beliefs, and understanding of current medical condition, including potential for death.
- Situate the current illness within the context of chronic disease and the long-term prognosis when appropriate. Address the possibility or probability of the patient dying, using clear simple language, e.g. 'your father may well die during this admission.'
- Determine if an advance care plan or living will exists if the patient is not competent.
- Explain a willingness to provide other potentially effective treatments and talk about the importance efforts to maintain comfort. Explain that CPR would not be effective due to illness severity and diagnosis.
- Establish goals of care. Consider offering purely palliative care and emphasize a focus on comfort when life-sustaining treatments are burdensome and likely to fail and/or pre-existent quality of life was poor.
- Do not say CPR is unlikely to work unless you are willing to provide CPR.
- Inform family members that a 'no code' order will need to be written in order to meet institutional policies (the situation in North America, but not necessarily in Europe).
- Early involvement of palliative care, social work, and spiritual care may all be helpful. Do not wait until death is certain to prepare family members for it.
- Ask family members to explain to you what you have told them to ensure you have been understood.
- Patients and/or family members must be encouraged and given the opportunity to ask questions.

Consider the consequences of specifically seeking consent to withhold CPR

- The consent process exists to facilitate choice, not to narrow it. Whenever consent for treatment or consent for withholding treatment is sought, decisional authority resides with patients or their decision-makers.
- Vigorous efforts to help people make the 'right' decision, commonly to forego CPR, can be coercive, disrespectful, and ultimately damaging to the doctor-patient relationship. Conversely, respectfully providing choices to patients and their families can enhance and enrich the doctor-patient/family relationship.

- Advice can be provided openly:
  - 'I think it is important that you understand that some families would choose CPR and others would not, and I would like to explain what I see as the consequences of both options … In my experience, the best option would be … However, the decision is yours to make.'

CPR potentially effective, but likely not

(For example, an intubated patient with advanced heart failure and a recent myocardial infarction.)

Goals: educate about the chance of dying, assess understanding of the medical situation and the potentially life-threatening nature of the illness. Ensure that if CPR is wanted, an informed decision has been made. Establish goals of care and expectations of treatment.

- Establish rapport and expectations, as above. If death is a likely outcome, prepare family members for this possibility and provide emotional support to help them accept this possibility early on.
- Assess if the patient is capable of being involved in discussions about his future care and if he would want CPR to be attempted. If the patient is incompetent, ask the family members if they think the patient would want a trial of CPR and admission to an ICU.
- Family members should be helped to recognize the illness trajectory and be made aware that death is possible, probable, and/or certain within the clinical trajectory. Be concrete—help them to understand the symptoms or signs of deterioration that the team will be watching for.
- Physicians must describe treatments that could be effective. Identifying long-term goals and establishing expectations for treatment can help to frame decision-making.
- Emotional support and palliative care services should be included in the care process.
- The risks and benefits of providing CPR should be described along with the possibility of CPR prolonging the final stages of the dying process. Patients and/or family members must be encouraged and given the opportunity to ask questions. ('Can we do anything more to help you understand? Please ask any questions at all.)
- Inform family members that the prognosis may change over the course of the illness and that all treatments, including CPR, will be reassessed on an ongoing basis in order to be sure that treatments are appropriate or effective and in keeping with patient wishes.
- Consider making a recommendation to provide or withhold CPR.

Death unexpected, patient might not want CPR to be provided

(For example, a patient with pneumonia and a past history of coronary artery disease, in whom sudden cardiac death is possible, but at this point unlikely.)

Goal: determine if a trial of CPR is desired.

- Explain that death from this sudden severe illness is possible, but unlikely, but that if the patient did become severely ill or (even) die suddenly, CPR would be initiated unless there was an order on the chart not to do so. Ask if the patient has ever thought about the kinds of treatment he would want if he suddenly became very ill and needed to go on life support. Be prepared to describe what life support means and the short- and long-term benefits and risks. Discuss the possibility of a trial of treatment as an option. This in itself might help to reduce feelings of guilt.

- If patients do not want CPR, explore the reasons why. It is just as important to ensure that there has been an informed refusal as it is an informed choice. In general, physicians should recommend that undecided patients remain full code and offer to revisit the decision with them in a few days after they have had time to think and potentially discuss their preferences with family members. Such a recommendation is a respectful acknowledgement of the sanctity of the patient's life as well as their right to choose.

CPR indicated

(For example, acute myocardial infarction or a patient with status asthmaticus and an increasing $PaCO_2$.)

Goals: allow patients or their family members an opportunity to forego CPR if that is their choice. Ask for a full family conference to be sure that there is agreement within the family. Ensure that such a decision is full and informed. Acknowledge that the patient's death is likely preventable.

- For patients in this category, it may not be appropriate to open 'code status' discussions and full code would always be the default choice. For others, given their age, injury or illness, it may be appropriate to present CPR as a form of treatment that is clearly indicated and potentially effective (informed consent with a recommendation for treatment).

- Patients preferring not to receive CPR should have the reasons for their preferences explored and the rationale for providing CPR should be given with a recommendation. Check that the patient fully comprehends the implications of not having CPR.

- Some patients may present unconvincing reasons for not wanting a trial of CPR: 'I'm too old', 'it sounds like too much bother.' Physicians should explicitly state that their preference would be to try to save the patients life if this is clearly possible: 'you are worth keeping alive and I think we should!' Within this process of negotiation, it is also important to recognize that a well-thought out, rational refusal must be respected.

- Patients and their family members should be reassured that trials of life-sustaining treatment can be stopped if they fail to reach desired goals and that patients rarely survive CPR with severe brain damage. It will be important to develop and understanding of what will be acceptable outcomes for the patient.

- In order for patients to competently refuse treatment, they must understand their illness, their treatment options, and the consequences of their choices.

Problem areas

Demands for treatment (see 📖 in 'Difficult cases' p200 and 📖 'Conflicts, negotiations, and resolution: a primer' p202)

Goals: maintain or establish a therapeutic relationship. Explore deeper issues, meanings, and values. Separate intentions and abilities. Develop a shared prognostic understanding.

- No matter what communication approach is taken, demands for CPR may arise. Such demands must always be carefully assessed. Attentively listening to the concerns of family members and patients is central to avoiding damaging conflict and an important step in negotiating any agreement. Satisfaction of family members increases as they are allowed more time to express their concerns. Asking about core values, fears, and goals may help in generating mutual respect and understanding.

- Emotions, not misunderstanding, are likely to drive unrealistic hopes and treatment demands. Consequently, decision-making must address emotions as well as facts.

- Physicians should strive to separate their intentions from their capabilities. Clearly, the goal to save the patient always remains, but medically, the ability to do so may not exist or be very uncertain.

- Sustained conflict over life-sustaining treatment can be very distressing to health care workers and patients and their family members. Conflict should ideally consist of considered disagreement between two caring parties about what is best for the patient.

- Physicians must demonstrate a willingness to involve external parties. Obtaining other medical opinions, ethics consults, and involvement of pastoral, palliative, and social services may all help. Physicians known and trusted by family members may also be of help.

Medical staff disagreement

Goal: privately resolve the disagreement or present any disagreement to family members as openly as possible and in a positive light.

- Multiple physicians and other health care professionals may be involved in the care of a particular patient, have differing perspectives, and make differing recommendations. Families and patients rightly find conflicting medical opinions confusing and stressful so disagreements should be resolved 'behind closed doors', whenever possible. Communication within the whole treating team is essential to diminish the possibility of 'mixed messages'.

- Delivering prognostic information should never be done in an offhand or casual manner. When multiple physicians are involved in the care of a patient, ideally all prognostic information should be given by one physician who can provide consistency.

- When interphysician agreement cannot be reached, the disagreement and the reasons for it can be presented to patients and their family members clearly and objectively. Such disagreements should be presented as a relatively common occurrence, especially in tertiary care centres, and as a sign that excellence in care is being pursued by ensuring that all available expertise is being utilized. That a medical consensus about treatment may be reached in the future should be explained.

- When there is medical disagreement about the appropriate level of care, patients and families are entitled to receive the 'most aggressive' level of care that is presented to them.
- Structured communication within a particular ICU should ensure that junior physicians and nursing staff must have the opportunity to voice their opinions and impressions and concerns. Ideally, decision-making about difficult cases will incorporate consensus building whenever necessary or possible.

Previous determinations of 'code status' did not consider prognosis
Goals: establish a shared understanding of prognosis, then provide an explanation for apparent change in treatment options.

- Preferences for CPR are routinely assessed prior to a clear determination of prognosis and without regard for efficacy. ICUs may receive patients that are full code by preference, but in whom it is clear or becoming clear that CPR could never be effective. The family should be kept informed on an ongoing basis of how the team's thinking is changing and why so that they are aware of the potentially life-threatening situation and how the treatments need to change.
- Preparing family members and patients for the possibility or probability of death is an essential aspect of advancing discussion about CPR. Once this has been done, the 'bad news' that CPR is no longer an effective option can be given to them and further decision-making can proceed.
- It may be necessary to explain that sometimes, preferences for CPR are discussed without careful consideration of whether or not it could be effective or that the prognosis and treatment options are changing as the disease evolves.

Avoiding damaging disagreement within the treating team

- One of the most significant factors in moral distress for residents and nurses is being asked to carry out medical care that they do not agree with or when they feel that they have had their opinions ignored.
- Challenging or difficult cases may require further discussion or debriefing after issues have been resolved and emotions have subsided.
- Planned family meetings with multiple team members are essential to developing consensus and a shared understanding by team members. There should always be a nurse present who will support the family during and after the meeting. Agreement about the goals of the meeting and specific information to be provided should be established before the meeting.
- Documentation is essential to avoid misunderstanding and assist with continuity of message and care. For any meeting carefully document:
  - Purpose of meeting or discussion.
  - Who was involved (names of professionals and family members with relationships to patient).
  - What was discussed.
  - Reactions.
  - Decisions made with rationale.
  - What follow-up steps are to be taken.

Further reading

1. Workman S (2007). A communication model for encouraging optimal care at the end of life for hospitalized patients. *QJM* **100**, 791–7.
2. Workman S (2006). Cardiopulmonary resuscitation: charting a course for the future. *QJM* **99**, 711–5.

Cardiopulmonary resuscitation: an overview of outcomes

Introduction

CPR can prevent and/or defer an otherwise inevitable death. Sadly, it can also significantly prolong the dying process, and increase family duress and patient suffering. Attempts to revive the failing heart and lungs date back hundreds of years. However, it was not until the 1960s that CPR was formalized. Fifty years on, it remains a topic of intense study, impassioned debate, divisive opinion, and legal consequence.

The 'special status' of CPR is emphasized by the fact that it is the only medical intervention that requires explicit documentation not to be performed. This challenges our normal mode of communication with patients and families. While the technicalities of CPR—as outlined by the guidelines for Advanced Cardiac Life Support (ACLS)—are easily taught according to accepted algorithms, discussions of the appropriateness of CPR in diverse clinical settings are much more complex and challenging.

In this chapter, we will focus on those factors that can help in prognosis and promote communication and advocacy. Provision of CPR has significant implications for ICU care and needs careful consideration, particularly for patients approaching the end of their disease trajectories. Our intent is not to dictate who should or should not receive CPR. Instead, our intent is to help deliver empathetic patient-centred care, even where the research is imperfect or the emotions extreme.

Background

- Up to 750,000 CPR attempts occur annually in the US.
- The cost of unsuccessful efforts exceeds $1 billion US.
- At least 70% of North Americans die in hospital and 25% of these deaths occur in ICUs.
- CPR is an expectation for anyone without explicit contrary documentation.
- Many physicians feel pressured to offer CPR.
- Equally, many are reluctant to stop CPR once they have started.
- However, reliable prognosticators are available.

The greatest determinants of outcome are:
- CPR for >20 minutes without return of spontaneous circulation (ROSC) is associated with decreased survival.
- An arrest that is unwitnessed, began as asystole, and had no ROSC after 10 minutes of CPR has a predicted mortality of 100%.
- As such, physicians can estimate non-survival.
- Overall, patient factors (i.e. 'who' is resuscitated) currently have a greater influence upon survival than resuscitation technique or technology (i.e. 'how' they are resuscitated).

Patient factors

Initial cardiac rhythm

- The order of 'survivability' is consistent between several studies.
- The likelihood of survival is ventricular fibrillation (VF) > ventricular tachycardia (VT) > pulseless electrical activity (PEA) > asystole (ASY).

- Strong co-linearity exists between the arrest type and whether an arrest is witnessed:
  - Most ASY/PEA are unwitnessed.
  - Most VF/VT are witnessed.
  - More in-hospital arrests are witnessed than out-of-hospital arrests.
- Of concern, two thirds of in-hospital arrests are currently ASY/PEA (see below).

Primary respiratory arrest (RA) vs primary cardiac arrest (CA)
Survival rates following primary RAs are higher than following primary CAs.
- >40% of RA patients (i.e. intubation, but no need for chest compressions/defibrillation) survive to be discharged home.
- 15% of patients are discharged home, following an unwitnessed CA.
- This difference is presumed because by responding to RA, cardiac collapse is avoided.
- Therefore, for some patients, it is appropriate to recommend only pulmonary resuscitation (i.e. intubation and mechanical ventilation), but not full CPR (i.e. chest compressions and defibrillation).
  - This means patients still receive rapid attention (and ICU transfer).
  - This facilitates treatment of reversible illness and discomfort.
  - This also prevents a DNR order being misconstrued as 'do not respond'.
  - This 'middle ground' may be reassuring to families.
  - This 'middle ground' also avoids therapy unlikely to improve survival.

Advanced age/medical comorbidities
- Several studies have reported an association between advanced age and poor survival following CPR, but just as many have not.
- However, several studies have found an association between being housebound/functionally dependent and significantly decreased survival following CPR.
- However, studies have failed to show a consistent association between specific comorbidities and decreased survival.
- Overall, age and comorbidity have not been shown to consistently predict survival.
- Therefore, insufficient evidence currently exists to make resuscitation recommendations solely based upon age and comorbidities.

Paediatric CPR
- Children (compared to adults) have a higher percentage of primary RAs.
- They also have a higher overall survival following CPR and superior survival following ASY/PEA (11% vs 24%).[1]
- Following paediatric in-hospital CA, ROSC was achieved in almost 75% of children.
  - 36% of children survived to discharge.
  - 34% are alive at one year.
- As with adults, survival following out-of-hospital paediatric CA is lower.
  - 29% achieved ROSC.
  - 25% survived to hospital admission.
  - Only 8.6% survived to discharge.
- Similarly, survival to discharge is higher if arrests are witnessed.

Location of cardiac arrest

Out-of-hospital cardiac arrest

- Out-of-hospital CA has significantly lower survival compared to in-hospital CA.
- This is likely because delay in CPR is a significant predictor of death.
- Therefore, if patients arrive in ASY despite out-of-hospital CPR, many have advocated stopping CPR.
- Similarly, there are recommendations to withhold CPR or not to exceed 10 minutes for unwitnessed out-of-hospital ASY.
  - Similarly, unwitnessed out-of-hospital PEA with CPR >5 minutes appears uniformly fatal.
- The Ontario Pre-hospital Advanced Life Support (OPALS) study:
  - Largest out-of-hospital CA multicentre study (17 cities, 18,000 cases).
  - Studied combination of advanced life support and rapid defibrillation.
  - Survival to hospital discharge was roughly 5.0%.

Nursing homes (NH)

- In elderly, NH patients, most studies report <5% survival.
- CPR for unwitnessed NH arrests results in <1% survival.
  - However, almost 30% of NH patients receive CPR following unwitnessed arrests.
- On-site, ACLS-trained physicians and the use of defibrillators have not increased survival.
- Therefore, some have recommended not offering ACLS in this setting.

In-hospital cardiac arrest

Survival to discharge following in-hospital CPR is typically <15%.[2] In addition, Canadian data showed that, despite 40 years of medical advances, survival following in-hospital CPR has not significantly improved:

- 13.4% survived to hospital discharge, 11.3% discharged to home.
  - Even this may represent a 'best case scenario', reflecting 24 hour code teams, and ICU and Coronary Care Unit (CCU) backup.

However, in survivors, neurological recovery is often acceptable:

- >50% of both adult and paediatric survivors maintain satisfactory cerebral performance.

Of note and as expected, survival following CA in ICU/CCU is higher than for non-monitored inpatients.

- 15–30% survival to discharge (because resuscitation begins almost immediately).
- As such, many hospitals are increasing the number of monitored beds or ensuring earlier intervention for patients exhibiting signs of early deterioration.
- Regardless, this emphasizes the importance of whether or not an arrest is witnessed.

Witnessed arrests vs unwitnessed cardiac arrests

- Survival is significantly higher following a witnessed (as compared to an unwitnessed) CA.

- Overall, when witnessed and unwitnessed arrests were combined:
  - Approximately 1 in 3 had ROSC, 1 in 7 survived to hospital discharge, but only 1 in 10 returned to independent living.
- For witnessed arrests alone:
  - Approximately 1 in 2 achieved ROSC, 1 in 3 survived to 24 hours, 1 in 4 survived to discharge, and 1 in 5 was able to return home.
- For unwitnessed arrests alone:
  - Only one fifth was successfully resuscitated (RA and CA combined).
  - **For unwitnessed CAs alone, nobody survived to discharge.**
- Of concern, >40% of in-hospital arrests are typically unwitnessed.

Special circumstances
- Up to 15% of patients with DNR orders receive surgery.
  - Reasons include relief of obstruction/pain, feeding tubes, tracheostomies.
- Appropriately, DNR orders can/should be suspended for the perioperative period after discussion with patients, families, anaesthesia, and surgery.
- Therefore, pre-emptive communication is recommended to ensure:
  - Patients' wishes are respected.
  - The operating room staff feel comfortable to proceed.

Conclusions

Only three factors have been consistently associated with increased survival: witnessed arrest (vs unwitnessed CA), VF/VT as initial cardiac rhythm (vs ASY/PEA), and restoring spontaneous circulation within 20 minutes (i.e. not offering prolonged CPR).

While laudable efforts to increase survival continue, this mandates empathethic discussions with our patients and families about allowing a natural death and/or optimizing the use or limitation of technological interventions, including CPR as patients approach the end of their lives.

References
1. Nadkarni VM, Larkin GL, Peberdy MA, Carey SM, et al. (2006). First documented rhythm and clinical outcome from in-hospital cardiac arrest among children and adults. *JAMA* **295**, 50–7.
2. Brindley PG, Markland DM, Mayers I, Kutsogiannis DJ (2000). Predictors of survival following in-hospital adult cardiopulmonary resuscitation. *CMAJ* **167**, 343–8.

A decision aid for communication with hospitalized patients about cardiopulmonary resuscitation preference

Introduction

- Discussions about CPR are an important component of end-of-life care in many settings, and become particularly important during illnesses that might progress towards the consideration of intensive care. Empathetic, timely, compassionate, yet explicit, discussions about CPR should enhance the provision of quality end-of-life care/palliative care, both before and during an ICU admission. However, the reality is somewhat different.
- Discussions about CPR preferences with hospitalized patients and their families occur in less than 30% of admissions.
- When it does occur, communication about resuscitation preference between the physician and patient or family is often misunderstood or overly optimistic.
- Patients and family members may have little prior accurate knowledge about CPR, its treatments and outcomes, or about the process of decision-making.
- Consequently, they may not have the necessary information to make a quality decision and they may not appreciate that CPR often mandates a subsequent admission to an ICU.
- There are no clear guidelines on optimal strategies for these discussions with hospitalized patients, and strategies to improve knowledge of CPR and assist patients and families in the decisional process are needed.
- In this chapter, we discuss the development of a decision aid and its role in clarifying preferences for or against the provision of CPR in a hospital setting in Canada.

Decision aids

Patient decision aids are 'tools that help people become involved in decision-making by providing information about the options and outcomes and by clarifying personal values. They are designed to complement, rather than replace, counselling from a health practitioner.' The CREDIBLE criteria have been developed to assess decision aids:

- **C**ompetently developed.
- **R**ecently updated.
- **E**vidence-based.
- **DI**sclosure of conflict of interest.
- **BaL**anced presentation.
- **E**fficacious at improving decision-making.

Although decision aids have been used in other clinical situations, there were no previously published decision aids to assist with discussions about CPR preferences.

We developed a decision aid to assist health care professionals with the discussions, deliberations, and decisions about CPR preferences with patients and their families.

• The decision aid reviews the advantages and disadvantages of CPR, the outcomes associated with its use, the process of decision-making, and some questions for users to consider helping clarify patient preferences.

• Hospital staff involved in the development and evaluation was supportive of the document. They felt that staff nurses could also use the aid to discuss the topic with appropriate patients to enable better decision-making with the attending physician or with medical house staff.

• In our evaluation work, the decision aid was shown to be acceptable to patients and families and useful in helping them clarify their preferences. It did not appear to bias users towards a specific decision.
  • The decision aid met the majority of the CREDIBLE criteria. Further evaluation on the impact on 'quality' of decision-making is needed.

Important considerations

• This decision aid reviews CPR decision-making because this is often the initial focus of end-of-life care discussions during admission to an acute care hospital. However, discussions about CPR often lead to communication about other treatment options such as intubation/ventilation, ICU admission, etc., and effective communication and decision-making related to CPR may impact decision-making about other end-of-life care issues.

• Our decision aid was developed for use within a shared approach to decision-making. In some circumstances, different approaches may be needed and the decision aid may be less helpful.

• The decision aid is designed to augment information sharing, but it also provides information to help patients understand the decisional process. This is relevant in CPR communication, particularly in settings where patients believe (perhaps erroneously) that they have complete autonomy in the decision without any input or decision-making role by the physician.

• Please see the next section for the decision aid that we developed for use at the Kingston, General Hospital, Ontario, Canada.

Further reading

1. Heyland DK, Frank C, Groll D, et al. (2006). Understanding cardiopulmonary resuscitation decision-making: perspectives of seriously ill hospitalized patients and family members. *Chest* **130**, 419–28.
2. Liddle J, Gilleard C, Neil A (1993). Elderly patients' and their relatives' views on CPR. *Lancet* **342**, 1055.
3. Ontario Health Research Institute (2006). Ottawa decision aids. Available from: http://decisionaid.ohri.ca/resources.html.
4. Frank C, Heyland DK, Chen B, et al. (2003). Determining resuscitation preferences of elderly inpatients: a review of the literature. *CMAJ* **169**, 795–9.

Cardiopulmonary resuscitation: a decision aid for patients in hospital and their families

The goal of this pamphlet is to provide information about CPR so you can be adequately prepared to participate in decisions about your care.

Questions and answers

1. What is CPR?

Cardiopulmonary resuscitation (CPR) is the term used to describe the treatments used to try and restart a person's heart after it has stopped beating. The heart may stop for many reasons and when the heart stops and is not restarted again in a couple of minutes, the person will die.

The heart may stop beating due to unexpected or expected circumstances.

- Unexpected circumstances would include healthy people with no history of serious illness such as younger people who are victims of drowning or traumatic injury.
- Expected circumstances that would cause the heart to stop would include people with serious illnesses. Heart disease, for example, directly affects heart functioning whereas other illnesses such as kidney failure, pneumonia, severe infection, or terminal cancer indirectly affect the heart.
- In patients with chronic illness such as cancer or severe heart failure, CPR may help extend life. In patients with an unexpected and reversible illness such as a heart attack, CPR may be life-saving.

When someone's heart stops beating, they become unconscious within a few seconds because there is not enough blood going to their brain. During this time, they are not aware of things around them and do not likely experience pain.

CPR was initially developed to restart hearts that had stopped because of sudden unexpected heart attacks. Later, it was used in all situations where someone's heart stopped and in many of these situations, CPR was not successful. With experience, we now have a better understanding of who is likely to benefit from this treatment.

Patients and families should be aware that CPR and resuscitation will only, at best, bring the patient back to how they were before their heart stopped and will not improve any of the illnesses that caused the cardiac arrest.

2. What happens during CPR?

If a person's heart stops while he/she is hospitalized and the decision is made to attempt CPR to resuscitate them:

- An emergency call goes out to a team of doctors and nurses.
- They rush to the patient's room and begin to try keeping the blood circulating around the body by pushing hard on the patient's breastbone.
- They try to help the person breathe by putting a breathing tube through the mouth to the lungs.

- They may use an electric shock (cardioversion) to try getting the heart restarted.

You may have seen resuscitation such as this on television programmes, although in real life, it may not be the same. Certainly, CPR is not always successful in restarting the heart, even though it commonly is on television.

3. Why is the doctor asking me about CPR?
- The physician wants to ensure that your thoughts about important **medical** decisions are taken into account when planning your care.
- It is important to note that the discussion around CPR may occur even if your risk of needing it is low.
- Like other treatment options being considered, patients and families should be participants in the decision-making. However, CPR is a treatment decision made with the doctors where the patient's input is crucial. Just as the surgeon would not operate without discussion with and consent of the patient, doctors should not decide about resuscitation without the input and opinions of their patients.
- It is important that you discuss your thoughts, concerns, and wishes with your family or power of attorney for health and personal care. Their input can be very useful to you. Your family or power of attorney for health and your doctors and nurses should follow those decisions if you are unable to speak for yourself.
- Doctors may wish to discuss with you other treatment options in case a serious illness develops, including your thoughts about admission to an intensive care unit (ICU) or a breathing machine (machines to help you breathe with a tube down to your lungs).

4. How well does CPR work?
The effectiveness of cardiac resuscitation varies, depending on the medical condition of the individual. Studies have found the following chances of success with CPR (Table 8.1):

Table 8.1

Disease causing the heart to stop	Approximate chance the person will recover and leave hospital (out of every 100 receiving CPR)
Heart attack	15
Severe kidney failure	5
Cancer	2
Heart failure	2
Serious infection (sepsis)	1

5. Are there any limitations or side effects from CPR?

The following are possible consequences due to the procedures used in cardiac resuscitation:

- Broken breastbone and rib bones from pushing down hard on the chest during the procedure. This is particularly problematic in people who have brittle bones or osteoporosis.
- Bruised or punctured lungs from pushing on the chest.
- Impaired mental functioning is the most concerning effect. This may occur because the brain has not received enough oxygen during the time the doctors were trying to restart the person's heart. The possibilities include a stroke, which may leave the individual with paralysis or speech problems as well as more subtle memory, language, and personality problems. These mental impairments may have an impact on a person's ability to live at home without a lot of care from family and caregivers. Severe forms of mental disabilities occur in 25–50% of survivors.

6. What other things should I consider?

As with all medical decisions affecting us, it is important to think about everything involved. In discussions around resuscitation, religious and personal beliefs and values will play a large role.

Personal beliefs

Many people may not want doctors to try to resuscitate them because of the serious and incurable nature of their primary health problems, or because they feel they are older and have lived a long life. Other personal beliefs may include:

- 'Even if it is only a 2% chance, that is enough for me' (risk/odds).
- 'I have lived a good life and when it is my time … ' (life is complete).
- 'Nothing is worse than death' (fear of death).
- 'I want to see my daughter married and then I can go' (unfinished business).

Religious beliefs

- Some people believe life is sacred and that maintaining life at any cost is a priority.
- Some people believe their death is God's will and it is appropriate to accept death.

Personal experiences

- People may have seen a family member with a DNR order not receive other appropriate treatments (such as antibiotics).
- Some people may have observed a family member being resuscitated and found it to be traumatic.

7. What happens if I don't have this discussion and I am unable to communicate my wishes because I am too sick?

It is important for you to know that if there is no discussion of these treatments and you were to have a heart attack, the doctors and nurses must try to do all they can to resuscitate you, even if that was not what you would want.

8. What will happen after I speak to the doctor about CPR?

- The outcome of your discussion will be documented in your chart to guide doctors and nurses if you are unable to speak due to your condition. If you and the doctors feel CPR and resuscitation is not the most appropriate treatment for your situation, this will be written as a 'No CPR' order. Medical and nursing staff are aware of these orders and patients' resuscitation preferences, and use them to guide care if the person's heart stops.
- If it is decided that CPR is an appropriate treatment, this will be documented in your chart.
- If you and the doctor decide on other life-sustaining treatments such as being on a breathing machine, this will also be noted as an order in your chart.
- Your discussion regarding whether you want or do not want CPR will not affect other aspects of your care. It does NOT mean that no other treatments would be provided. If antibiotics, intravenous fluids, or other medical treatments are appropriate, they will still be discussed and offered to you. It does mean staff will focus on helping you to remain as comfortable as possible while providing care.

A summary of what's involved in a decision about CPR (Table 8.2)

Table 8.2

Choice	What is involved	Possible advantages	Possible disadvantages
CPR	• Chest compression. • Electric shocks to restart the heart. • Tube down the throat to assist with breathing. • Possible ICU stay.	• May prevent immediate death. • Chance of returning to near previous function. • Chance of returning home from hospital.	• Low proportion of patients able to return home from hospital. • High rate of stroke and brain injury. • Risk of broken breast or rib bone and bruised lung. • Does not improve other health issues if successful at resuscitation. • Possible need for significant care from family members in order to return home.
No CPR	• Other active medical treatments (e.g. antibiotics, ICU admission) may be given, depending on treatment choices. • Comfort measures only may be provided, depending on treatment choices.	• May be less traumatic for family members at the time of cardiac arrest. • Death with less likelihood of discomfort from tubes, procedures, or fractured ribs.	• Death occurs at the time of cardiac arrest. • Patients may be concerned **'no CPR'** means no other treatments will be provided.

Important things to consider about CPR discussions and your CPR treatment decision

- Studies have shown that physicians do not always initiate discussions with patients in hospital about this treatment decision. Please consider asking your physician to discuss this with you.
- Share your views about CPR and other life-prolonging treatments with your family. We encourage you to share this document with your family so they can be informed.
- Discuss the role your power of attorney for health would play in the event you are mentally incapacitated to make these decisions for yourself.
- If you change your mind about the decision concerning CPR, be sure and let someone on the health care team know so that this can be discussed and documented on your chart.

CPR treatment decision process:

- Consider the possible outcomes of CPR.
- What are the possible advantages and disadvantages of CPR for me?
- Do I have other questions that need answering?
- Who should participate in the decision-making?
- What are my thoughts about this decision? (Which way am I currently leaning in my decision?)
- Discuss your decision with your doctors (hospital and GP) and with your family.

If you have questions or concerns about the information provided in this pamphlet, please feel free to discuss it with a staff member such as your doctor. Other staff members such as a nurse, bioethicist, or staff from spiritual and religious care may be helpful for some patients. Your family physician may also have a helpful perspective.

Withholding and withdrawal of life support

Discussions about withdrawal of life support in the ICU:
    a perspective from the UK 242
Simon L Cohen

Decisions to forgo life support: a perspective from Europe 246
Thomas Fassier, Elie Azoulay

Limitation of life support in an Australian ICU 250
Malcolm Fisher

ICU care during withdrawal of life support: a personal
    perspective from Canada 252
Graeme Rocker

Withdrawal of ventricular assist device support 258
Jane MacIver, Heather J Ross

Life support after cardiac arrest 262
Virginie Lemiale, Nancy Kentish–Barnes, Alain Cariou

Withholding and withdrawing life support:
    Muslim perspectives 268
Fekri Abroug, Lamia Ouanes Besbes

Withdrawal and withholding of life-sustaining therapies:
    protocolized approaches 274
Judith E Nelson

The Liverpool Care Pathway for patients dying in intensive care
    in the UK 276
Jane Harper, Laura Chapman

Discussions about withdrawal of life support in the ICU: a perspective from the UK

Introduction

This chapter reflects on best practices from a UK/European perspective and provides personal insights into particular situations that have been influential in my own career. While there may be some overlap with other contributions that focus on communication, the editors feel that this is justified in the context of the need to emphasize the importance of effective planning and the conduct of discussions that will be remembered by families for years after a death in the ICU.

Preparing for the family conference

- All the key interested parties should be invited to the family conference. On the medical side, this must include the nurses as well as the doctors—there is evidence to suggest that the nurses are better at communication than physicians at this time. Other professionals who have a lot of contact with the patient such as physiotherapists and dietitians may also be included and students in these disciplines should be invited to help them in the learning process of what is an essential part of intensive care.
- All the interested parties in the family should be invited and they may wish to include some significant outsiders such as their religious advisor or general practitioner.
- The timing of such a conference will depend on the clinical situation and the certainty or otherwise of the caring team. There is a case for holding such a conference at the earliest opportunity. However, at that time, the response to treatment and prognosis is always difficult to predict and may not be clear.
- The meeting should be held in a quiet room, usually away from the bedside where the relatives hopefully will feel comfortable and able to ask their questions.
- Ample time should be allocated to such meetings. The degree of satisfaction on the part of the family may well depend on how much time is allocated.

Conducting family conferences

- Those conducting the conference should be sure they are fully aware of all the facts of the case. It is common in the ICU for there to be at least two teams of carers, namely the admitting physicians and the ICU team involved in any one patient, and it is very important that their views are integrated and respected.
- The clinician conducting the conference should allow ample time for the family to participate and present their concerns. This is facilitated by making sure that the clinicians do not monopolize the meeting.
- A useful way of insuring family satisfaction is to speak in relatively short and clear sentences, leaving intervals of silence between inviting comments. The clinicians should understand that the family may not

be aware at all of the medical details and these should be explained in simple, clear language.

- It should be emphasized repeatedly that although some forms of treatment such as antibiotics, pressor agents, dialysis, or mechanical ventilation may be withheld or withdrawn because they are not achieving any benefit for the patient, this does not mean that care is being withdrawn. It should be explained that the emphasis of care is switched from cure to palliation.
- Many families may have anxieties that if they agree to a 'not for CPR' order, this implies that they are agreeing that their patient will not be cared for. The importance of stressing the continuation of care and indeed, the integration with palliative care cannot be over-emphasized.
- The clinicians conducting the meeting must be continuously aware of the distressing mix of emotions among the family members. These include distress at the prospect of the impending loss of a loved one, guilt that is frequently irrational, anxiety that they may not have done the best for the patient, anger, particularly if the admission to the ICU follows what was thought to be a routine procedure.
- There may also be conflict between family members who may be distressed that their loved ones are dying in an alien environment and where they are offended by the paraphernalia of medical technology.
- It is important that at all times, the family is told the truth. In particular, if there have been any errors in care such as it may frequently occur with drug administration, these are clearly explained.
- As with any other clinical procedure or assessment, there should be full notes of the meeting in the patient's chart.

Checklist for the communication of end-of-life decisions at the family conference

- Master the medical facts of the case.
- Ensure that the whole team agrees with the management plan.
- Give ample time for the meeting.
- Allow the family to attend and bring any other interested parties.
- Select a quiet, undisturbed room for the meeting.
- Explain the medical facts.
- Explain that the decision to withdraw modalities or change the emphasis of care is a medical responsibility.
- Try to obtain the family's understanding of and assent to the treatment plan.
- If there are points of disagreement or distress, arrange to repeat the conference.
- Do not forget to make full notes of the proceedings.

Pitfalls and difficulties in end-of-life communication

Here are a few vignettes from my own experience to illustrate some of the difficulties that may occur in the course of communication of end-of-life decisions.

Culture

- Families may hold strong views about treatment limitation, often on religious grounds, thought it may be difficult to differentiate religious from cultural views. I have come across cases where families were totally against the concept of treatment limitation when the question was discussed initially. There may be elements of distrust or fear of the medical team. However, with time and repeated discussions, some families will come round to accepting the situation. An unusual case of my experience was that of the tragic story of a young Chinese student who came to the UK and suffered a massive subarachnoid haemorrhage. She fitted all the criteria of brain death. There were no family members to ask about organ donation, so we contacted the Chinese Embassy and were firmly told that in their view, organ donation was against the culture and wishes of the patient. The nurses found it difficult to care for a brain-dead patient in the ICU for days until the family arrived.

Guilt

• I have many cousins, most of whom I rarely see or know. The mother-in-law of one such cousin was admitted to our unit. Fortunately, I did not take part in her care. She had multiple problems and eventually, treatment was withdrawn. I met this cousin by chance a few months later. When he reminded me his mother-in-law had died in our unit, I asked him how his wife was feeling about her bereavement. He replied, 'She can't get over the fact that she pulled the plug.' Clearly, the clinicians who had presented the case to her had not explained effectively enough that the decision to withhold all treatment was a medical one and not one for which any family member should take responsibility. Getting this wrong is too easy a trap to fall into, but it leaves devastating memories for family members.

Truth-telling

• I was responsible for the unit when a patient was returning from the operating theatre. In the elevator, the patient suffered a cardiac arrest when her endotracheal tube became misplaced. Efforts at resuscitation in the elevator were somewhat limited at first and she came to the ICU in a very critical state. I explained the situation to the family and told them that we had been responsible for the fact that the tube had fallen out, and we would investigate as to why and how this had happened so it should not happen on a future occasion. The family accepted my explanation and reassured me by telling me that they had given up hope when she was admitted to the ICU! Nevertheless, I am sure that telling them the truth contributed to their acceptance of the situation.

False hope

• It is always pleasing to give a good prognosis to family members and it is very easy to see other peoples' errors. I have seen many patients with haematological malignancies following unsuccessful bone marrow transplantation, where trivial rises in cell counts are presented to the family as a major progress only for this false hope to be dammed.

Trust

• I have overheard conversations in the relatives' rooms between different families where they have warned each other to be careful because the doctors in the unit kill people. Clearly, any explanations had been insufficient to earn the trust of the families.

Facing the inevitable

- It has been my experience that sometimes, relatives and nurses are aware of the need for treatment limitation because of a lack of progress, long before the physicians who may have invested emotional energy into the patient's success and in so doing, may have lost sight of the overall prognosis.

Conflict

- Conflicts in the ICU are common and should be avoided at all times, but especially when presenting the case to the family. Another pitfall I have met occurred in relation to an elderly lady with multiple organ failure. We held a properly constituted family conference with her two daughters explaining the situation and they agreed with our treatment plan. One month after her death, a complaint was made to the ICU by her husband. The daughters felt he was too frail to come to the hospital, but he very much resented the fact that he had not been consulted about his wife's death. Fortunately, I had recorded full details in the patient's record and we were able to go over the facts again, and I at least felt that he had some satisfaction.

Education

- It is important that people working in the ICU, all of whom in one way or another may take part in the communication of end-of-life decisions, hone their communication skills. There are various ways in which this can be done. There are courses on the communication, trainees can have their conferences video-recorded and indeed, may improve at their skills by practising with actors, acting as family members. It is useful to discuss the results of the conference with colleagues.

Do not denigrate colleagues

- I have often heard unfortunate remarks passed about colleagues who send their patients to the ICU after a crisis, occasionally iatrogenic. Describing other doctors as idiots or worse does not help and only creates an atmosphere of mistrust and disrespect.

Conclusion

In today's European ICU, families should be fully informed in an honest and clear non-judgemental manner by a representative team who should be ready to answer and explain any problems arising. This will facilitate the acceptance of what is often a tragic situation, helps to ensure satisfaction with care while hopefully, facilitating as good a death as possible for the patient and a less stressful bereavement for the family.

Decisions to forgo life support: a perspective from Europe

Introduction
The conduct of end-of-life care, and the provision and limitation of life support varies across the globe. Our handbook is international in scope and in Europe, a change to a more patient- and family-focused model of care is underway.

Prevalence of life support decisions
Decisions to forgo life-sustaining therapies (DFLSTs) are common in modern ICU practice and are supported by European intensive care medicine societies, as they are in Canada and America. However, the frequency and nature of the decision-making processes vary across different European countries, as evident in recent studies and questionnaire-based surveys:
- ETHICUS: this international multicentre study was conducted in 1999–2000, involving 37 ICUs in 17 European countries. Of more than 31,000 ICU patients, 13.5% died and DFLSTs were made for 73% of these dying patients (10% of admissions). There was considerable geographic variation in the frequency of DFLSTs and between participating physicians according to their religious affiliations. In general, compared to Northern Europe, DFLSTs were less common in southern European countries. In addition, the mode of death varied. For example, the provision of unsuccessful CPR was more common in southern Europe.
- LATAREA: this was a nationwide, prospective, multicentre study in France (conducted over two months in 1997) and involved 113 ICUs and more than 7,000 patients. Among 1,165 dying patients, DFLSTs occured in 53% of deaths (11% of admissions), with most of the decisions being made by the medical team. Families were involved in 44% of the decision-making process.

Legal frameworks
- DFLSTs are legal in France, according to the professional code of ethics.
- The surrogate decision-maker has a legal status in most European countries, but there are differences between countries in the designation process for the surrogate and the extent of their legal power. Most often, the surrogate decision-maker is seen as an adviser, not as a primary decision-maker.
- Whereas euthanasia is illegal in the UK, Canada, Australia, and the US, euthanasia (and physician-assisted suicide) are legal in the Netherlands and in Luxembourg, and euthanasia in Belgium (see 📖 Palliative care in the ICU through a legal lens p190, and 📖 'Euthanasia: the Belgian experience' p214).

End-of-life decision-making in European countries
Although physician paternalism persists, the shared decision-making model is gaining ground and increasingly supplants the more traditional model of physician paternalism.

- Nevertheless, DFLSTs remain, most of the time, the sole responsibility of physicians; this strategy has the strength of alleviating relatives' guilt or the burden of decision-making, and the weakness of sometimes bypassing the respect for the patient's autonomy.
- The 'paternalistic' attitude of European physicians is underpinned by the ethical principle of non-maleficence, seeking to avoid additional pain, stress, and anxiety to family members.
- Advance care planning and advance directives, the designation of surrogates, and various models of patient–family–physician relationships have been used as alternatives to physician-based decision-making.

Advance plan planning

- Advance care planning is legally valid in Belgium (2002), Denmark (1998), France (2004), Germany (2003), the Netherlands (2002), Spain (2002), the UK (2005), and Switzerland (under debate in 2009), although with varying interpretations.
- However, the use of advance directives as a component of advance care planning to guide DFLSTs varies widely in Europe, but remains rare overall (affecting some 10–15% of DFLSTs).
- Surrogates are becoming involved more frequently in DFLSTs than they were ten years ago, but this approach and the use of advance directives remain overall less common than in North America.

Multidisciplinary care in Europe

- The physician-nurse partnership in Europe remains at the core of multidisciplinary care near the end of life, but many aspects of this partnership need to improve with the recognition that:
  - Nurses' opinions are a mandatory component of the DFLST decision-making process and should be sought.
  - Nurses' professional expertise is crucial for optimal pain and other symptom management and for family support.
  - Gaps between nurses' and physicians' perception of collaboration in end of life and suboptimal communication can lead to misunderstandings, divergent practices, and conflicts near the end of life.
  - Decision-making processes that involve other caregivers (family doctor, attending physicians, psychologist, etc.) should be utilized when required.
- Ethics committees and consultations have been shown to be useful in clinical studies (resulting in improved communication, fewer conflicts, and shorter length of stay), but they are rarely used in practice (see ☐ 'The ethics consultant and clinical ethics committees' p208).

The need for culturally competent care

- Within Europe, the north to south gradient in the frequency of DFLSTs suggests the need for a better understanding of the strong influences of cultural differences that influence end-of-life care in various countries.
- Cultural backgrounds, ethical perspectives, and religious differences among and between physicians, and between physicians and their patients and caregivers can have profound influences on the provision and limitation of life support.

- More effective cross-cultural care near the end-of-life will help to meet the needs of patients and families, and improve the dying experience and mourning process that vary from one culture to another.
- Similarly, understanding and respecting cultural differences that exist between care teams and families, and also between caregivers themselves will help to avoid misunderstandings and conflicts.
- Culturally competent care that starts from the ICU admission and persists throughout the ICU stay should help ICU teams:
  - To tailor the process of making decisions about life support to the individual needs of each patient and family.
  - To provide comfort care, in the event of a decision to forgo life support, that meets the cultural and religious needs of patients and families near and at the end of life.

Further reading

1. Sprung CL, Cohen SL, Sjokvist P, *et al.* (2003). End-of-life practices in European intensive care units: the Ethicus Study. *JAMA* **290,** 790–7.
2. Carlet J, Thijs LG, Antonelli M, *et al.* (2004). Challenges in end-of-life care in the ICU. Statement of the 5th International Consensus Conference in Critical Care, Brussels, Belgium, April 2003. *Intensive Care Med* **30**, 770–84.
3. Fassier T, Lautrette A, Ciroldi M, Azoulay E (2005). Care at the end of life in critically ill patients: the European perspective. *Curr Opin Crit Care* **11**, 616–23.

Limitation of life support in an Australian ICU

In most western societies, the processes that surround withholding and withdrawal of life support are similar to those in Australia.

Australian society permits families and medical practitioners to work together to determine, as best they can, what the wishes of the patient would be if the patient were able to participate in the discussion.

If there is consensus that continuation of treatment would not be in keeping with the patient's wishes, then treatment may be withdrawn on the basis of 'presumed refusal of consent'.

Even if such withdrawal is directly related to death, the patient is presumed in law to have died from their disease, and the act of withdrawal is legal.

Australian society also permits the use of 'double effect', where drugs may be given to control painful suffering even if such administration shortens life. In practice, we try to avoid withdrawal that may be associated with a precipitous demise, both to allow families to spend time at the bedside and to emphasize the process is one of allowing the patient to die.

Palliative care vs withdrawal of treatment

Reaching a point where cure is impossible should never lead to withdrawal of 'care', but to the institution of a different form of care in which the goals are:
- Alleviation of suffering.
- Provision of a quiet and dignified environment.
- Encouragement of patient and family to communicate, touch, and deal with 'unfinished business'.

Patients and relatives constantly impress us with the wisdom, dignity, and stature they display when they are provided with a supportive environment. Caring for the family unit as a whole assumes a higher priority than caring for the patient alone.

Particular attention should be paid to:
- The removal of unnecessary equipment/monitoring which may impair the patient's appearance.
- The provision of unrestricted visiting.
- The elimination of unnecessary procedures or investigations (particularly those which may cause discomfort).
- The determination and fulfilment of the needs of the group collectively and individually.
- Unnecessary drugs are withdrawn and analgesia optimized.

Artificial forms of life support are maintained until the patient and relatives have had time together. Often, people ask whether they should go or stay. They are to be encouraged by us to do whatever they feel most comfortable with.
- It is important that the doctor leading the process regularly visit the patient and relatives at the bedside. Opportunity is provided for exposure to pastoral and social workers, if desired.
- When the physician is comfortable that the patient, relatives, and staff have had sufficient time to accept the inevitability of death and the patient is pain-free, supportive therapy may be withdrawn, preferably

in a manner in which a single action is not followed by an immediate demise.
- In most cases, the removal of inotropic agents or reduction of inspired oxygen concentration will lead to death over a period of time.
- Formal disconnection of patients from ventilators is more likely to be followed by rapid demise.
- Patients who are to be disconnected from artificial ventilation should be sedated rather than permitted to experience discomfort and acute breathlessness.
- We discourage patients who wish to be disconnected from artificial ventilation while awake and without sedation as this causes more distress to the patient, relatives, and staff.

Three enquiries are common before and after a death:
- Whether small children should see the relative before and/or after death.
- Whether relatives should view the body after death.
- Whether family members and others should stay till death occurs or make their farewell and leave.

While there is considerable opinion about the benefits of viewing the body after death, which is not supported by data, our attitude is to encourage the participants to decide themselves, and to both support their decision and encourage them to support each other. We explain that there are no rules or right and wrong, and people may feel comfortable doing different things. Family groups are encouraged to discuss what their wishes are, and during these periods and waiting periods, to 'tell the good stories.' In particular, we are impressed by the consequences of suggestions that children of all ages should be asked what they wish to do, and if they wish to see the patient, what they will see should be explained prior to the visit.

After death
- Families should be able to contact the physician or other staff if problems arise related to bereavement or unanswered questions become a problem.
- In addition, it is usual for our social workers to contact families after an interval.
- Families in Australia are particularly grateful if staff members attend patients' funerals.

Looking after each other
- Dealing with death causes stress and suffering in those delivering care as well as those who are receiving or observing the care.
- The key to managing staff problems is prevention by adequate support at the time, but after the event, the effects upon staff and the need for support should be considered.
- Such support may range from a session at the local pub to a formal debriefing with a skilled counsellor.

Further reading
1. Logan RL. Scott PJ (1996). Uncertainty in clinical practice: implications for quality and costs of health care. *Lancet* **347**, 595–8.
2. Gillett G (2001). The RUB. Risk of unacceptable badness. *NZ Med J* **114**, 188–9.
3. Cassell EJ (1982). The nature of suffering and the goals of medicine. *N Engl J Med* **306**, 639–45.

ICU care during withdrawal of life support: a personal perspective from Canada

Introduction

Most deaths in the ICU follow decisions to withdraw life-sustaining therapy (WLST). Comfort with the process of life support withdrawal is a necessary skill for all who practise in an ICU setting.

There is no one correct way to manage WLST, but if the ICU team keeps their focus primarily on the needs of the patient while maintaining support for the family at the bedside and through bereavement, it should be possible to provide a comfortable death for most patients and families within practices that are in keeping with local professional and legal requirements.

There should be no unseemly rush, nor should the process be unnecessarily prolonged. Canadian and US data show that for most patients and families, we met these goals. The goal should be a death that is as natural and free of technical support, if possible, and in all other ways in accord with what most of us would consider a 'good death' (see below).

The ICU administration should acknowledge that excellent care of the dying patient is a high acuity assignment and as high a priority as the care of other critical care patients. Nurses providing care for the patient undergoing WLST should not have to accept additional patient assignments.

Checklists

In Halifax, Nova Scotia, many years ago, we found that a WLST checklist was helpful, primarily to avoid overlooking important components of a life support withdrawal process (e.g. informing colleagues from consulting services or those who provided significant care prior to the ICU admission, exploring needs for spiritually and culturally sensitive care, organ donation preferences, etc.). (See 📖 p274 for a link to the most recent iteration of this form.)

Principles of a good death[1]

In an article in the BMJ in 2000, Richard Smith, the editor, set out the principles of a good death as follows:

- To know when death is coming and to understand what can be expected.
- To be able to retain control of what happens.
- To be afforded dignity and privacy.
- To have control over pain relief and other symptom control.
- To have choice and control over where death occurs (at home or elsewhere).
- To have access to information and expertise of whatever kind is necessary.
- To have access to any spiritual or emotional support required.
- To have access to hospice care in any location, not only in hospital.

- To have control over who is present and who shares the end.
- To be able to issue advance directives which ensure wishes are respected.
- To have time to say goodbye and control over other aspects of timing.
- To be able to leave when it is time to go and not to have life prolonged pointlessly.

While the above principles apply to deaths in general and some might not apply in the ICU setting, nevertheless, most do and those deaths that occur in the ICU that do not meet these goals could adversely affect both families and ICU teams, but will remain in the memory of families long after the ICU team moves on.

Principles that apply to all clinical situations in the ICU

- Reinforce with families that a withdrawal of life support is a shared decision—physician's expertise and concern for the patient combined with their love and concern—so that they do not feel the full responsibility of what they often describe as 'pulling the plug.' Spend time validating their decision so they gain comfort that it is the 'right' decision.
- It is extremely difficult to predict how long it will take for patients to die after WLST. Families should know this. Several studies point to a median time of about four hours. It will likely be quicker for patients who have been on multiple life support modalities and slower for those on single modalities.
- On rare occasions, a patient may not die following life support withdrawal.
- The point is not how long it takes or when death occurs, but that we ensure comfort throughout the dying process.
- Anticipation is key. It is the unexpected or unanticipated event that causes distress at the bedside, both for patients and their families.
- We should advise families that:
  - We cannot predict accurately the timing of death.
  - Our role is to prove comfort whatever the duration.
  - Death will likely occur somewhere between a range of minutes to hours or even days (e.g. if dialysis has been the primary life support modality).
  - Families should also be aware that sometimes events proceed much faster or slower than anticipated.
  - In some situations (e.g. acute brain injury), patients may not die as anticipated.
- Discuss in advance with patients (where this would be possible and acceptable to them) and with families how the process of WLST will proceed (what is being taken away, and when and how).
- Be honest, yet empathetic, and use straightforward language with no acronyms, abbreviations, or jargon.
- In general, put the patient's and family's preferences before your own, but explain why it is that you might advise against proceeding as a family might wish, if that situation arises.
- Explain what will happen and do not be afraid to warn those who sit at the bedside about skin colour changes and noises. They are all part of a

natural process of dying. Sometimes, patient appearances suggest stress or pain, but we can reassure families we eliminate or minimize any chance of pain or discomfort by the use of comfort medications.

- For patients where mechanical ventilation (MV) is the primary mode of life support, explore with those involved (nurses, respiratory therapists, and family) whether an extubation would be best (assuming an endotracheal tube is in place) or whether a transition to a T-piece would be preferred (in settings where there is high risk of pulmonary haemorrhage or airway obstruction).
- Discuss with more experienced colleagues if you have any doubt about how to proceed in a given circumstance.
- Be visible. Always be available to patients, families, the nurses, and respiratory therapists in the ICU during the dying process.
- Recognize that the focus of care now shifts to encompass the family unit as the 'patient.'

Medication

Provide comfort medication prescriptions in advance of the first step of a life support withdrawal process and be sure of patient comfort before the first and subsequent steps. Patients with severe brain injury or in deep coma for other reasons will not in general need pre-sedation. Providing individualized and appropriate doses of comfort medication in advance of a reduction in life support (in anticipation of, and to prevent/reduce any subsequent distress) is accepted practice in the UK and Canada.

The drugs chosen and the dosages to be used will be dependent on the prevailing levels of analgesia/sedation at the time of the life support withdrawal decision. If using an opioid, it would be reasonable to provide an initial intravenous bolus of twice the prevailing hourly dose with an prescription for a range within which to initially titrate comfort medication and a provision to increase this as necessary (see also 📖 in 'Symptom relief for the imminently dying patient' p54).

How and in what order should we withdraw various life support modalities?

In Malcolm Fisher's section on life support limitation in this chapter, he makes the point that in his unit (Sydney, Australia), they are careful to avoid changes in mechanical ventilation and other modes of life support that would precipitate a crisis and sudden distress.

There is no single answer to the question of the order in which WLST occurs because it depends on many factors:

- Those modalities that prevail at the time of the life support withdrawal decision.
- Whether and to what extent patients are vasopressor-dependent.
- Whether they have an endotracheal tube or a tracheostomy.
- Whether they are on mechanical support for the circulation.
- Whether they might die several days after dialysis is withdrawn if they are otherwise on minimal support of other organ systems.

High-dose vasopressor dependence plus mechanical ventilation

Generally. it would be reasonable to reduce/withdraw vasopressors first before moving to changes to mechanical ventilation. Some patients will die without ventilator changes or before all changes to mechanical ventilation/oxygen are made. Again, all this can and should be discussed in advance with all who are involved.

When extubation is not recommended

• High risk of pulmonary haemorrhage.
• Expected airway obstruction.

If the former is likely, linen, and preferably, green towels should be placed in anticipation.

When extubation is the plan

To reach the point of extubation, I think it is wise to ensure comfort prior to taking what might be a one-step change for patients with lower levels of respiratory support or perhaps each of up to three to four steps at short intervals (~10–20 minutes) when reducing high levels of mechanical ventilation/pressure support ± high FiO_2.

It is important to consider whether a precipitant drop from a high FiO_2 to 21% is optimal (I do not think that in general it is) or whether a stepwise, but not a drawn out process, would be best in the circumstances. Provision of oxygen is a form of life support, but can also provide comfort from the distress of a hypoxic death. The key issue is to provide as natural a death as possible and one that is free from unnecessary distress caused by precipitant changes in levels of support.

Remember, sedating drugs (opioids or benzodiazepines) generally do not have an immediate onset of action (e.g. intravenous morphine might take 15 minutes to achieve a desired effect).

Be willing to adapt your own practices

There is and always will be considerable practice variation in the provision of end-of-life care. Styles of practice are personal, and may be positively informed or biased by particularly seminal events.

My own practice changed after I conducted some simple surveys of colleagues in Canada. Given the same scenarios, ICU clinicians (respiratory therapists, nurses, and physicians) were more or less equally divided on whether to extubate, reduce mechanical ventilation, use a T-piece, or extubate.

I subsequently moved several years ago from using a T-piece to try to extubate wherever possible as the goal of reducing and removing mechanical ventilation (after listening to colleagues whose preference was to go that route). I never regretted that decision.

Seek feedback

Physicians tend to think they do a better job in these situations than do their colleagues and their assessment of the quality of the process of dying and death might be an overestimate. Nevertheless, it is important to seek feedback and act upon it. We can ask our colleagues in the ICU and, after a reasonable time frame (a month or more), the families who sat at the bedside. The results of these kinds of surveys can and should be illuminating and help to improve practice.

Specifically, have an ICU team meeting after the patient dies to be sure everything went well from their perspective and to address any of their concerns and learn from their observations.

References

1. Smith R (2000). A good death. An important aim for health services and for us all. *BMJ* **320**, 129–30.

Further reading

1. Gerstel E, Engelberg RA, Koepsell T, Curtis JR (2008). Duration of withdrawal of life support in the intensive care unit and association with family satisfaction. *Am J Respir Crit Care Med* **178**, 798–804.
2. Sprung CL, Ledoux D, Bulow HH, *et al.* (2008). Relieving suffering or intentionally hastening death: where do you draw the line? *Crit Care Med* **36**, 8–13.
3. Wall RJ, Curtis JR, Cooke CR, Engelberg RA (2007). Family satisfaction in the ICU: differences between families of survivors and non-survivors. *Chest* **132**, 1425–33.
4. Cook DJ, Rocker G, Giacomini M, *et al.* (2006). Understanding and changing attitudes toward withdrawal and withholding of life support in the ICU. *Crit Care Med* **24**(Suppl), S317–23.
5. Rocker GM, Cook DJ, Shemie SD (2006). Practice variation in end-of-life care in the ICU: implications for patients with acute brain injury. *Can J Anaesth* **53**, 814–9.
6. Rocker GM, Cook DJ, O'Callaghan C, *et al.* (2005). Canadian nurses' and respiratory therapists' perspectives on withdrawal of life support in the intensive care unit. *J Crit Care* **20**, 59–65.
7. Rocker GM, Heyland DK, Cook DJ, *et al.* (2004). Most critically ill patients are perceived to die in comfort during withdrawal of life support: a Canadian multicentre study. *Can J Anesth* **51**, 621–30.

Withdrawal of ventricular assist device support

Introduction

Ventricular assist devices (VADs) are mechanical pumps that are surgically implanted to improve the performance of the damaged left (LVAD), right (RVAD), or both (BiVAD) ventricles. VADs are indicated for patients with advanced heart failure who are at risk of imminent death either from an acute event or chronic decompensation of existing heart failure. VADs can be used in the short term as a bridge to recovery, long term as a bridge to transplant, or as a destination therapy, an alternative to transplant. Results of the REMATCH trial suggest that patients with advanced heart failure who are treated with an LVAD live longer and have a higher quality of life than patients receiving optimal medical management.[1]

VADs are a treatment and not a cure, and mortality on device support remains high. The risk of death is highest immediately following implantation with an expected survival of 50–70% at one year. In general, treatment goals are discussed with the patient and family, and agreed upon prior to device implantation. These goals include extending the survival time, improving the quality of life, and most importantly for patients, going home. If the continued use of VAD support will no longer meet these goals, e.g. if there is multisystem organ failure or an overwhelming infection, discussions regarding the potential for device withdrawal are initiated. This approach relies heavily on informed consent, advanced care planning, and discussions with the patient and family regarding the potential for device withdrawal, prior to device implantation. We discuss our overall approach in more detail[2] (see 'Further reading') and focus here on the potential for device withdrawal.

Potential for device withdrawal

Engaging in discussions about the potential for device withdrawal prior to device implant allows the team and family to understand the patient's wishes and serves to direct decision-making should device withdrawal need to take place. In our experience, patients usually want their families to know that it is okay to withdraw support if they have no reasonable chance of recovery. If the need to withdraw support becomes a reality, families take comfort from knowing what the patient's wishes are and use this information to guide decision-making. Following lengthy discussions and prior to device implant, we ask both the patient and substitute decision-maker to read and sign a document that states 'device withdrawal will be considered when despite all efforts, the patient has no reasonable chance of receiving a heart transplant, surviving to leave the hospital or continued device use will no longer be serving the purpose for which it was originally placed' (see appendix).

Stopping the VAD

Given the high mortality associated with VADs and the increasing use of such devices, critical care physicians need to be comfortable with the need to withdraw such devices as they would other modalities of life support when goals of care cannot be met. Our practice at the Toronto General Hospital is as follows:

- The decision to withdraw support is made by the transplant team, the patient (when able), and the patient's family or surrogate decision-maker using objective criteria established as part of our programme mandate.
- Once discussions regarding the potential for device withdrawal are initiated, at least two members of the transplant VAD team meet with the family to discuss the patient's situation.
- The discussion includes a review of the events to date, patient prognosis, and indications for device withdrawal.
- Where possible, discussions are framed within the patient's stated goals of treatment.
- The family are allowed time to ask questions.
- Typically, the decision is made over several days to allow time for reflection and acceptance by the family and team members.

Once the decision is made to withdraw device support, a member of the VAD team communicates the decision to the ICU staff. A team member remains with the patient to coordinate care, and assist with communication and decision-making between family and nursing staff. At the outset, the team member communicates the wishes outlined in the advance directive to the nursing staff. The family is encouraged to create an environment the patient would find comforting including:

- Music.
- Storytelling.
- Prayer or quiet.

Our ICU provides the opportunity for observance of cultural or religious practices that may be important to the patient or family, and asks clergy with whom there is a personal relationship to be present as needed to support the patient and family. Decisions regarding the use of cardiac monitors during device withdrawal are made in consultation with the family and nursing staff. When withdrawal of the VAD is planned, we first discontinue neuromuscular blocking agents and ensure that there is no residual blockade. In our experience, severe heart failure and acute pulmonary oedema occur rapidly after VAD withdrawal, accompanied by dyspnoea, air hunger, anxiety, or other distress. Accordingly, it is our practice to consider anticipatory opiate treatment, with appropriate adjustment of dose based on the circumstances, symptoms, signs, and current regimen of medications of the individual patient. When all these steps have been taken and the family signals readiness, we silence alarms and discontinue the VAD, remaining close to the patient's bedside to attend to the patient's and family's needs.

The VAD coordinator, in collaboration with the directors of the heart transplant programme, conducts post-mortem debriefing for staff in the ICU. Debriefing occurs after the family has left the patient's bedside and again in one week. During these discussions, staff are encouraged to share their experience and support each other to work through their feelings. Usually, these sessions are adequate for staff support. If necessary, the transplant psychosocial support team or clinical bioethicist can be approached for more in-depth debriefing.

Conflicts

Disagreements regarding device withdrawal, either between the ICU staff and the transplant team or members within the transplant team, can occur. The first step to resolve differences is to discuss the issue with the larger transplant team. All members of the team participate and the decision is reached through consensus. The majority of disagreements are resolved with this approach. If consensus cannot be achieved, consultation is sought from the hospital ethics committee and other relevant experts outside the university health network. In our experience, disagreements centre around two main issues, the timing of device withdrawal and who actually stops the pump.

Turning the pump off

This requires knowledge of how to silence alarms, cease pump operation, disconnect the equipment, and turn the power unit off. We have found it supportive to have at least two transplant team members in attendance during device withdrawal and make this a responsibility of the transplant team, not the ICU team. This sharing of responsibility has been beneficial to the individuals involved by allowing them to support each other, the family, and the team during this very difficult time. We follow this up with small group debriefings to help the individuals manage the feelings around device withdrawal.

Deactivating implantable cardio-defibrillators and pacemakers

We use a similar discussion process for deactivation of implantable cardio-defibrillators (ICD). The majority of our heart failure patients have ICDs either as primary or secondary prophylaxis against sudden death. ICDs reduce sudden death through anti-tachycardia and/or pacing programmes or internally defibrillating the heart when they sense a potentially lethal arrhythmia. While this therapy can be life-saving in the earlier stages of the disease, it can become problematic for patients dying from refractory heart failure. When extending life is no longer a treatment goal, we engage in discussions with the patient, surrogate decision-maker, and family about deactivating the ICD. Discussions include prognosis, information on how patients with heart failure die, and indications for ICD deactivation. We have found some patients prefer the possibility of a sudden death vs the progressive symptoms associated with terminal advanced heart failure. Other patients prefer a death that is anticipated, allowing them time to get their affairs in order and say goodbye. Discussing ICD deactivation allows the patient to direct not only how they live, but also potentially how they will die. When a heart failure patient decides to deactivate their ICD or their pacemaker, a member of the team contacts the electrophysiology service to discuss the decision and arrangements are made to have the ICD turned off, pacing functions remain activated for symptomatic relief or may also be turned off at the patient's request.

For patients with pacemakers/ICDs in the ICU undergoing withdrawal of other life support modalities, strong consideration should be given to contacting cardiology or electrophysiology to turn pacemakers off prior to treatment withdrawal. This prevents unwanted internal defibrillation at end of life.

Conclusion

Establishing a process for device withdrawal is an increasingly important issue in the management of advanced heart failure. It has been a key factor in the success of our VAD programme. Our approach is based on informed consent, advance care planning, and the potential for device withdrawal (VAD) or deactivation (ICD). An atmosphere of open and honest communication can help patients and families understand the indications for device implantation and the potential for device withdrawal. Disagreement can occur and any process must include strategies for conflict resolution. Using our process as a framework may be beneficial to other programmes that are adding VAD support to its repertoire of treatment strategies for patients with advanced heart failure. Our process for device withdrawal is documented in our programme mandate and has been communicated to all staff working in areas caring for VAD patients.

Further reading

1. Rose EA, Gelijns AC, Moskowitz AJ, *et al.* (2001). Long-term use of a left ventricular assist device for end-stage heart failure. *N Engl J Med* **345**, 1435–43.
2. MacIver J, Ross HJ (2005). Withdrawal of ventricular assist device support. *J Palliat Care* **21**, 151–6.
3. Singer PA, Robertson G, Roy DJ (1996). Bioethics for clinicians: 6. Advance care planning. *CMAJ* **155**, 1689–92.
4. Powell TP, Oz MC (1997). Discontinuing the LVAD: ethical considerations. *Ann Thorac Surg* **63**, 1223–4.
5. Bramstedt KA, Wenger NS (2001). When withdrawal of life-sustaining care does more than allow death to take its course: the dilemma of left ventricular assist devices. *J Heart Lung Transplant* **20**, 544–8.
6. Goodlin SJ, Hauptman PJ, Arnold R, *et al.* (2004). Consensus statement: palliative and supportive care in advanced heart failure. *J Card Fail* **10**, 200–9.
7. Wiegand DL, Kalowes PG (2007). Withdrawal of cardiac medications and devices. *AACN Adv Crit Care* **4**, 415–25.

Appendix

Consent for treatment for VAD

The goal of mechanical circulatory support is to support the failing ventricle(s) to allow patients to recover end organ function and improve physical conditioning while waiting for either recovery or a donor heart to become available. If despite all the efforts, the patient has no reasonable chance of receiving a heart transplant, surviving to leave the hospital or continued use will no longer be serving the purpose for which it was originally placed, and the device will be discontinued. This will occur only after the transplant team caring for the patient are in agreement that the goals for mechanical circulatory support cannot be met, and after consulting with the patient or if the patient is too ill, with the family or substitute decision-maker.

'My signature herewith confirms that I have read and understood the contents of this message and I voluntarily agree to be bound by its terms. I also acknowledge that I have been afforded an opportunity to ask any questions I might have related to the use of the ventricular assist device and that _____ has answered all my questions to my satisfaction.'*

* Adapted from Columbian–Presbyterian Medical Centre

Life support after cardiac arrest

Introduction

Out-of-hospital cardiac arrest (OHCA) is a leading cause of death in western countries. Despite recent advances in the management of cardio-pulmonary arrest (CPR), the survival rate of OHCA patients still remains very low, even after the return of spontaneous circulation (ROSC). The vast majority of OHCA patients subsequently suffer from a post-anoxic encephalopathy, leading to a post-resuscitation neurological deficiency that is either transient or definitive, and represents the major cause of death in these patients. Currently, apart from moderate, induced hypo-thermia, no other treatment has shown any ability to decrease the conse-quences of cerebral ischaemia due to cardiac arrest.

With increasing public education in basic life support and with the widespread use of automated defibrillators, post-cardiac arrest coma has become an increasingly common clinical syndrome, and after brain trauma and drug overdose, the third most common cause of coma in western countries.

Unlike traumatic or focal ischaemic causes of coma, cardiac arrest presents a global ischaemic insult to the brain. The extent of cerebral damage is largely influenced by the duration of interrupted cerebral blood flow and subsequent metabolic derangements.

- Cerebral oxygen stores are lost within 20 seconds of the onset of cardiac arrest.
- Glucose and adenosine triphosphate stores are lost by five minutes.
- Then, a cascade of complex chemical derangements ensues, which leads to neuronal death and culminates in the post-cardiac arrest coma.

The majority of patients in whom ROSC has been obtained on site are comatose during the next hours and admitted to an ICU. At that time, for most of them, it is impossible to predict outcome (ranging from complete neurological recovery to death or persistent vegetative state, but it is pre-dictable that a large proportion will never regain consciousness (Fig. 9.1). In admitted patients who survive the initial cardiac arrest, rates of mean-ingful neurological recovery range approximately from 20% to 30%. This uncertainty increases the relatives' emotional suffering. Thus, it is impor-tant for families and physicians to have an estimate of the patient's chance of neurological recovery.

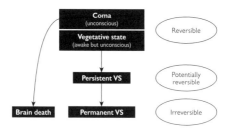

Fig. 9.1 Post-anoxic neurological abnormalities (VS=vegetative state).

The need for a waiting period

- Immediately after cardiac arrest, no clinical signs or investigations accurately predict the patient's outcome. After ROSC, accurate prognostication can only occur after 72 hours have elapsed from all confounding factors that may influence neurological evaluation. This last point is of particular importance if sedation and neuromuscular blockade were used in conjunction with therapeutic hypothermia. This treatment strategy mandates extending the waiting period.
- Awakening generally takes place within three to four days after ROSC, and neurological impairment is expected if a patient fails to do so. These patients are often left in a severely cognitively disabled and fully dependent state; some remain in a minimally conscious or vegetative state, and very few awaken neurologically intact (Fig. 9.2).
- During the first hours and days after ROSC, half of these patients will subsequently suffer from a post-resuscitation syndrome that could include severe shock leading by itself to death. This shock should be treated without limitation during the very first hours and days in order to reach the appropriate window for neurological evaluation.
- The absence of clinical improvement during the waiting period may help families and physicians reach a common understanding of the patient's prognosis. This waiting period is important in our understanding of how families can deal with decision-making after cardiac arrest. If given time to watch for change in neurological condition, most families will agree with decisions to withdraw life support if patients deteriorate or if there is no improvement.
- Finally, brain death will occur in about 10% of these patients a few days after cardiac arrest because of cerebral oedema due to initial cerebral anoxia. Those patients are dead, and life support will be stopped after completion of organ donation-related processes if organ donation is the wish of patient and the family.

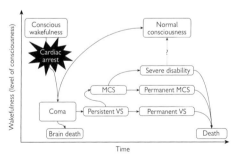

Fig. 9.2 Range of consciousness disorders after cardiac arrest (MCS=minimally conscious state; VS=vegetative state).

Tools to predict outcomes during ICU stay

It is reasonable to estimate the probability of poor neurological outcome at about 70–80% in the population of patients admitted to an ICU after a cardiac arrest. No variable (anoxia time, duration of CPR, cause of cardiac arrest) can reliably discriminate accurately between patients with poor and those with favourable outcome. Thus, while these variables should be considered, decisions about life support withdrawal should not be based on these elements.

Prognostication should always be based on a rigorous clinical evaluation that should include detailed neurological examination. There are no specific clinical signs that can predict outcome in the first few hours after the ROSC. Absence of motor response to pain at 72 hours remains the best supported clinical predictor. Several additional clinical findings accurately predict poor outcome:

* Myoclonus.
* Status epilepticus within the first 24 hours.
* Absence of pupillary responses within days 1 to 3 after CPR.
* Absent corneal reflexes within days 1 to 3 after CPR.
* Absent or extensor motor responses after three days.

The prognosis is invariably poor in comatose patients with absent pupillary or corneal reflexes, or absent or extensor motor responses three days after cardiac arrest. On the other hand, single seizures and sporadic focal myoclonus do not accurately predict poor outcome. In the same way, although permanent status epilepticus is associated with a mortality approaching 100%, exceptions to this dismal outcome have been reported.

Effects of hypothermia
The use of therapeutic hypothermia can complicate the clinical evaluation for prediction, especially if sedation and neuromuscular blockade are employed. All other usual factors (medications, temperature, concomitant disease processes) must be considered before any prognostication process.

Effects of age
While the mortality rate increases with age, age alone does not appear to predict poor neurological outcome, nor slower neurological recovery. There is no evidence that post-ischaemic encephalopathy or severe neurological residual impairment is more prevalent in the elderly. Chances for survival are mainly affected by pre-existing medical conditions combined with prolonged arrest and CPR time. As for other patients, the use of life-sustaining therapy after cardiac arrest for elderly patients should be realistic, individualized, and serve to preserve the patient's dignity.

Investigations that may enhance prognostication
In addition to physical examination, various methods have been evaluated for assessing the neurological prognosis of unconscious cardiac arrest victims, including:

* Electrophysiological tests.
* Biochemical markers.
* Neuroimaging techniques.

Electrophysiological tests
Electrophysiological tests in coma consist of electroencephalogram (EEG) and evoked/event-related potential studies. Systematic reviews of

outcome prediction in comatose patients post-arrest have concluded that somatosensory evoked potentials (SSEPs) are the best diagnostic method for predicting outcome. Bilateral absence of the N20 component of the SSEPs with median nerve stimulation recorded on days 1 to 3 or later after CPR accurately predicts a poor outcome. Conversely, the presence of the N20 response is not helpful in predicting outcome as many patients who fail to recover could have preserved N20 responses.

The use of routine EEGs is not recommended, but should be used if ongoing seizure activity is suspected. Generalized suppression pattern, burst suppression pattern with generalized epileptiform activity, or generalized periodic complexes on a flat background are strongly, but not invariably associated with poor outcome. Burst suppression or generalized epileptiform discharges on EEG predicted poor outcomes, but with insufficient prognostic accuracy.

Circulating markers

Anoxo-ischaemic cerebral insult is associated with the blood release of various biochemical markers and the peak plasma level is thought to be correlated with the amount of neuronal definitive death. A large peak of serum neuron-specific enolase and/or S-100 protein concentration is a highly specific, but only moderately sensitive marker for a poor neurological outcome after CPR. The search for a simple, reliable, and readily available biological test remains an exciting challenge, but clinical decisions with potentially irreversible consequences should never rely on a single marker, but can only be made in the context of all available prognostic information.

Imaging

Routine CT scan imaging does not add to clinical assessment unless stroke, bleeding, or trauma is suspected on the basis of history or clinical examination.

Providing end-of-life care after cardiac arrest

In a small number of distressing cases, patients regain spontaneous circulation, but remain in a persistent vegetative state or are seriously neurologically impaired. In this situation, when care providers and families or proxies reach consensus, end-of-life care can be considered: this consists of withholding/withdrawing all invasive support (mechanical ventilation, circulatory assistance, renal replacement therapy) and, in some cases, in withdrawing food and fluids. These are profoundly difficult decisions, but generally relatives, doctors, and nurses reach an agreement on the course of action. In these cases, decisions can be made without the need for legal intervention. Difficulties arise if there is a disagreement or conflict between caregivers and relatives, or simply amongst relatives.

Most of these neurologically impaired patients are mechanically ventilated and it is reasonable to plan for an extubation and the definitive withdrawal of respiratory assistance. This should be performed in conjunction with all comfort care that can be provided in such a situation.

Good relationship with the family is important to optimize end-of-life processes.

- Information given to the family must be clear at admission to the ICU and neurological impairment should be explained empathetically soon after admission.
- Families should understand that outcomes include survival with seriously impaired neurological function or a persistent vegetative state that would necessitate constant care.
- The burdens of the decision to withdraw life support treatments should, in our opinion, be mostly borne by the ICU team and where possible, we should minimize that burden on the family. However we recognize that in other countries/jurisdictions, more of that burden may have to be accepted by families (e.g. in US).
- The way in which life support is withdrawn should be clearly explained to the family and the plans clearly documented. Individualized palliative measures should begin in advance of withdrawal of life-sustaining therapy in situations where any distress is anticipated, and include analgesia, sedation, or oxygen, if needed. Relatives should be allowed to stay with the patient without any limitation of visiting time.
- Families should be made aware that the timing of death after the withdrawal of life support is difficult to predict and that there is a possibility (however small) that some patients may continue to breathe without the assistance of mechanical ventilation and may need additional care away from a critical care setting.

Conclusion

The physical examination is the strongest predictor of death or poor neurological outcome in comatose survivors of cardiac arrest. Pupillary light response, corneal reflexes, motor responses to pain, the search for myoclonus status epilepticus, and SSEPs studies can be reliably combined to predict outcome in comatose patients after CPR for cardiac arrest. Although decisions to withdraw life-sustaining treatment may be delayed for a variety of reasons, the most useful signs occur at least 24 hours and, in the case of motor response, at 72 hours post-cardiac arrest. This time window should be extended if confounding factors interfere, particularly when hypothermia has been used in conjunction with sedatives and/or neuromuscular blockades. The existing literature does not allow for an earlier prognosis to be made. We need more precise clinical studies on brain monitoring and neuroimaging to provide data to support or refute their usefulness in prognostication.

Table 9.1 Glasgow–Pittsburgh cerebral performance categories

Level 1: good cerebral performance.	Conscious: alert, able to work and lead a normal life. May have minor psychological or neurological deficits (mild dysphasia, non-incapacitating hemiparesis, or minor cranial nerve abnormalities).
Level 2: moderate cerebral disability.	Conscious: sufficient cerebral function for part-time work in a sheltered environment or independent activities of daily life (dressing, travelling by public transportation, and preparing food). May have hemiplegia, seizures, ataxia, dysarthria, dysphasia, or permanent memory or mental changes.
Level 3: severe cerebral disability.	Conscious: dependent on others for daily support because of impaired brain function (in an institution or at home with exceptional family effort). At least limited cognition. Includes a wide range of cerebral abnormalities from ambulatory with severe memory disturbance or dementia precluding independent existence to paralytic and able to communicate only with eyes, as in the locked-in syndrome.
Level 4: coma, vegetative state.	Not conscious: unaware of surroundings, no cognition. No verbal or psychological interactions with the environment.
Level 5: death.	Certified brain dead or dead by traditional criteria.

Further reading

1. Meynaar IA, Oudemans–van Straaten HM, van der Wetering J, et al. (2003). Serum neuron-specific enolase predicts outcome in post-anoxic coma: a prospective cohort study. *Intensive Care Med* **29**, 189–95.
2. Chan PS, Krumholz HM, Nichol G, Nallamothu BK; American Heart Association National Registry of Cardiopulmonary Resuscitation Investigators (2008). Delayed time to defibrillation after in-hospital cardiac arrest. *N Engl J Med* **358**, 9–17.
3. Hypothermia After Cardiac Arrest Study Group (2002). Mild therapeutic hypothermia to improve the neurologic outcome after cardiac arrest. *N Engl J Med* **346**, 549–56.
4. Grubb NR, Elton RA, Fox KA (1995). In-hospital mortality after out-of-hospital cardiac arrest. *Lancet* **346**, 417–21.

Withholding and withdrawing life support: Muslim perspectives

Introduction

Literature about the frequency of end-of-life decisions and practice patterns in American and European countries is growing, but data on the behaviour of Muslim physicians and families remain scarce.

End-of-life decisions are a concern for all religions and cultures, but the issue is of particular importance for Islam because it is one of the fastest growing religions nowadays and spreading throughout the world. Despite the fact that Islam has its roots in Arabia, it is not an 'Arab' religion. Islam counts 1.1 billion Muslims around the world, of whom only 18% live in the Arab countries. The majority of Muslims worldwide are Asian or African. Indonesia has around 200 millions Muslims while India counts 133 millions. Twenty million Muslims live in China, 27 million in Russia, 10 million in the European Union, and 10 million in North America.

Physicians practising in a multicultural environment may one day have to make end-of-life decisions about a Muslim patient and therefore, need to understand the perception of end-of-life decisions from the perspective of the Muslim patient and family within the context of the Islamic faith.

Foundational values in Islam

Islamic bioethics is an extension of Sharia which is based on Quran (the holy book of Muslims) and Sunna (Prophet Muhammad's words and acts).[1] Because the Quran is seen as an eternal truth, the framework and principles of the law are thought immutable. However, the application and interpretation of the law changes with each age. Islamic law (Sharia) allows and encourages interpretation (ijtihad) and renewing of the law (tajdid).

Major branches of Islam

The two major branches of Islamic faith, the Shia and the Sunni, may differ somewhat in interpretations, methodology, and authoritative systems, but not fundamentally in bioethical rulings. Although some differences among Muslims exist and are attributable to differences of opinion by various schools of jurisprudence, Muslims are expected to be moderate and balanced in all matters, including health. Islam has the flexibility to respond to new biomedical technologies. In the absence of an organized 'church' and ordained 'clergy' in Islam, the determination of valid religious practice and the resolution of bioethical issues is left to qualified scholars of religious law. To respond to new medical technologies, Islamic jurists, informed by technical experts, have regular conferences to discuss and seek consensus statements on emerging issues. Recent conferences have dealt with issues such as organ transplantation, brain death, assisted conception, and technology in the ICU.

Similarities of monotheistic religions

The three monotheistic religions, Judaism, Christianity, and Islam, believe in the same god (the God of Abraham). As a monotheist religion, Islam shares many foundational values with Judaism and Christianity. Although Islam has some doctrinal differences from Judaism and from Christianity, it shares essentially the same code of morality. Hence, Islamic bioethics will appear familiar to many occidental physicians, wherever they practice.

Sanctity of life

In Islam, life is sacred. The saving of life is a duty and the unwarranted taking of life is a grave sin. Accordingly, Islamic bioethics teaches that the patient must be treated with respect and compassion. The physical, mental, and spiritual dimensions of the illness should be taken into account.

The four main concerns of Islamic ethics

These are similar to those of other ethical systems: autonomy (the right of patient's self-determination), beneficence (patient's benefit and well-being), non-maleficence (physician's obligation to not injure patients, '*primum non nocere*'), and justice (personal justice, but also social justice corresponding to the obligation made to the physician to spare ineffective treatments in health systems with limited resources).

However, Islamic bioethics puts more emphasis on beneficence over autonomy, particularly at times of death. Indeed, many ICU patients are incapable of making decisions. Family members may prefer not to be involved in end-of-life decisions. They also may disagree among themselves or may not be aware of patient's wishes. Therefore, physicians have the obligation of making end-of-life decisions. They do so on the basis of the principle of paternalism which gives physicians the moral authority to decide for the patient's best interest.

The rationale of Islamic bioethics can be summarized as follow 'everything possible must be done to prevent premature death, but not at any cost'.[2] Life-sustaining treatments can be withheld or withdrawn in terminally ill Muslim patients when the following conditions are fulfilled:
- The physicians are certain about the inevitability of death.
- When certain that treatment in no way will improve the condition or quality of life.
- In addition, the intention must never be to hasten death, only to abstain from overzealous treatment.

The Islamic principle of 'istislah', which corresponds to the seeking of the best interest of the patient and his family, allows a collective decision not to prolong the life of a terminally ill patient through consultation of all those involved in providing health care and of patient's family. This principle underlies many of the end-of-life decisions in Islam. Administering a drug with the explicit intention to relieve pain, a drug administration that in the same time may shorten life (the rule of double effect in Catholicism), does not result in criminal charges.

The reason in this instance is that delaying the inevitable death of a patient through life-sustaining treatment is not in best interest of:
- The patient.
- The family.
- The community.

The decision to withdraw futile treatment is seen as allowing death to take its natural course in these conditions. However, such decision should be collective, taken on the basis of:
- Informed consent.

- Following a consultation with the patient's family.
- Concerns all those involved in providing health care, including the attending physician.

However, basic nutrition should not be discontinued because such a withdrawal would be perceived as starving the patient to death, a crime according to the Islamic faith.

The Quran also emphasizes that 'it is the sole prerogative of Allah to bestow life and to cause death', and therefore, euthanasia is never allowed.

End-of-life decisions in Muslim physicians' practice

Little is known about Muslim physicians' practice with regard to end-of-life decisions. A questionnaire was addressed to 439 anaesthesiologists in Turkey, 90% of whom were Muslims. Sixty-six percent of physicians who answered the questionnaire revealed that they have previously made DNR orders at least once. In 94% of cases, this was not a documented order and it was only a verbal order. In 83% of such instances, DNR orders were made after discussion with colleagues. Discussion took place with families in 14% of cases and with the institutional ethics committee in 2% of such cases. The majority of respondents indicated that the decision to limit life-sustaining treatment should be made by consensus among physicians, patients' relatives, and the ethics committee.[3] This interesting study was obviously limited by the fact that these were stated intentions of physicians rather than their real practice.

In a prospective one-year observational study conducted in the medical ICU of a Lebanese university hospital (a Christian hospital, but caring for both Muslim and Christian Lebanese):[4]

- 46% of all deaths recorded in their ICU were preceded by one kind of end-of-life decision.
- In 86% of these cases, such decisions corresponded to withholding of life-sustaining treatments.
- Withdrawal of treatments occurred in the remaining 14%.

The main reasons underlying end-of-life decisions were 'futility of care' in 88% of cases and/or poor quality of life in 53%. Families were involved in the decision process in 79% of cases.

Physician behaviours

In a large European survey regarding physicians' behaviour, life-sustaining treatment was more often withheld (63%) than withdrawn (37%) if the physician was Muslim.[4,5] This pattern was similar to that of Jewish or Greek orthodox physicians. It differed from that of Protestant physicians who equally practised withholding or withdrawing active treatments. It was also in contrast with the practice of Catholic physicians who more often withdrew than withheld treatments. Active shortening of the dying process, defined as a circumstance in which a physician performed an act with the specific intent of shortening the dying process, which is overtly not advisable by Islam bioethics and corresponds to a crime in the Islamic faith, was never practised by Muslim physicians. Few Muslim physicians adhere to the view that patients' wishes are crucial in end-of-life decision-making. It is not even an everyday issue of discussion among Muslim families where discussion about death is considered taboo.

Islam allows end-of-life decisions to be held by ICU physicians provided that the decision:

- Relies on certitude of inevitable death.
- Follows discussion with the primary physician, the other ICU physicians, and nurses.

Patterns of paternalism

Of interest, within the European survey led by Sprung,[5,6] Muslim ICU physicians had one of the highest rates of discussion with ICU nurses. On the other hand, Muslim physicians had the lowest rate of discussion with patients' families, either because of 'a lack of patient responsiveness to therapy' or because 'the family would not understand'. The latter reason reflects the paternalistic attitude that characterizes the usual relation between Muslim physicians and patients or families. This attitude contrasts with recommendations of Muslim bioethics and qualifies as misconduct since bioethics strongly recommends:

- Consultations between all the parties concerned about the well-being of the patient (between physicians, nurses, families).
- A collective decision not to prolong the life of a terminally ill patient through an explicit informed consent of the family, and consultation with care givers, including the attending physician, nurses, and family.

Despite clear shortages of ICU beds and health care allocations in the majority of Muslim countries:

- A deliberate policy restricting ICU admission is rarely practised in Muslim ICUs.
- Even patients with very bad prognoses are usually admitted to ICUs.
- These patients are generally given maximum treatments initially.
- This attitude allows, in general, some time to confirm the severity of the illness.

The medical team subsequently discusses the prognosis with patients' families and gives them one of two options when the prognosis is hopeless with certitude:

- Either let the patient die in the hospital.
- Or help him to return to die at home.

The majority of Muslim patients wish to die at home, in their own bed. This practice is common in some ICUs where as many as 10% overall ICU deaths occur in the patients' home.[7] Technically, the patient is transported home in an ambulance. He/she is placed in his bed and subsequently, all life-sustaining treatments (mechanical ventilation, central venous lines, and vasopressor infusion) are removed. Death is allowed to take its natural course.

This practice has several advantages:

- First, it respects patients' wishes to die at home. This also meets families' needs to maintain close contact with loved patients.
- This procedure also allows some cultural and religious rituals while dying persons are surrounded by their families and friends.
- One additional benefit of this procedure is that it avoids all administrative procedures when death occurs at hospital, especially for families living far from the hospital.
- One of the peculiar aspects of end of life in Islam is that a rapid funeral is strongly desired by our religion (usually on the same day of death).

References

1. Sachedina A (2005). End of life: the Islamic view. *Lancet* **366**, 774–9.
2. Bulow HH, Sprung CL, Reinhart K, *et al.* (2008). The world's major religions' points of view on end-of-life decisions in the intensive care unit. *Intensive Care Med* **34**, 423–30.
3. Iyilikci L, Erbayraktar S, Gokmen N, Ellidokuz H, Kara HC, Gunerli A (2004). Practices of anaesthesiologists with regard to withholding and withdrawal of life support from the critically ill in Turkey. *Acta Anaesthesiol Scand* **48**, 457–62.
4. Yazigi A, Riachi M, Dabbar G (2005). Withholding and withdrawal of life-sustaining treatment in a Lebanese intensive care unit: a prospective observational study. *Intensive Care Med* **31**, 562–7.
5. Sprung CL, Cohen SL, Sjokvist P, *et al.* (2003). End-of-life practices in European intensive care units: the Ethicus Study. *JAMA* **290**, 790–7.
6. Sprung CL, Maia P, Bulow HH, *et al.* (2007). The importance of religious affiliation and culture on end-of-life decisions in European intensive care units. *Intensive Care Med* **33**, 1732–9.
7. Boussarsar M, Bouchoucha S (2006). Dying at home: cultural and religious preferences. *Intensive Care Med* **32**, 1917–8.

Further reading

1. Hedayat KM, Pirzadeh R (2001). Issues in Islamic biomedical ethics: a primer for the paediatrician. *Pediatrics* **108**, 965–71.
2. Daar AS, al Khitamy AB (2001). Bioethics for clinicians: 21. Islamic bioethics. *CMAJ* **164**, 60–3.

Withdrawal and withholding of life-sustaining therapies: protocolized approaches

Introduction

A number of institutions/organizations have developed and successfully implemented protocols and order sets for use by ICU clinicians and others in withdrawal or withholding of life-sustaining therapies. Below are links to some of these, which can be adapted by other institutions according to local standards and specific needs.

UK

- Liverpool Care Pathway. From link below, choose non-cancer option and then intensive care.
- ⊕ www.mcpcil.org.uk/liverpool_care_pathway

Canada

- Withdrawal of life support checklist: Queen Elizabeth II Health Sciences Centre, Halifax, Nova Scotia.
- ⊕ classic.aacn.org/PalCare/pdfs/withdrawal_support_qeII.pdf

USA

- Principles and physician orders for withdrawal of life-sustaining measures.
- ⊕ depts.washington.edu/eolcare/instruments/wls-orders2.pdf
- EPERC (end of life/palliative education resource centre)
- ⊕ www.eperc.mcw.edu/ff_index.htm

The website provides the following three-part series:

  - Fast fact and concept #033: ventilator withdrawal protocol (part I).
- ⊕ www.epcrc.mcw.edu/fastFact/ff_033.htm
  - Fast fact and concept #034: symptom control for ventilator withdrawal in the dying patient (part II).
- ⊕ www.eperc.mcw.edu/fastFact/ff_034.htm
  - Fast fact and concept #035: information for patients and families about ventilator withdrawal (part III).
- ⊕ www.eperc.mcw.edu/fastFact/ff_035.htm
- Ventilator withdrawal guidelines—Massachussetts General Hospital.
- ⊕ www.massgeneral.org/palliativecare/WithdrawalProtocol.pdf
- Procedure for withdrawal of life support in the MICU—Johns Hopkins
- ⊕ www.aacn.org/WD/Palliative/Docs/withdrawal_procedure_jhopkins.pdf
- ⊕ www.aacn.org/WD/Palliative/Docs/withdrawal_support_jhopkins.pdf
- Do-not-resuscitate orders—guidelines for physician staff, Froedtert Hospital, Milwaukee, WI.
- ⊕ www.capc.org/tools-for-palliative-care-programs/clinical-tools/policies-procedures/dnr-orders.pdf
- Adult ICU comfort care orders for the withdrawal of life support, UCSF
- ⊕ http://nursing.ucsfmedicalcenter.org/docshares/ComfortCareOrders.pdf

The Liverpool Care Pathway for patients dying in intensive care in the UK

Introduction
Rationale for a standardized approach
- Of patients dying in our hospital in the UK, approximately 10% die in ICUs.
- In the UK, for general ICUs admitting adult patients, mortality rates are about 20%, with an additional 10% of patients dying in hospital after ICU discharge.[1] Up to 70% of those patients who die have life support treatments withheld or withdrawn.[2]
- In the UK and elsewhere in Europe, there is large variation from ICU to ICU, both in the proportion of patients for whom treatment is withheld or withdrawn and in the way patients are managed during the dying process.[2]
- Families describe patients frequently suffering pain and discomfort in the days before death, and there are large differences reported in the doses of analgesic medication or sedatives administered to dying patients.[3]
- Currently, a standard care approach to death and dying does not exist in UK critical care units.

Differing approaches
Different members of the ICU team will approach end-of-life care from different perspectives.
- Nursing staff are dedicated to caring for patients and have a holistic view of the needs of the patient and the family unit.
- Doctors are more frequently engaged in problem-solving centred around the primary physiological problems of the disease.
- Conflict may arise from different perceptions about the reversibility of disease and the burden of treatment.
- Staff may be uncomfortable about the temporal relationship between discontinuing inotropes and ventilation and the time of death.
- Additionally, the medico-legal environment of the early 21st century may make doctors and nurses feel increasingly vulnerable about withdrawing and withholding treatment.
- Some clinicians worry about the 'double effect' of giving sedative and analgesic medications that may hasten the moment of death.
- Good and open communication within the team, ensuring that all views are heard, and clear standardized guidance on treatment is essential to maintain confidence of everyone involved in the process.

The transition towards a predominantly palliative approach
- Even when the clinical staff agrees about the prognosis and the need to change emphasis from intensive treatment to calm palliation, there is a vast difference in the way that doctors approach withdrawal of treatment in these critically ill patients.

- A lack of protocol and guidance at this difficult time can lead to reduced confidence in the proactive management of dying patients. This in turn can impact on the information and support given to families and the symptom control offered to patients.
- Patients, families, and medical staff may have different focuses at the end of life, but with a common overall aim to provide compassionate care.
- Patients may have concerns about being a burden to their families and do not want to be alone.
- Families want their relatives not to suffer.
- Sometimes they want to be intimately involved in end-of-life discussions and care giving, and sometimes they do not.

The Liverpool Care Pathway for the dying patient

- The goals of care for patients dying on ICU are no different than for patients dying elsewhere. The important issues to address are symptom control, psychological insight, spiritual support, and communication.
- The Liverpool Care Pathway for dying patients (LCP) was developed at the Royal Liverpool University Hospital and the Marie Curie Hospice in Liverpool initially for patients dying from cancer and has been adapted to address issues in the intensive care environment.
- The LCP is a document that is multi-professional in approach and incorporates appropriate guidelines related to end-of-life care. It provides a template for the process of care and replaces all other documentation in this phase of illness. It provides specific instructions for rationalizing interventions and for prescribing analgesia, sedation, and other medications for symptom control, and has proved helpful for patients, families, and staff.
- The development of an LCP specific to the needs of the critical care environment has allowed palliative care principles to guide end-of-life care in the ICU.
- The LCP ICU is currently being rolled out nationwide and studies are ongoing (available from: http://www.mcpcil.org.uk/liverpool_care_pathway/non-cancer/lcp_-_intensive_care_unit).

Initial assessment and care of the dying ICU patient

- As the focus of care changes from hoping for cure to comfort care, good communication is essential. Thus, the first item to be documented in the pathway is that 'the multidisciplinary team agrees that the patient is dying'.
- A judgement that the patient is, in fact, dying relies on good communication between all professionals dealing with the patient and may take several days, with discussion from all members of the multi-professional team, taking into account physiological, biochemical, and any other prognostic indicators. The family and, if possible, the patient are involved in these discussions.
- Once the decision has been reached that a patient is dying, the LCP identifies that the active care of the patient should include the goals described in Table 9.2.

Table 9.2 Initial assessment and care goals

Psychological insight

- Patient/family's ability to communicate in English assessed.
- Insight into condition assessed.
- Plan of care explained/discussed.
- Family/other expressing understanding of planned care.

Comfort measures

- Current medications assessed and non-essentials discontinued.
- PRN medication SC/IV written up according to agreed guidelines.
- Discontinue inappropriate interventions.

Religious/spiritual support

- Religious/spiritual needs assessed with the patient/family.

Communication with family/other

- Identify how the family is to be informed of impending death.
- Family/other given hospital information.

Comfort measures (continued)

- Discontinue inappropriate nursing interventions.
- Syringe driver to be set up once prescribed by physician.

Communication with primary health care team

- GP practice is aware of the patient's condition.

Ongoing care

While the provision of comfort is important at all stages of a critical illness, when it is agreed that the patient is dying, treatment refocuses from 'aggressive' intervention to preserve life to that of ensuring comfort during the dying process, for both patient and family. Explanation and communication with the family and, where possible, the patient is vital. The fact that the patient is now dying, the likely course of the illness, the DNR order, and the plan of care, as described in the LCP, are explained in as sensitive and understandable a way as possible.

- Spiritual needs of the patient and family are addressed. They should be able to discuss any outstanding issues about care and about their feelings about their role in treatment limitation. The family should be prepared for uncertainty about the precise time of death after treatment withdrawal. Nursing support is vital during the interview with medical staff and during the process of dying.
- The family should be given written documentation about the process and any relevant hospital information. When possible, the GP practice should be informed that the patient is dying as they may need to support other members of the family.

Documentation

- The underlying diagnosis is documented, as is the baseline physical condition of the patient.
- Investigations and interventions are discontinued, as are non-essential medications, including fluids and nutrition; there is an inclusive tick box list of items that allows exclusions (e.g. some families may wish fluids continued and their wishes are respected).
- We do not feel that 'staged' withdrawal is generally in the patient's or family's best interest and simply increases distress, unless there are specific reasons to justify this approach. We also recognize that the actual process of treatment withdrawal is a very contentious subject, with individual units and clinicians having their own approach. Variance is documented and reasons for variance given so that the pathway can be audited and adjusted, if necessary.
- Sedative medications are continued or infusions prescribed and started. They are titrated to effect, with the goal that the patient is comfortable, not agitated, nor excessively tachypnoeic. Analgesics are similarly titrated if required, to ensure the patient does not appear to be in pain. Muscle relaxants have no place in this situation.

Further care

- Nasogastric tubes are removed, unless the clinician anticipates that this will lead to vomiting.
- Because of the possibility of air hunger in dying patients, we normally maintain mechanical ventilation, but without positive end expiratory pressure (PEEP) and without added oxygen.
- Implantable cardiac defibrillators are deactivated.
- Nursing staff are encouraged to remove monitoring devices to allow the family the opportunity to sit with their relative, to touch, and to communicate as naturally as possible. If the nurses find it necessary to continue electronic monitoring, the bedside monitors are switched off when possible, so that the patient's signs can be observed at the nursing station only.
- Where possible, the patient is nursed in an isolation room or a separate part of the unit so that families can have unrestricted access and other patients may not be distressed.
- Observations should be less frequent and should focus on symptom control rather than physiological parameters. Nursing staff should continue to tailor medications to ensure patients are pain-free, not agitated, not vomiting, dyspnoeic or otherwise uncomfortable. Consideration should also be given to mouth care, bowel care, pressure areas, and micturition problems.
- In some cases, patients are extubated if they are not ventilator-dependent. This must be discussed with and described to the family so that they are prepared for signs of respiratory obstruction and respiratory secretions.

Care after death
- After death, the doctor documents the fact of and time of death, and staff speaks to the family; the patient is laid out according to hospital policy and cultural requirements, and the general practitioner informed.
- When appropriate, the coroner is informed.

Conclusion: role of the LCP in the ICU
The LCP ICU provides a template for the delivery of optimal end-of-life care, as it does in other environments. It also improves documentation of this aspect of care, allowing data collection and audit of care given. Experience in Liverpool shows that in the ICU, more than in any other care setting, the LCP plays a vital role in challenging the death-denying culture and raising the profile of end-of-life care. The LCP ICU encourages clinical staff to see the value in providing excellent care at the end of life; it increases confidence and reduces the stress related to this aspect of work, previously caused by a lack of clear guidance on practical matters.

References
1. Intensive Care National Audit and Research Centre (2006). Case mix programme summary statistics, 2006–7. Available from: http://www.icnarc.org/documents/Summarystatistics2006-7.pdf.
2. Sprung CL, Cohen SL, Sjokvist P, et al. (2003). End-of-life practices in European intensive care units: the Ethicus Study. *JAMA* **290**, 790–7.
3. Sprung CL, Ledoux D, Bulow HH, et al. (2008). Relieving suffering or intentionally hastening death: where do you draw the line? *Crit Care Med* **36**, 8–13.

Lessons learnt

Hope and caring amidst prognostic uncertainty: a physician's
    perspective *282*
John E Heffner

Don't rush to a bad decision *286*
Duncan Young

'I am sorry, but I have no idea who you are.' *290*
John Myburgh

Hope and caring amidst prognostic uncertainty: a physician's perspective

A sudden and devastating illness

David presented at 35 years of age with shortness of breath, right calf pain, and bilateral lung infiltrates after several weeks of generalized weakness. Lung biopsy demonstrated pathologic features of bronchiolitis obliterans with organizing pneumonia (BOOP) and leg ultrasonography detected deep venous thrombosis. Steroids and anticoagulant therapy were initiated. Five days later, David developed massive haemoptysis and severe respiratory failure with dense bilateral pulmonary consolidation. David required intubation for mechanical ventilation. Bronchoscopy confirmed diffuse alveolar haemorrhage.

David's family

David had a devoted wife, Cyndi, and three young children who visited their father daily in the ICU where he was being treated for severe acute respiratory distress syndrome. The family struggled with how their father could have suddenly become so devastatingly ill. The initial fear of losing their father and husband and suspicion of his physicians transformed slowly to an awareness of the seriousness of the illness, acceptance of the physicians, and understanding of the disease. Subsequent investigations established that David had an underlying connective tissue 'overlap' condition that had caused his lung disorder.

Clinical course

Despite plasmapheresis, management of ensuing pneumonias and episodes of sepsis with protracted periods of hypotension, repeated courses of steroids, cytotoxic therapy, and antibiotics, profound hypoxia persisted. David spent weeks at a time on 100% oxygen with high levels of positive end expiratory pressure. He required sedative and paralytic drug therapy to control his ventilation. As weeks turned to months, intervals of lucidity with brief interruptions of sedation progressed to deep coma despite the discontinuation of sedative drugs. Neurologists evaluated David with visual and auditory evoked potentials and brain imaging studies, sharing with the family a bleak prognosis. David was unlikely to survive and if he did survive, he would have at best cortical blindness and at worse poor cognitive capacity.

Devotion

Cyndi and her family demonstrated love, devotion, and concern for David, tinctured with the compassion that compels families to want desperately their father/husband to survive, yet would not commit him to a severely disabled life he would not want for himself. David's interdisciplinary ICU team had extensive discussions with the family, listened to their concerns, learned their values, and patiently awaited the important decisions about life support to emerge. Each day, hope danced with medical realities of a grave prognosis—science interweaved with love. No one was ready to make the necessary decisions. Inexplicably, and despite the intensivists' certainty that there was no reasonable chance of response to continued curative care, they could not bring themselves to encourage the withdrawal of support. But after four months in the ICU, a timetable was set for the decisions to be made over the coming days.

Skipping ahead to today

Now eight years later, David visits his pulmonary and rheumatology physicians every three months for adjustment of his azathioprine therapy that controls his connective tissue disease.

- He lost a toe to vasopressor vascular constriction and has mild muscle weakness from prolonged steroid and paralytic therapy.
- He runs his rapidly growing hotel business himself although he has to use reading glasses for the fine print of financial spreadsheets.
- Only a small peripheral visual field deficit exists in one eye.
- His pulmonary function tests demonstrate only mild restriction, but he performs all of his needed activities without limitation.
- His children busy themselves with the usual issues facing college-aged students and Cyndi has a look when she gazes at her husband that every day with him is a wondrous blessing.

What happened?

We, intensivists, practise in a world of uncertainty where life and death decisions must be made, yet our ability to predict the future is sorely limited.

Empiric studies demonstrate that critical care physicians can predict the outcome for critically ill patients within days of ICU admission in a statistically valid way. However, these predictions are not sufficiently reliable to justify irrevocable life and death decisions for individual patients in the first days of ICU care. Data are lacking for predictive abilities later in the course of ICU stays.

Making predictions

However, critical care physicians have more accurate prognosticating skills as compared with non-intensivists. Expertise and experience do matter.

Despite limitations for predicting patients' eventual outcomes, intensivists' prognostications have been shown to represent one of the most important factors in determining family decisions for the withdrawal of life support.

Because of the importance of physicians' influence, intensivists must recognize how they employ 'probabilistic thinking' in predicting the future, considering the inherent inaccuracies in existing objective prediction models.

'Probabilistic thinking' identifies the factors that influence a decision, considers the importance of each, and then determines the individual contribution of factors to the final estimate of outcome. In David's instance, disparate factors (well- to poorly defined) contribute to group decision:

- Prognosis.
- Brain imaging results.
- Consultants' opinions.
- Clinical course.
- Family hope.
- Contextual caregiver instincts.

Although efforts have focused on objectifying life-supportive decisions in the ICU, real-life ICU care requires many subjective judgements. Final decisions for withdrawing life support usually reflect:
• A great amount of personal instinct.
• Experience.
• Sharing of values with our patients and families.

Conclusion

For intensivists, predicting the future in order to formulate recommendations for withdrawal of life support will always remain a highly complex, personal, and frequently humbling experience.

Further reading

1. Knaus W (2004). Probabilistic thinking and intensive care: a world view. *Crit Care Med* **32**, 1231–2.
2. Rocker GM, Cook DJ, Sjokvist P, *et al.* for the Level of Care Study Investigators and the Canadian Critical Care Trials Group (2004). Clinician predictions of intensive care unit mortality. *Crit Care Med* **32**, 1149–54.
3. Cook D, Rocker G, Marshall J, *et al.* for the Level of Care Study Investigators and the Canadian Critical Care Trials Group (2003). Withdrawal of mechanical ventilation in anticipation of death in the intensive care unit. *N Engl J Med* **349**, 1123–32.
4. Barrera R, Nygard S, Sogoloff I I, *et al.* (2001). Accuracy of predictions of survival at admission to the intensive care unit. *J Crit Care* **16**, 32–5.

Don't rush to a bad decision

Robert was a 58-year old engineer who was transferred to our tertiary care ICU from a nearby district general hospital. He had a 5-year history of bulbar-predominant myasthenia gravis and a thymoma. The tumour had been debulked surgically, and then treated with radio- and chemotherapy, which had brought his malignancy under control, but had left him with a left phrenic nerve palsy. A localized recurrence of the thymoma had been seen on a computerized axial tomogram a few months previously and further chemotherapy was planned. A month previously, he had been admitted to his local hospital with a severe chest infection requiring mechanical ventilation, but had recovered well and returned home. He then presented again to his local hospital with severe type 2 respiratory failure, was reintubated, and transferred to our ICU for expert neurological opinion.

He rapidly improved over the next two days on standard myasthenia treatment and antibiotics. As his lung fields cleared, the chest radiographs revealed extensive changes suggestive of local and metastatic spread of his thymoma. This was confirmed with a computerized axial tomogram of his chest. Expert opinion from his oncologist reinforced our view that he had untreatable malignant disease.

On day 3, Robert was awake and alert, communicating with writing and a letter board. He could tolerate the endotracheal tube without any sedatives. Although his oxygen requirements were modest, he required significant inspiratory pressure support and attempts to wean him failed. Measurement of his respiratory mechanics suggested he had a very poor respiratory compliance, probably caused by pleural and lung involvement with the thymoma.

'How long do I have?'

Roger asked us for his diagnosis and prognosis, if he was going to live and for how long. We explained that he had an untreatable progression of his thymoma, that he had at best weeks to live, and if we could not wean him, his life expectancy was a few days at best.

Non-verbal signals

Three of the intensive care consultants involved in his treatment arranged a case conference to discuss options for palliative care, and the discussions were repeated with Roger, his family, and the hospital palliative care team. Extubation to non-invasive ventilation was considered, but the intensive care team thought it was likely to be ineffective and cause acute distress. Roger did not wish this, even with opiates to manage the distress. A tracheostomy was considered, but the intensive care team was unwilling to anaesthetize and operate on a patient, only for him to wake up again to die. There was no immediate need for a tracheostomy anyway as he was very tolerant of the endotracheal tube. We must have conveyed our anxieties about a surgical procedure used for palliative care in a non-verbal way to Roger, who subsequently became very 'anti' tracheostomy whenever it resurfaced in discussion.

Over the next two weeks, Roger gradually improved in every respect except for his dependency on assisted ventilation. He remained orally intubated, but wide awake and remarkably cheerful. The intensive care team at his local hospital had agreed to take him back so he could be closer to his family, and after a long delay (it was mid-winter and beds were at a premium), he returned to their unit.

Differing policies

Our ICU and the unit in Roger's local hospital generally have very similar policies and protocols. However, in the case of tracheostomy, practices differ markedly. Our policy was at that time very conservative with 'late' tracheostomies performed by the surgical team in the operating theatre. The policy at Roger's hospital was 'early' tracheostomy using percutaneous techniques. Given these differences in the use of tracheostomies, it is perhaps unsurprising that the consultants caring for him rapidly decided that a tracheostomy was an appropriate and a humane part of their palliative care plan. After a few days, the team had gained Roger's confidence and convinced him and his family that a tracheostomy was in his best interests. This was performed uneventfully under general anaesthetic.

ICU to home

Roger stayed in the ICU at his local hospital for another month by which time, the team had managed to wean him back to spontaneous ventilation. Roger's local hospital has a national reputation for the care and support they provide to critically ill patients after they are discharged from the unit and hospital. This expertise allowed them to discharge Roger home directly from the ICU with a comprehensive support package in place. He died peacefully in his own bed a month later.

Lessons learnt

- Patients with untreatable, but undiagnosed malignancies, will occasionally present as acute emergencies and will be resuscitated and admitted to ICUs before the diagnosis is made. Normally, these patients require sedatives for endotracheal tube tolerance and mechanical ventilation, and in the UK, when the terminal diagnosis is made, sedatives are often increased and ventilatory support withdrawn. This would have been Roger's fate had he not been so remarkably tolerant of the endotracheal tube and so had no requirements for sedatives, and he would not have had the time with his family or the option to die in his own bed. Perhaps an early managed withdrawal of treatment in the ICU is not always the best option for 'untreatable' conditions.
- Keep the patient's best interests at the core of decision-making. In Roger's case, the real risks of a tracheostomy were very small in appropriately skilled hands and the benefits clearly substantial. We did not perform one primarily because of an ill thought-through prejudice against anaesthetising a patient only to have them wake to die. Our colleagues at the referring hospital had a much clearer view of the risk/benefit balance. We also compounded the error by making Roger aware of our anxiety, so when we tried to revisit the possibility of

tracheostomy, we had lost his trust and he simply would not consider having the procedure.

• High-quality end-of-life care can be started in an ICU and carried on in a patient's home if the team has the will, experience, and organizational skills.

• There are always lessons to be learnt from colleagues elsewhere, and it is important to be aware of one's own personal and institutional biases and whether these biases support or compromise high-quality end-of-life care.

'I am sorry, but I have no idea who you are.'

The impact of the stress on relatives following the unexpected death of a loved one was exemplified in a case that I recall from some years ago.

A sudden tragedy

The patient was a 27-year old man, Dino. He collapsed whilst writing his final university law degree exams. He was admitted to the hospital, profoundly comatose with fixed and dilated pupils.

Initial CT scan confirmed widespread subarachnoid haemorrhage with acute hydrocephalus and evidence of severe intracranial hypertension. He was admitted to the ICU following placement of a ventricular drain. I met with his mother, Maria, to explain the nature of his condition and to prepare her for a likely bad outcome. Maria was understandably devastated at the situation, particularly as her husband had died from a similar event almost 20 years previously, soon after they had arrived in Australia from Italy. She had struggled to come to terms with his death and had single-handedly raised her only child since her husband's death. As expected, Dino did not respond to treatment and progressed to become brain dead 36 hours after admission. I met with Maria frequently during this period and explained in detail the course of his illness, the process of certification of brain death, and that he was now legally dead. I was fortunate to have an experienced and highly skilled social worker to attend all of the conference sessions. The social worker gently affirmed what we were discussing.

Inconsolable grief

During our meetings, Maria was inconsolable with grief, but maintained an appearance of control and dignity, speaking little, but nodding her acceptance and understanding whilst quietly weeping. The discussion moved onto organ donation. I established that Dino had indicated his wish to be an organ donor from his driver's licence and whilst Maria appeared to struggle with the concept, primarily on the grounds of her religious beliefs, she accepted Dino's decision and wanted to accede to his wishes. We discussed the benefit to others of her decision at length and I emphasized that she had the ultimate say in the decision to proceed to organ donation. I introduced her to the organ donation coordinators following which she consented to the procedure.

Last few hours

She had no relatives and few friends. During the last few hours in the ICU, she was comforted and supported by the attending nursing staff, the social worker, and the local Catholic priest. Her goodbye to Dino was heart-wrenching, with many of the staff in the ICU crying or fighting back tears, myself included. As Dino left the ICU to go to the operating theatre, Maria walked slowly past my office and I spoke to her. I expressed my condolences and sadness at her loss, but also gently thanked her for the decision to give consent to organ donation and praised her strength and dignity at such a difficult time. As is my practice, I gave her my contact details and said that should she have any questions or concerns in the future, she could come and see me at any time. I also asked our social worker and organ donation coordinator to let me know how Maria was coping during their follow-up meetings with her. Something about her loneliness and palpable sadness struck a chord with me …

Some months later

Six months later, our social worker contacted me to arrange an appointment with Maria. She had struggled to cope with the loss of her son and wanted to talk to someone in the ICU to explain to her what had happened. I remembered Maria immediately and arranged an appointment the following day. I was pleased to have the opportunity to speak to her again and possibly help her through a difficult time. She arrived at the meeting. She had aged substantially in the six months, but still maintained an air of dignity and control. She walked into my office and extended her hand. 'I am pleased you came to see me again, Maria,' I said. 'I have thought about you a lot over the last six months and wondered how you were getting on since Dino passed.' 'I am sorry, but I have no idea who you are,' she replied. 'Have we met before? Can you please tell me what happened to my son?'

Lessons learned

- The sudden, unexpected death of a beloved parent, spouse, or child is a devastating human experience.
- In the ICU, the time available to understand and accept the enormity of this is invariably far too short, no matter how much time the attending physician spends with the surviving family.
- Keep a record of these cases and always offer to speak to the family in the future.
- Few will come back, but for those that do, the opportunity to reconnect with the carers that were closest to their loved one during the process and at the end is often a vital link in understanding and accepting their loss.

Personal reflections

A sister's tale *294*
Vicki Guy

A Vietnam veteran's story *298*
Harold MacAloney

Hope—a wife's perspective *300*
Alison McCallum

Organ and tissue donation: a mother's plea for
  'a gentle ask' *302*
Denice Klavano

Personal reflections

Both contributors are current or retired nurses. Each went through an ICU experience as: (1) a sister of a dying patient, and (2) as a patient who survived. Their shared experiences and the lessons to be learnt shed light on where we need improve care for all critical care patients.

A sister's tale

I have been on both sides of the health care system. I am a registered nurse and from a family that lost one of its own after five long months in the hospital. My sister died of alcoholism. If the story were that simple, there would not be much to discuss.

Hard lessons

Those things that we know as health care professionals that we fail to educate our patients about compromise our integrity as a medical community. My sister had an alcohol withdrawal seizure at home. In the emergency room with our mother, no member of the health care team addressed the fact that my sister was the colour of a lemon nor did they ask about an advance directive or health care wishes should she rapidly get sicker than she already was. The chance was missed to actually talk to my sister about what she wanted and that chance never came again.

The first time we were approached as a family, my sister was in the ICU. She was intubated and 'knocking on death's door'. We did not know that her chance of survival was slim and should she survive, her quality of life would likely be greatly diminished. I have never questioned that the attending physicians wanted her to live as few doctors enter the medical field to do otherwise. The problem here was the lack of information given to our family to make the appropriate choice to sustain life.

Physicians change, plans change

The physicians in the ICU change weekly, which disrupts the continuity of care for a family staying for months. Each physician has an area of special expertise and tends to focus on different systems.

Back at the beginning of this journey, in our first family meeting with the ICU physician, we learned that my sister could recover, but she might not. We discussed the quality of life she would have if we needed to continue life support or if she recovered. The physician, Dr #1, reminded us that death is not the worst outcome and reassured us that no decision would be made without prior family consultation. We left feeling some hope that 'our patient' might get through this situation, but if not, we would be consulted and supported as a family.

The next week, my brother-in-law got a call from the next ICU staff physician, Dr #2, to discuss 'code status'. Her kidneys were shutting down. The decision was made, at Dr #2's suggestion, that if things 'got worse,' they would not intervene, but would continue to treat my sister until that point.

Sudden changes of direction

During week 3, Dr #3 called a family meeting. My sister was not improving; he thought her body was giving up and it was time to stop treatment. A family conference was set for the next morning to make decisions about withdrawing life support. The following day, we each had a moment with my sister before meeting with Dr #3. As I looked into the eyes I had known for 30 years, I felt incredibly guilt ridden. I did not want the responsibility of making the decision to stop life support. I did not want to always wonder if I had made the correct decision. My sister smiled when I said 'hello'. I do not know if she knew who I was or if it was a reflexive smile, but that did not matter. Suddenly, I did not know what was 'best'.

Meanwhile, Dr #3 thought my sister had improved overnight despite a gastrointestinal bleed and discussions then proceeded along a path we had not expected. Dr #3, who had consulted with the gastroenterology team, now informed us that a liver would need at least six weeks to recover, and although it was our decision to remove life support, he thought it was unfair to do so at this point in time. We suddenly felt like we were making a choice to 'kill' my sister as opposed to 'letting her die'. Dr #3 indicated that my sister had not yet signalled that she was giving up. With this sudden change in approach three weeks into her hospitalization, we could not make the decision to stop treatment. We were frightened and unsure of the decisions the health care team and we were making.

Dr #4 recommended an immediate tracheotomy. There were more differences of opinion without discussion among colleagues. We had already discussed the pros and cons of intubation vs tracheotomy with Dr #1 during week 4, and we decided to keep the endotracheal tube. My sister would not have wanted a hole in her throat. After talking with Dr #4, we felt we had made the wrong decision because this doctor was distressed that she still had an endotracheal tube and felt it had more negative consequences than a tracheotomy. A tracheotomy was placed the next morning.

Stepping down to ward care

My sister was transferred to a step-down unit soon after being weaned from the ventilator, and shortly after that, we were back on a ward unit. This time period is blurred. Days came and went, and my sister just lay in bed. She looked pregnant with ascites; the hepatic encephalopathy had progressed to ensure that each day included delusions and general confusion between some periods of lucidity. There seemed to be no treatment plan. No tests were done, no progress made.

Four months after her admission, my sister developed squamous cell carcinoma in her mouth. She deteriorated quickly before starting radiation. She was in pain and unable to talk. The doctors again had differing opinions. One did not want to give her pain medications because of her liver function; another thought it reasonable to relieve the pain. No plan of action was discussed.

At last, I realized with absolute certainty, and for the first time, that we were no longer helping my sister. I refused to watch her whimper and cry in pain any longer. I decided to be her advocate. I requested palliative care's involvement and morphine was ordered. The palliative care nurse was excellent. Comfort care was implemented and arrangements were made to try to move my sister home. With confidence, I told my sister we were trying to get her home as she wished and had been asking for months. This never happened. My sister died in the hospital four days later at the age of 46.

Lessons and hindsight

After this ordeal of life and death, I can reflect on what happened and what I think should have happened.

- My mother and sister should have been asked in the emergency room, when my sister was still conscious and alert, what her wishes were should she get sicker.
- It would have helped in the second or third week to hear about mortality statistics; we could have made more realistic decisions.
- The last five months of my sister's life were not lived in quality, nor beyond the first week in the ICU were we asked what quality of life meant to her.
- Ordinary people need to understand what the life support 'package' means and that it does not always work.
- I understand that many people choose life support and life-sustaining measures when clinicians may choose otherwise, but I think we fail to educate people appropriately and fail to ask about their wishes in a timely or meaningful manner.
- Treating teams need to understand the wishes of their patients as soon as they enter the hospital system.
- We need to learn to set goals of care in real time. There is so much to lose when these discussions do not occur.[1]
- Excellent frameworks are available as guidelines.[2]
- A choice for palliation is not a sign of failure.

Structural problems that we need to fix

Team and hospital structures created problems. As Bowman has noted,[3] 'large health care teams with shifting and inconstant members, each trained in separate professions with separate working cultures, often fracture communication and make for an environment that is not conducive to balanced discussion'.

- The weekly changeover in staff physicians creates great challenges for much needed continuity. The result in our case was shifting and conflicting information.
- Families of critically ill patients need open communication with medical teams that share similar philosophies of care and are prepared to continue that philosophy at handover time.[3,4]
- Perhaps too many teams were involved. Perhaps too few remember to look at each person as a whole instead of a collection of individual systems or body parts.

'There are worse things than dying'

My sister stated that she just wanted to go home, and I think she knew if she went home, she would die, and I also think she was OK with that decision. Though there was no way to know when she would die, it seems obvious that her death was prolonged. If frank discussions regarding prognoses were discussed earlier, perhaps more people could die at home, as many wish.[5] There are worse things than dying, as Dr #1 suggested.

Dual roles

Was it my responsibility to ask for palliative care and insist on adequate pain relief? Being a nurse created expectations of me on the part of both family and the clinicians that I found extremely difficult. In this situation, I was not a nurse—I was a sister. I should have known to call in palliative care sooner, and put an end to my sisters suffering. But we made the best decisions we could at that time, as a family, and maybe the physicians feel that way too. We all needed to retain some hope. There were many ups and downs over many months. I desperately wanted my sister to live. I wish I had known earlier how unlikely that was.

A more detailed account of this experience was published in: Guy V (2006). Liver failure, life support, family support, and palliation: an inside story. *J Crit Care* **21**, 250–2.

References

1. Quill T (2000). Initiating end-of-life discussions with seriously ill patients: addressing the elephant in the room. *JAMA* **284**, 2502–7.
2. Curtis R (2000). Communicating with patients and their families about advance care planning and end-of-life care. *Respir Care.* **45**, 1385–94.
3. Bowman K (2000). Communication, negotiation, and mediation: dealing with end-of-life decisions. *J Palliat Care* **16**, S17–23.
4. Rocker GM, Cook DJ, O'Callaghan CJ, et al. (2005). Canadian nurses' and respiratory therapists' perspectives on withdrawal of life support in the intensive care unit. *J Crit Care* **20**, 59–65.
5. Heyland DK, Lavery JV, Tranmer JE, Shortt SE, Taylor SJ (2000). Dying in Canada: is it an institutionalized, technologically supported experience? *J Palliat Care* **16**, S10–16.

A Vietnam veteran's story

Background

I served as a nurse in many military hospitals in the US and overseas, including one year in Vietnam during the war (1969–1970). I retired from the military in 1976 and went to work as a registered nurse in a German hospital. I worked as a staff nurse, unit manager, and finally as director of care and administrator of a 139-bed nursing home, retiring and returning to Canada in 1990.

I suffered a myocardial infarction in mid-June 2006. After a work-up at a regional hospital, I was transferred to the tertiary referral centre for a triple bypass. Things did not go as planned and I was not fully conscious for a few weeks.

The ICU experience: key memories

- I was given medication that caused me to have nightmares so intense that I had difficulty determining what was real or not.
- Many dreams involved me being prepared for burial, others were of war scenes in which I either felt danger or that I was captured.
- Later, I came to realize that I had been restrained. I felt that this was not right, I was not dead and my wife would not let these things go on.
- I became afraid to sleep at night. Now, two years later, these dreams are vivid in my memory as if they occurred only yesterday.

After a tracheotomy, I was eventually transferred to the step-down unit.

- I was unable to speak and although I mouthed words slowly, some doctors and some nurses told me that they could not lip-read. Others tried, mostly successfully.
- Much of the time, I had to resort to writing what I was trying to say. This became very frustrating.

In the step-down unit, I had a particularly bad spell that lasted one day and night.

- I dreamt that a new nurse had showed up and I could not determine if she was male or female.
- I saw what appeared to be a large tracheotomy scar on her neck.
- I realized that she had had a computer implanted and was programmed for nursing care.
- This was so real that several days later, when this nurse came back on duty, I was looking for that scar on her neck.
- Finally, I realized that this now was reality and the rest had been a dream.

Things that caused fear

- I was surprised to learn that on the step-down unit, we did not have call bells.
- The patients verbally called the nurse, but as I could not talk, I had to find some way to make a noise. I used a piece of plastic to tap against the bed rail.
- One nurse took this away while others saw to it that I had some way to call for them.

- Doctors who entered the unit, stood with a chart in their hands and looked at a patient from a distance, but gave no sign of greeting or of what was going on.
- I feared being sent back to the cardiovascular ICU. This was an experience that I would like to forget, but cannot.

The nurses at the tertiary referral centre all introduced themselves. Some of the younger doctors did not bother to do this, which made me feel that they may have been insecure. Sadly, at the regional hospital, the nurses did not introduce themselves.

I received good care from the majority on the step-down unit and enjoyed sharing some humour with the people there. The physiotherapist, most of the nurses, the dietitian, and most of the doctors were able to answer my questions, allay many of my fears, and give me hope of recovery.

Lessons to learn: my suggestions to improve care

- Install call bells for the patients in the unit or at least provide one for patients who are mute.
- Remember that patients not only have illness to deal with, but day-to-day worries about home and family.
- When a doctor enters a unit, a smile and a general greeting to all would be welcome.
- Have patience with your patients. Remember your patients are the reason you have a job.
- Do not tell a patient that you are going to do something and then not do it. The patient lies there and waits for you to come back.
- Don't be afraid to use some humour when dealing with your patients.

The expression 'laughter is the best medicine' is not off-key. An example of this is when I was transferred back to the regional hospital. We were unsure about whether I would need to remain on oxygen therapy, whether I would need to use a walker, and if the tracheotomy site would heal over. My family physician entered my room and said, 'Man, you're hard to kill.' This joking statement was better than any tranquilizer I could have received. In less than a week, I was able to walk without assistance or the need of oxygen.

- When a patient wants to go home, there is a reason for this. Some want to die among their loved ones as opposed to strangers. In my case, I was glad to return to the regional hospital as it meant that my wife, who was my main support, was only a five-minute drive away instead of having to make a round trip of two and a half hours to see me. This eased a worry and helped greatly in speeding up my recovery.

I am thankful for the care that I received and now two years later, I am still able to look down at the grass instead of up at the roots.

Further reading

1. Dodek PM, Heyland DK, Rocker GM, Cook DJ (2004). Translating family satisfaction data into quality improvement. *Crit Care Med* **32**, 1922–7.

Hope—a wife's perspective

I am a family physician. The setting is the final stage of my husband's long and very complicated illness. Along the way, David had been an ICU patient.

Hope is something I learned a lot about from David these last few months. Hope trumps all other sentiments as the brutal reality of a deteriorating situation emerges.

David was mystified by medicine and the medical 'system', yet he trusted implicitly that everything that was done to him was to increase his odds of survival or to teach someone something. He relied on me to be his gatekeeper.

David hoped, even on his last day, that his treatment was working and asked me to call his office for him one more time to explain he was not feeling up to talking that day, hopefully tomorrow ... He had to maintain that daily routine. He hoped to hear one more favourable outcome from one of Elizabeth's soccer games, and he hoped that one of his treating team would actually tell him the results and significance of any of the endless tests he was put through.

David did not want to die. He wanted to live another day, to be there for his children and enjoy their accomplishments and know what becomes of them. He also felt enormous responsibility for the ongoing financial stability of his three office staff and realized his office provided a refuge to them from a seemingly never-ending list of domestic woes that they had to deal with. He also enjoyed their chit-chat and laughing banter as they dealt with legal office routine. He also felt needed in his career as he knew he had the expertise ('most of it is in my head') to provide solid, accurate, honest, and fair legal counsel.

David also appreciated being needed and used as a teaching patient as, once again, he was able to feel useful in some way despite his rotten body, and hoped students would learn from his condition.

As his physical abilities fell away, he resorted to a more supervisory role. He described in great detail—and with great effort—to one of his children how the windows should be taken down, cleaned, re-glazed, re-puttied, window frames re-insulated, and finally, windows replaced. He could not understand why this was not done as soon as he asked for it to be done. His tolerance and patience ebbed as he became weaker, but seldom let his frustration be known, even in his tight circle. He was a listener, I was a talker, but he corrected me if I was inaccurate or embellished. He was a fountain of knowledge, winning all trivia games we ever played, yet he was not intellectual and not interested in listening to or reading analyses of world or political events.

David hoped, always, that his lot would improve. This is when I understood how powerful hope is as he requested more chemotherapy treatments when many of us would have expected him to throw in the towel, accept defeat, and head for the route of palliative care. Not David, he would not give up. I gave him up when I believed he finally hoped for comfort.

Organ and tissue donation: a mother's plea for 'a gentle ask'

In Canada, the word 'inukshuk' has several different meanings, but most of us recognize the arrangement of stones that represent an inukshuk. There are several interpretations of inukshuk. Inukshuks were sometimes seen as memorials to mark a place of respect or to show direction to travellers. We are all travellers. Please let me take you on my journey.

I am appealing to you as a parent. As a mum. Leave your white coats and uniforms behind and put yourself in my shoes. Reflect on the gift that is life and consider how you can share that gift at death.

'There has been an accident ... '

'Do you have a son named Brad Howell?' I could not identify the voice on the other end of the phone. I thought he said it was the Halifax regional police, but that could not be. I confirmed that Brad was my son, a reservist with the Princess Louise Fusiliers. The officer said there had been an accident at the Halifax armouries. I was confused. How could there have been an accident at the armouries?

He must mean a car accident as Brad should be driving home right about now. I was advised to come immediately to the hospital. I called to tell my other children that Brad had been in an accident and I was going to the hospital. I reassured them that it was probably nothing, may be a broken leg or something, something fixable, and I would call them as soon as I knew. It was 12.20 a.m.

I did not yet know that my son, my precious son, had just been pronounced dead.

The police were waiting for me in the parking lot at the infirmary. I thought that was unusual. An officer, clearly with tears in his eyes, took me into the hospital. They walked me to the 'family room'.

My heart stopped—not the family room—this cannot be happening. A feeling of dread began to work its way into my consciousness. Soon a nurse came in and asked if I had been told what happened ... I told her I only knew there had been an accident.

She told me that Brad had been crushed between a forklift and a truck. She had no word on his condition. The doctor would be in to speak with me shortly. My mouth went completely dry. Crushed? Crushed? One word. One single word.

Then, I saw the priest. My God, please not the priest ... Please God, please ... not my son ...

... I don't remember much after that

The doctor was kind. He had nice shoes. I remember the pattern of the floor tiles. Funny, the things you might notice when your life has just fallen apart.

No parent is ever prepared for this. I have just heard the worst news possible. It just does not get any more terrible than this. The devastation is total.

As you read this, you need to know that you need to ask the family to consider organ or tissue donation. Perhaps you are a parent yourself.

Anyone can identify with this devastation. You are, at best, uncomfortable about asking about donation, particularly at this terrible moment.

How do you approach a mother who has just found out her beloved child is dead. Don't be afraid … I am that mother.

How can anyone offer any meaningful comfort? You can. Ask about donation. It is the gentle ask.

I challenge you to let go of your own discomfort and approach this family about donation. You may be concerned about intruding upon a shock and grief of shattering proportions. I have just heard the worst possible news. You cannot make it any worse.

In the hours and days ahead of that point, I will have to make dozens of decisions; none of which I feel equipped to make and never thought I would have to. What would you like him to wear? Cremation or burial? Which cemetery? Who has to be notified? Which church? What hymns? The decisions are endless. The FIRST question that should be asked, the first of those many decisions to make should be 'would your loved one have wanted to be an organ or tissue donor?

The decision to donate is the only decision that may have the power to comfort in the days ahead. The only straw to grasp at when searching for meaning in a meaningless and senseless event.

The silent and heartfelt plea that another life may be lived through this gift. Another family spared this grief.

Be brave—ask about donation

Brad and I had discussed donation shortly before his death. His health card had come in the mail and we talked about donation. I told him to do as he wished, that just because I worked in donation, to not let that influence him. He shrugged and gave me that easy smile of his. 'Mom,' he said, gesturing to his body … 'This is only a rental.'

The gift of organ and tissue donation can give another dimension of meaning to a life too briefly lived. A newborn baby, a preschooler, a teenager. To give that family the comfort, and yes, the gift of a legacy for that precious life.

I cannot describe the comfort of knowing that my son's eyes continue to see the world, although through a different lens. The games of rugby he so loved to play will continue with the gift of tendons into another athlete or weekend warrior. Heart valves will save the life of a child with a heart defect. These are gifts of comfort to a grieving mother, to a devastated family. To know that our precious child lives on through the gift of life or mobility to others. To feel that his death was not completely in vain. Truly, a living legacy. Please, allow us, allow me, the privilege of leaving my child's footprints on the hearts of others. Even in anonymity. I will know.

Please help me honour …

Please help me honour Brad, the others who have gone before him, and those who will follow. If your loved one passes away and you are not asked, please do the asking. Could my loved one be an organ or tissue donor? Discuss donation with your families. Sign your donor cards. Share the gift of life.

Brad enriched our lives with his love, humour, and belly laughs. I believe that in the lives of those recipients as they live and love, there is a legacy. And when they laugh, I am sure there is an echo to Brad's spirit. And he is smiling.

Brad made a difference in life and also in death. Brad left his footprints on the hearts of others. My favourite meaning for inukshuk? I was here.

Thank you.

Special situations

Chronic critical illness *306*
Judith E Nelson

Ventilatory support and palliative care in amyotrophic lateral
  sclerosis *312*
*Jesus Gonzalez Bermejo, Amélie Hurbault, Christophe Coupé,
  Vincent Meininger, Thomas Similowski*

Cystic fibrosis *318*
Walter Robinson

Integrating paediatric palliative care into the paediatric intensive
  care unit *322*
Stephen Liben

Palliative care in the trauma intensive care unit *328*
Anne C Mosenthal

Non-invasive positive pressure ventilation for acute respiratory
  failure near the end of life: overview and outcomes *334*
Tasnim Sinuff

Use of non-invasive positive pressure ventilation for
  patients who have declined intubation: controversy
  and justification *338*
Tasnim Sinuff

Chronic critical illness

Advances in ICU care have enabled more patients to survive acute critical illness, but have created a new population of those who are 'chronically, critically ill.' In the US, where clinicians' authority to withhold or withdraw life-supporting ICU treatments is most closely limited, this patient group is large and growing.

How do we define chronic critical illness?

- Chronic critical illness can be identified by the placement of a tracheotomy for prolonged mechanical ventilation along with other treatments.
- Definitions based on the duration of mechanical ventilation are also used, but the time period varies and this approach may not convey the multiorgan and syndromic nature of chronic critical illness.

With ongoing catabolism and complications, including neuropathy/myopathy, anaemia, pressure ulcers, and recurrent infections, chronic critical illness is a devastating condition, imposing heavy burdens on patients, families, professional caregivers, and the health care system. Symptom suffering is common, hospital stays are long, return to the community is rare, and six-month mortality rates exceed those for most malignancies. Unquestionably, the chronically critically ill need excellent palliative care.

Integrative palliative care approach

For chronic as for acute critical illness, an integrative approach to palliative care is most appropriate, i.e.:

- Palliative care is provided as part of comprehensive intensive care to all patients, including those continuing on life-supporting therapies, and is given from the outset rather than deferred until death is clearly imminent.
- Optimal palliative care for the chronically critically ill would actually begin during the acute phase of critical illness, including early and ongoing communication about the patient's condition, treatment, prognosis, and care goals, along with the alleviation of the patient's distress, attention to family needs, and transitional planning.

Communication

After initial efforts to liberate the patient from mechanical ventilation have failed, clear communication about potential burdens and benefits of continuing critical care therapies is essential. Research has revealed that at this juncture, patients and families generally lack information that both they and their ICU caregivers agree is relevant and important for decision-making.

When critical illness is becoming chronic, what do patients and families want and need to know?

- Whether the patient is likely to achieve ventilator liberation, how long this is expected to take, and what complications can be anticipated as the treatment goes on for a prolonged time.
- What the prospects are for hospital survival, and for functional and cognitive recovery.
- In addition, they want to know about withholding or withdrawing life-prolonging treatment as an alternative approach.

Challenges for communication

Communication about chronic critical illness involves several special challenges:

- Survival of the acute phase of critical illness—although without real recovery—may create unrealistic expectations about the outcome of ongoing treatment. With the stabilization of haemodynamics and, as usually occurs after tracheotomy, lower doses of sedating medications, the patient may seem to be improving while the prospects for meaningful survival and functional recovery are actually dimming.
- Despite less pharmacologic sedation, brain dysfunction remains highly prevalent and prolonged among the chronically, critically ill, impairing their ability to participate directly in discussions and decision-making.
- Endotracheal intubation is another continuing impediment to communication, even after tracheotomy.
- Over a protracted period of hospital and ICU treatment for complex illness, the number of specialty clinicians typically increases while the role of the original primary care physician may recede. The risk of conflicting and confusing information in this situation is high.
- At the same time, high levels of anxiety and depression, as are common among ICU families, interfere with comprehension and processing of medical information.

To meet these challenges, treatment of patients with chronic critical illness and their families calls for leadership of the clinical team by a physician with advanced communication skills, a strong fund of knowledge about chronic critical illness, and an ongoing commitment to meet informational needs and coordinate care. Institution-based palliative care clinicians are increasingly available to play this role as primary caregivers or to assist other physicians with communication and care coordination.

Strategies for communication

The evidentiary foundation for specific communication strategies has not yet solidified. However, existing data and clinical experience suggest that an incremental approach, implemented as a sequence of discussions over time, is likely to be effective.

- Although it is common to defer discussion of prognosis, treatment preferences, or care goals until the futility of further treatment is obvious, and then pressure the family for a rapid reversal of direction, this approach can breed distrust, distress, and anger, and actually delay the implementation of an appropriate plan of care.
- Patients, families, and even clinicians themselves need time to consider the changing clinical course, to process and comprehend relevant information, to re-order priorities among care goals, and to prepare for and accept loss if this is unavoidable.
- When information is provided incrementally and sequentially, starting early and continuing across a series of discussions, with updates as the clinical situation evolves, this time is afforded. Ideally, decision-making in chronic critical illness occurs as a process rather than a pivotal event.
- Recent research in the setting of acute critical illness also supports the use of printed materials (e.g. brochure or leaflet) to communicate information that is relevant for medical decision-making and for

emotional and practical support of families. A brochure for distribution to families of the chronically, critically ill is under development and expected to appear in prototypical form in the near future.

Sources of suffering

Symptom suffering is highly prevalent among chronically, critically ill patients. Potential sources are many and varied, including the following:

- Underlying illness, comorbid conditions, complications (e.g. pressure ulcers).
- Diagnostic and therapeutic interventions (e.g. endotracheal suctioning, intravenous or urethral catheterization).
  - A key observation of recent research is that severe pain and discomfort are associated with non-invasive interventions such as turning in bed or moving from bed to chair, rated by patients at levels of distress similar to or greater than those for arterial blood gas puncture and central venous catheter insertion.
- Physical environment in which care is provided (e.g. loud alarms and other noxious stimuli).
- Psychological stressors (e.g. inability to communicate verbally due to endotracheal intubation, social isolation and depersonalization, and sleep deprivation).

These factors, which are known to cause distress during acute critical illness, are likely to have a cumulative impact over a prolonged period of treatment when critical illness becomes chronic.

Common symptoms in chronic critical illness

Chronic critical illness is associated with a significant burden of physical and psychological symptoms.

- Common physical symptoms include pain, dry mouth, difficulty sleeping, and dyspnoea.
- Dyspnoea is reported during full ventilatory support as well as during weaning from mechanical ventilation.
- Common psychological symptoms include feeling sad, nervous, and worried.
- Nearly all patients are greatly distressed by the inability to communicate during endotracheal intubation.

As self-reported by chronically, critically ill patients who are symptomatic, the intensity of physical and psychological symptoms is high.

Treatment of symptoms during chronic critical illness: basic premises

Existing evidence suggests that symptom treatment of chronically, critically ill patients is generally inadequate. Although effective therapies are available, the view is still widespread that their use might compromise restorative care, including efforts to liberate patients from mechanical ventilation and prolong their lives. This view is without evidentiary support. In fact, data indicate that:

- Symptom distress is associated with unfavourable outcomes, including higher mortality.

- The appropriate use of medications and non-pharmacologic techniques for analgesia and control of other distressing symptoms may actually improve physiology and outcomes, besides furthering the fundamental goal of compassionate care.

Treatment of selected symptoms

Since empirical evidence in this area is scant, recommendations for symptom treatment in chronic critical illness are derived from research in other settings and from clinical experience.

Pain

- In general, opioids are more useful for analgesia than any other class for reasons of efficacy as well as safety. There are many choices, and the drug and dose can be adjusted to address dysfunction of multiple organs as is so common with chronic critical illness.
  - Knowledge of equianalgesic dosages of various opioids is important.
  - Except for the management of procedure-related or infrequent pain, these analgesics should generally be prescribed on a standing schedule, with 'rescue' medications provided for 'breakthrough' pain.
  - In patients with renal dysfunction, the accumulation of active metabolites of morphine and meperidine are often problematic (myoclonus, prolonged sedation), indicating the preferential use of another opioid such as hydromorphone.
  - The use of a short-acting opioid such as fentanyl (or morphine) is encouraged prior to procedures that may be painful or uncomfortable, including pressure ulcer care and turning or repositioning of patients for whom this has previously been distressing.
  - Close monitoring of effectiveness and side effects of the analgesic regimen is required.
  - Side effects of opioids should not deter their use as they are needed to relieve pain that is refractory to treatment of underlying causes. These effects can usually be managed by clinicians with the appropriate knowledge and skills such as those trained in palliative medicine.

Dyspnoea

- Dyspnoea is commonly experienced by mechanically ventilated patients, even during periods of 'full' ventilatory support. Clinicians may hesitate to treat dyspnoea with opiates except when death is imminent, but this reluctance is not supported by existing evidence.
  - Opiates offer the most effective relief of dyspnoea.
  - Data suggest that the appropriate use of opiates, which reduce exertional dyspnoea and improve exercise tolerance, may actually facilitate liberation from mechanical ventilation and overall recovery.
  - In cancer patients, low doses of opiates (e.g. 5mg for opioid naïve patients) can relieve dyspnoea without lowering the respiratory rate or oxygen saturation, or raising CO_2. Safety in tracheotomized patients should be even greater since they can be immediately returned to full mechanical ventilation at any time.

Inability to communicate

- Among patients requiring prolonged mechanical ventilation via any route of endotracheal intubation, including tracheotomy, distress due to inability to communicate is highly prevalent. Every effort should be made to facilitate patient communication, both to relieve this distress and to permit greater participation in establishing a care plan that respects the patient's preferences, values, and goals.
  - Valved or fenestrated tracheotomy devices can be used to augment speech.
  - Other techniques such as picture-letter boards and writing should be used liberally to promote non-verbal communication.
  - Use of physical restraints should be minimized as these impede gesturing, which is an important form of non-verbal communication, and may limit communication indirectly by increasing anxiety, frustration, depression, and social withdrawal.

Delirium

Brain dysfunction, including delirium, is now known to be a prominent feature of chronic critical illness. Not only is prevalence high, but the duration of delirium among the chronically, critically ill is prolonged—significantly longer than it is typical during acute critical illness, even though doses of opiates and sedatives are generally lower after tracheotomy—and is associated with longer lengths of stay in the hospital and poorer functional status for survivors.

- No published data have yet identified factors that are clearly associated with the onset of delirium during chronic critical illness, but research in other settings suggests that benzodiazepine administration and untreated pain may play a role.
- For treatment of delirium, major tranquilizers/antipsychotics such as haloperidol are preferred over benzodiazepines, which may actually worsen delirium.

Further reading

1. Camhi SL, Nelson JE (2007). Chronic critical illness. In: Vincent, JL (ed). *Yearbook of intensive care and emergency medicine*, pp 908–17. Springer–Verlag, Berlin.
2. Carson SS (2006). Outcomes of prolonged mechanical ventilation. *Curr Opin Crit Care* **12**, 405–11.
3. Nelson JE, Mercado AF, Camhi SL, *et al.* (2007). Communication about chronic critical illness. *Arch Intern Med* **167**, 2509–15.
4. Nelson JE, Tandon N, Mercado AF, Camhi SL, Ely EW, Morrison RS (2006). Brain dysfunction: another burden for the chronically critically ill. *Arch Intern Med* **166**, 1993–9.
5. Nelson JE, Meier DE, Litke A, Natale DA, Siegel RE, Morrison RS (2004). The symptom burden of chronic critical illness. *Crit Care Med* **32**, 1527–34.
6. Nelson JE (2002). Palliative care in chronic critical illness. *Crit Care Clin* **18**, 659–81.

Ventilatory support and palliative care in amyotrophic lateral sclerosis

Introduction

Patients with neuromuscular disease are sometimes managed in an ICU setting at some point in their clinical course. Decisions to withhold, provide, continue, or withdraw life support will become necessary for all such patients eventually.

In this chapter, we use amyotrophic lateral sclerosis (ALS) as an example and consider some facets of management that need to be understood by ICU clinicians (see also 📖 in 'Don't rush to a bad decision' p286).

Background

ALS is a degenerative motor neuron disease. The annual incidence of ALS is 1.5 to 2.5 per 100,000 with a prevalence rate of 6 to 8 per 100,000.

- Mean survival is 30 months from diagnosis and less than six months after the onset of diaphragmatic involvement. Death usually occurs from chronic progressive respiratory failure with respiratory muscle dysfunction.
- The terminal stage is accompanied by numerous symptoms: dyspnoea, weakness, physical fatigue, reduced activity level, mental fatigue, loss of motivation.
- More than half of patients complain of communication difficulties, pain, dyspnoea, and sleep disturbance.
- The disease is one of changes and losses that can lead to both physical and psychosocial decline for patients and to some extent, their families.
- In some studies, up to 50% of patients refused information on life-threatening complications of their disease, remained undecided, or did not complete any advance directives concerning treatment in the terminal stage.
- Denial may be part of the patient's defence mechanisms. This can hinder communication with clinicians on this anxiety-provoking subject and limit discussions about future care management (life with assisted ventilation).
- Sessions with a psychologist can/may be helpful and can provide an evaluation of the patient's ability to take in and understand such decisions, but not all patients will be willing to see a psychologist.

Who decides goals of care?

- Denial in the ALS population is more predominant than in cancer. Patients often do not discuss end-of-life issues and goals of care until a crisis occurs. That being said, we should do our best to move to a model of care that preserves patient autonomy and is family-centred.
- Decision-making is a process and should be shared by patients/families and health care providers. Patients and families rely on the health care team to give them all the information they need to make a decision and we cannot pass the entire responsibility for these decisions over to patients/families. We need to be clear in our language, realistic, and truthful.

Discussing the need for assisted ventilation

- Some reasonable goals: reverse what is reversible, enhance function when possible, provide comfort, and aim to optimize the patient's perceived quality of life for as long as possible.
- Values and therefore, choices change over time and illness. Health care teams need to facilitate communication in order to determine what is meaningful to patients and families.
- Truth-telling in difficult clinical settings is a skill and requires compassion and emotional intelligence. For example, it is okay to explain that every patient is unique and that we do not have a crystal ball, but that in our experience … 'This is what I can share with you that may help you to better understand and feel better about the decisions you may make … ' This kind of approach can facilitate discussions and decision-making.
- Ethics consultation/committee involvement may be helpful in especially difficult cases.

Discussing palliation

Clinical experience has shown that the term 'palliative care' can sometimes be difficult to accept for the patient. For the patient, it can be seen as the abandonment of any hope, defeat, etc. …

These feelings can be limited by following a few recommendations:

- Emphasis can be placed on the concepts of comfort and support.
- If the term palliative care is brought up by the patient or the family, the discussion should be resumed by asking what the term means to them. In this context, the following exchange is a suggestion: '*Patient*: Are you talking about palliative care, doctor? *Doctor*: Yes, that is one name for it. The term can have different meanings. I'd like you to tell me what it means to you … '
- Keep in mind that the patient's neurologist should continue to play a key role in the care management and continuing neurology consultations is a priority, even though the patient's respiratory condition makes this difficult (ventilator-dependent patient, patient in intensive care, patient in rehabilitation, etc.).

Discussions about assisted ventilation

Assisted ventilation becomes a consideration in hypercapnic patients, those with a vital capacity less than 50% predicted or with nocturnal SpO_2 <90% in the absence of other causes of hypoxaemia.

Mitsumoto and Rabkin provide this explanation: 'Many assistive devices can greatly help your breathing which, if left unassisted, may decrease your energy levels and impede your sleep at night. One such device is a non-invasive positive pressure ventilator. It includes an easy-to-use mask that fits on your face. It should increase energy and provide better sleep.' We would add: 'It may also relieve your shortness of breath when you use assisted ventilation, and probably also when breathing unassisted.' Mouthpiece ventilation can also be considered if the patient has enough bulbar function.

Discussions about assisted ventilation are a collective decision process. These points need to be considered:

- Assessment of ALS-induced handicap and rapidity of the disease progression.

- Assessment of patient comfort.
- Investigation of future treatment choices.
- Assessment of the patient's wishes (after they consider comprehensive information).
- Investigation of advance directives.
- Consultation with care providers involved in home care, the family doctor, consultant in charge, clinical psychologist, etc.
- Consultation with the health care proxy.
- Consultation with the family (psychological vulnerability).
- When relevant, check technical and financial feasibility of the possibility of a return home after initiating assisted ventilation.
- In their supporting roles, clinicians must fully respect the patient's preferences and values.

The need for ventilation (and possibly tracheostomy) should always be discussed in advance whenever possible

When respiratory failure occurs, discussions about ventilatory support should not be handled exclusively by the respiratory medicine specialist or the intensivist who will be initiating assisted ventilation. It requires multidisciplinary consultation and information-sharing to ensure a consensus view.

What kind of assisted ventilation in ALS

- Non-invasive ventilation (NIV) in ALS improves respiratory symptoms, fatigue, and sleep disturbance, and reduces the number of hospitalizations.
- NIV in ALS is both palliative care and life-supporting. High-level evidence shows that life is prolonged with NIV. From our own data on 150 ALS patients supported by NIV, the median survival is two years and three patients have been ventilated for more than five years.

Assisted ventilation through a tracheostomy allows easier suctioning of pulmonary secretions; it avoids repeated aspirations in patients presenting with sialorrhoea or bulbar ALS. However, whether tracheostomy meets palliative care objectives remains controversial.

The intubated patient

After initiating assisted ventilation, we advise:
- Retrieving the information listed above (advance information).
- Attempting early NIV; this will often require extubation of the patient and a decision that needs to be discussed collectively with the patient and with the family. If NIV proves unacceptable or ineffective, palliation should be provided for dyspnoea and sialorrhoea in the knowledge that death will likely follow before long.

When assisted ventilation is rejected in ALS

When assisted ventilation is unacceptable to a patient, the subject should not be raised again. This only increases anxiety unnecessarily. Respiratory symptoms are treated medically. Oxygen has unpredictable effects, is not very helpful, and for some, may be harmful (if it worsens alveolar hypoventilation) and cannot be routinely recommended.

Ventilation withdrawal
- As with any end-of-life situation involving dyspnoea, opiates and benzodiazepines, with or without oxygen administration, are effective in relieving symptoms when assisted ventilation is reduced/withdrawn. Their use should be individualized, based on prior needs, and where distress is anticipated, they should be started before reducing/stopping assisted ventilation. Temporary re-introduction of assisted ventilation with plans to reduce it more gradually can be defended if the sedative doses administered are not sufficient to provide comfort and peace.
- Clinicians should reassure the family concerning pauses in breathing or agonal gasps, which should not be misinterpreted as signs of pain/distress, but rather as features of a natural dying process.

Treatment of bronchial congestion in the terminal stage
- Bronchial congestion can be very uncomfortable in the absence of an effective cough. Manually assisted coughing, in particular, CoughAssist™ type devices, has never been shown to be effective in terminal stages, though they can be effective in earlier stages of the illness.
- Translaryngeal suction is invasive, painful, and only effective for a very limited period. It should not be used in the terminal stage.
- Medical treatments can be used to reduce secretions, e.g. glycopyrrolate, atropine and scopolamine.

Support of the family

It is important to realize that mourning begins even before the death of a loved one. Mourning is a normal and universal process that everyone will inevitably go through. According to E. Kübler–Ross, the resolution of mourning occurs in successive stages: denial, anger, bargaining, depression, then finally, acceptance.

However, individuals go through the process at their own pace and rely on different individual resources. The clinical psychologist can facilitate mourning. Support can be proposed through conversations, but people in mourning often prefer to work through the first stages alone. In these cases, it is important to let them know that a meeting can always be organized later, and that follow-up is possible in a setting of their choice.

Distress of teams managing the care of patients with ALS who present with respiratory failure

- It is important to remember that when an ALS patient arrives in the ICU, it is not always due to a failure of communication in another health care setting (remembering that patients/families are not always willing to discuss these difficult issues until a crisis occurs).
- Faced with the extreme physical dependence and psychological distress of patients/families living with this disease, clinicians can experience feelings of guilt, frustration, helplessness, and anxiety.
- Finding the right balance between maintaining a necessary distance and getting too emotionally involved can be difficult.
- Patient's dependence on mechanical ventilation is an additional source of anxiety if the team lacks expertise in using these devices.

It is important to have mechanisms in place to help support ICU staff so they can provide the best care to patients and families. Support groups and focus groups on clinical practice can enable the medical team to:
- Achieve a better understanding of ALS and its progression, and thus provide more empathetic care to patients and families.
- Share their experiences during a period of time set aside for reflection, specifically to restore communication and confidence within the team which is often adversely affected in the context of such distress.

Conclusions

Despite having a predictable disease course, many patients with ALS defer decision-making until a crisis and arrive in emergency rooms and ICUs. Decision-making is complex in these circumstances and effective communication is the only recipe that will yield success. There are assisted ventilation devices that have the potential to prolong life and more importantly, the quality of life and relief of dyspnoea. The initiation of these devices requires careful consideration. As in many chronic diseases with fatal outcomes, the management of quality palliative care in ALS can only result from group reflection and multidisciplinary teamwork; the doctor and the patient are only two members of this team.

Further reading

1. Lou JS, Reeves A, Benice T, Sexton G (2003). Fatigue and depression are associated with poor quality of life in amyotrophic lateral sclerosis. *Neurology* **60**, 122–3.
2. A consensus conference report (1999). Clinical indications for non-invasive positive pressure ventilation in chronic respiratory failure due to restrictive lung disease, COPD, and nocturnal hypoventilation. *Chest* **116**, 521–34.
3. Bourke SC, Tomlinson M, Williams TL, Bullock RE, Shaw PJ, Gibson GJ (2006). Effects of non-invasive ventilation on survival and quality of life in patients with amyotrophic lateral sclerosis: a randomized controlled trial. *Lancet Neurol* **5**, 140–7.
4. Van den Berg JP, Kalmijn S, Lindeman E, *et al.* (2005). Multidisciplinary amyotrophic lateral sclerosis care improves quality of life in patients with amyotrophic lateral sclerosis. *Neurology* **65**, 1264–7.
5. Mitsumoto H, Rabkin JG (2007). Palliative care for patients with amyotrophic lateral sclerosis: 'prepare for the worst and hope for the best'. *JAMA* **298**, 207–16.

Cystic fibrosis

Overview

Cystic fibrosis (CF) is a clinical success story of the 20th century. From a fatal diagnosis in infants in 1938, CF has progressed to a chronic, but manageable illness of adolescents and young adults. In North America, there will soon be more adults than children with CF. Unfortunately, the overwhelming majority of patients with CF will still die of respiratory failure in adulthood.

Prior to the 1990s, admission to the ICU for patients with CF was uncommon, and generally limited to infants or older patients with acute reversible problems such as rib fracture. However, with the advent of bilateral lung transplantation and the improving longevity of individuals with CF, admissions to ICUs are increasing. The number of patients who receive palliative care and subsequently die in ICUs is also increasing.

Advance care planning

Although one might expect that individuals living with a chronic and life-limiting disease would be more likely to have made advanced care plans, several aspects of CF care may act to limit the number of patients with documented DNR orders or advance directives:

- CF clinicians are often unreservedly optimistic, given their appropriate emphasis on the ability of the daily CF regimen to extend life and the rapid increase in life expectancy in the past decade.
- As a consequence, CF clinicians may be reluctant to discuss advance care planning with adults with CF. A recent US study of CF adults suggested that while two thirds wanted to discuss advance care planning with their clinicians, only one third have had such a discussion with CF clinicians.
- The availability of lung transplantation may also complicate advanced care planning. Many patients with severe CF lung disease may be listed for transplantation, and therefore, may desire more aggressive care to extend life in hope of an organ becoming available. As a result, patients and families with CF may want simultaneously to pursue aggressive restorative care and symptom relief, and this option should be offered.

For those on the transplant list, careful consultation with the transplant team will facilitate care planning. For example, there could be disagreement among transplant teams about the suitability of transplantation after endotracheal intubation for respiratory failure. Non-invasive ventilation earlier in the course of the admission, if it forestalls intubation, may help in maintaining transplant viability.

Prognostic indicators

Several studies of the outcome of ICU care in CF have been performed, yet institutional differences (such as the degree to which non-invasive ventilation is used) make comparison of these studies difficult. No single prognostic indicator has been found to predict survival to ICU discharge. However, patients having three or more of the following factors have a poor prognosis:

- $PaCO_2$ >50mmHg (6.7kPa).

- Lack of previous response to intensive multi-antibiotic therapy for an infective exacerbation.
- Multiply resistant organisms in the sputum.
- Portal hypertension secondary to CF liver disease.
- Nutritional failure to the degree that the patient is cachectic despite sufficient nutritional intake.

Only in one study was the pre-admission pulmonary function, as measured by FEV1, predictive of survival to discharge from the ICU.

Distinctive factors in CF care in ICU

Difficulty of maintaining airway clearance

Positive pressure ventilation, endotracheal incubation, and/or sedation will limit the ability to cough and cooperate with airway clearance techniques. No amount of tracheal suctioning can equal the airway clearing efficacy of chest physical therapy and coughing, and so regular chest physical therapy for airway clearance is an essential aspect of restorative or palliative care for CF in the ICU.

Patients, their families, and CF clinicians are likely to be experts in the various modes of airway clearance, and their experience should be solicited. Use of mucolytics such as hypertonic saline or Pulmozyme® may assist in airway clearance. Delivery of nebulized antibiotics such as tobramycin or aztreonam may enhance proximal airway clearance.

Abdominal pain

The presence of abdominal pain, absence of bowel sounds, or failure to pass stools should trigger abdominal X-rays to exclude distal intestinal obstruction syndrome (DIOS), which is the formation of obstructing stools in the small and large bowels.

Risk factors for the development of DIOS include:
- Dehydration.
- Missed doses of pancreatic enzyme supplementation.
- Opioid therapy.

Preventative use of lactulose or intestinal lavage with electrolyte solutions should be considered on admission to the ICU, and continuation of oral pancreatic supplementation is essential with any oral intake of fat. At a minimum, oral lactulose should be used with the administration of any opioids.

New onset diabetes

This may occur in patients with CF admitted to the ICU. Approximately 20% of all adults with CF will develop CF-related diabetes (CFRD). The onset may be more subtle than those with other types of diabetes. Early detection through glucose surveillance, and glucose control once diagnosed with CFRD, is essential in order to maintain good nutritional and pulmonary status.

Burkholderia cepacia infection

This can lead to the so-called 'cepacia syndrome', a sepsis-like picture with high fever and rapid decline towards multiorgan system failure. Fever and bacteraemia are uncommon in CF, so the presence of signs of bacteraemia in those with *Burkholderia cepacia* should trigger immediate and aggressive antibiotic therapy, with consultation of the infectious disease service to explore possible synergy between multiple antibiotics.

Massive haemoptysis

If greater than 240mL over 24 hours, it can be a terminal event in CF.

- Bleeding results from rupture of newly formed bronchial arteries near areas of bronchiectasis.
- Bronchial artery embolization, though not without risk, can be effective in controlling bleeding.
- Even after embolization, patients with a prior episode of massive haemoptysis have an increased risk of recurrence.

During a massive haemoptysis, rapid sedation may be effective in reducing the understandable fear and in limiting deep coughing, which may worsen the bleeding. Use of dark towels to minimize the visual impact of the expectorated blood may also minimize the understandable fear of the patient and the family during the episodes.

Symptom control in the ICU

Chronic pain is part of life for many patients with CF. Near the end of life, the frequency of headache and chest pain accelerates, compounding the distress due to worsening dyspnoea.

Headache

Two distinctive aspects of headache in CF patients should be mentioned.

- Many CF patients have long-standing sinusitis and nasal polyposis. They may have developed pain from erosion into the surrounding structures. ENT consultation with consideration of sinus lavage may be appropriate.
- Many CF patients may have developed chronic morning headaches secondary to hypoxaemia during sleep. Although analgesia is sometimes effective for these headaches, a more effective treatment is nocturnal, non-invasive ventilation to correct the gas exchange anomalies during sleep.

Chest wall pain

For many CF patients, chest wall pain can be severe. The most common sources of chest wall pain are:

- Anterior vertebral compression fractures secondary to osteoporosis.
- Rib fractures secondary to osteoporosis and chronic cough.
- Musculoskeletal pain such as trigger point pain—again due to frequent coughing and hyper-expansion of the chest wall.

Treatment of this pain with local musculoskeletal therapies as well as systemic analgesia is always appropriate and will facilitate airway clearance.

Dyspnoea

This is the hallmark of severe end-stage CF. Therapy for dyspnoea should be grounded in two approaches:

- Treat the underlying infective exacerbation with aggressive use of combination antibiotic therapy and airway clearance.
- Relieve the sensation of breathlessness, usually with opioid therapy.

Improved airway clearance, provision of supplemental oxygen, and respiratory support during sleep with non-invasive ventilation have all been demonstrated to improve the sensation of breathlessness in adults with severe CF lung disease. Therapeutic manoeuvres which are successful in other patients with dyspnoea due to end-stage chronic obstructive pulmonary disease (COPD), such as opioids, will also be effective in CF.

Anorexia and fatigue

These are common symptoms in end-stage patients with CF. Combined with difficulties with sleeping, these symptoms can be deeply troubling to patients and families. If opioid therapy for dyspnoea is sedating, consideration should be given to intermittent use of stimulants to maintain wakefulness so that communication with families is possible.

Summary

The ICU management of patients with CF presents many serious challenges. Overcoming these challenges requires close collaboration between multiple disciplines and specialties. Quality care at the end of life for patient with CF requires an ICU culture where all patients are valued, respected, and their dignity is preserved.

Further reading

1. Thomas SR (2003). The pulmonary physician in critical care. Illustrative case: cystic fibrosis. *Thorax* **58**, 357–60.
2. Texereau J, Jamal D, Choukroun G, *et al.* (2006). Determinants of mortality for adults with cystic fibrosis admitted in intensive care unit: a multicentre study. *Respir Res* **7**, 14.
3. Sood N, Padarowski L, Yankaskas J (2001). Outcomes of intensive care unit care for adults with cystic fibrosis. *Am J Respir Crit Care Med* **163**, 335–8.
4. Sawicki GS, Dill EJ, Asher D, Sellers DE, Robinson WM (2008). Advance care planning in adults with cystic fibrosis. *J Palliat Med* **11**, 1135–41.
5. Kremer TM, Zwerdling RG, Michelson PH, O'Sullivan P (2008). Intensive care management of the patient with cystic fibrosis. *J Intensive Care Med* **23**, 159–77.

Integrating paediatric palliative care into the paediatric intensive care unit

Communication: when done right, intensive care is indistinguishable from palliative care—the case of Carmen

Carmen, a 12-year old with severe cerebral palsy, seizure disorder, and dependent on g-tube feeding was admitted to the paediatric ICU (PICU) with her fourth episode of respiratory failure in two years, likely due to aspiration pneumonia. Weaning from each episode of mechanical ventilation had taken longer each time and she was oxygen-dependent at home for the past six months. Within the last year, her previously very good quality of life at home had declined as she became progressively distressed by increasing dystonia and difficulty with oral secretions (despite maximal treatment).

On this admission, her primary care physician, the hospital palliative care team, and the PICU team met first separately and then with her parents to discuss options and choices in her care.

After several discussions, a care plan was agreed upon that focused on Carmen's quality of life and symptom control while in the PICU as well as on activities that she would enjoy while being weaned from the ventilator (e.g. music therapy and massage therapy).

While it was agreed that she would receive neither chest compressions nor cardioversion in the event of a cardiorespiratory arrest, it was also agreed that she might benefit from BiPAP as a bridge to support her after extubation, but that in the event she was unable to breathe adequately with BiPAP, she would not be re-intubated and the focus would be on comfort.

The team and parents agreed to wean Carmen directly to BiPAP (rather than extubate her and wait to see how she did with oxygen alone). After ten days, she was extubated to BiPAP and initially did well, but over the next week, and despite maximal BiPAP support, she progressed to increasing respiratory distress and required a continuous infusion of morphine to treat her obvious dyspnoea. Her parents felt that she was uncomfortable with continuous BiPAP and they understood that she was likely dying. The BiPAP mask was removed, her dyspnoea was well controlled with medication, and she died two days later in her mother's arms.

Mortality in the PICU

- Depends on patient population (e.g. referral centres managing complex cardiac post-operative children have higher mortality rates than non-referral-based non-post-operative ICUs)
- Most of the children who die in the PICU are less than four years old and most die while still sedated and ventilated.
- In North American PICUs, the most common mode of death is after active withdrawal of 'life-sustaining treatment' therapy such as removing a ventilator or following decisions to not attempt cardiopulmonary resuscitation, The frequency of removal of life-sustaining treatment may be lower in South America and Europe.

Pain and symptom management

- Pain is difficult, but essential, to assess in critically ill neonates and children.
- Many children in the ICU receive continuous infusions of sedatives and analgesics started either post-operatively or at the initiation of mechanical ventilation. Some children are placed on continuous or regular intermittent doses of neuromuscular blockers that result in muscle relaxation and paralysis of skeletal muscle without any analgesic or sedative effects. Children on neuromuscular blocking drugs will not move and cannot breathe on their own. **In most circumstances, it is possible and desirable to intermittently interrupt the use of regular neuromuscular blockers in order to assess the level of comfort and sedation of the child.**
- After an acute neurological event, it may be difficult for both parents and staff to appreciate the level of neurological function in the presence of high doses of sedative/analgesics.
  - Carefully lower the amount of sedation to allow for a better evaluation of the level of consciousness and amount of pain. There is neither indication nor rationale for increasing sedatives just because the child 'has suffered enough'. Rather, the point of sedative/analgesic administration is to respond to pain by first assessing its cause and intensity and then to selectively apply pain management principles as would be done for any child in pain.
- Non-pharmacological pain management techniques can be adapted for use in the PICU.
  - Encourage parents to hold their critically ill child in their arms, even while the child remains connected to a ventilator and multiple infusion pumps.
  - Massage therapy.
  - Music therapy.
  - For older children who are conscious, art therapy, and even zoo therapy (interactive activities with animals) may sometimes be possible.

Maintaining hope and communicating with children and families

- Most children who die in the PICU do not have the ability to communicate verbally because they were either pre-verbal due to their young age or non-verbal because of their pre-existing medical condition.
  - For verbal children, communication is still very limited during their illness in the ICU, either because of the illness itself or the life support technology. This means that these children are often deprived of the opportunity to talk about their illness and impending death. These limitations also restrict these ill children's ability to communicate their fears, wishes, dreams, hopes and desires about their life in general and about their possible death in particular.
  - Non-verbal means of communication are thus often very important in communication with critically ill children.

- Siblings can be helped to cope with their brother's or sister's death by being given the opportunity to help with their care in a supervized manner. ICUs can facilitate this by having visiting policies that encourage parents to bring siblings for short visits.
- Maintaining hope is a cornerstone of paediatric palliative care and is a common and challenging task for children, parents, and professionals.
  - The difficult question is sometimes asked directly—'how can we maintain hope in the face of our child's death?'—or indirectly in other ways, e.g. 'what do we do now?', 'how can we go on?', 'what is the point of anything?' These questions speak to the need to maintain hope and the struggle to find meaning in the tragic loss that is the death of a child. In the face of such questions (which may be unspoken), the role and challenge for those working in paediatric intensive care are to assist in reframing what hope can be when a cure is no longer possible.
  - A starting point for the health care professional is to recognize his or her own need to maintain hope and to find meaning in the work that he or she does. 'Hoping' is understood to be distinct from 'wishing.' Hope is the understanding that things will somehow be all right, no matter what the outcome. Wishing may be another way to deny reality and is the insistence that, despite the facts, the outcome will somehow 'magically' be different.

A practical approach to maintaining hope is to:
- Accept that at times, loss of hope may be part of the process.
- Be an active listener as families may find their own way to meaning.
- Facilitate the process that leads to a shift from hoping for cure, to hoping for quality of life, to hoping that death will be as comfortable as possible. While dying 'healed' may be an unrealistic goal for many children in the PICU, there is still much to be gained by addressing issues related to the child and family's emotional and spiritual needs. The beginning of addressing these needs begins with an assessment of the child and family as whole persons. In practice, this evaluation of the whole person means asking questions not necessarily traditionally addressed in paediatric critical care such as:
  - What is the most important thing in your life right now?
  - What is happening in the ICU that is stopping you from making the most of the time you have with your child right now?
  - Are there important celebrations that you would consider having on the ICU very soon, even before the 'real' date (e.g. birthdays, Christmas, etc. …)?

Decision-making

- One challenge in paediatric palliative care is to help parents make decisions that respect what is in the best interests of their child vs those decisions that may help to alleviate their own legitimate suffering.
- When it is difficult to separate the non-verbal child's suffering from that of the parents, it can be helpful to reframe the situation by asking parents to try to interpret what their child may be 'telling' them in actions as opposed to in words.

- Some parents come to interpret repeated life-threatening episodes as meaning that their child is 'ready to go' and may find some solace in knowing that they have found a way to 'listen' to the non-verbal messages their child is sending.

Setting goals

- Acknowledging that a child is terminally ill is especially difficult in an intensive care environment. An advantage of doing so is that all diagnostic tests and therapies are directed towards a common goal: to increase the comfort and quality of life of the child (as opposed to the usual goal of striving to maintain life). For example, a child who suffered an anoxic insult with subsequent seizures will clearly be more comfortable not seizing and therefore, the use of anticonvulsants is indicated even if the child is terminally ill, but should the same child develop pneumonia, the question of the use of antibiotics is less clear and requires thoughtful and sensitive discussion about benefits and burdens of therapy. However, **one should avoid an order for 'no tests' or 'do not escalate' placed in the chart, but rather do everything possible to ensure maximum comfort and quality of life for the child**.

As the time of death approaches

- There are children who die in the ICU with little prior warning for parents. Examples are neonates born at term, but who unexpectedly die from birth complications, sepsis, or have congenital heart or other congenital abnormalities; in older children, it may be from severe trauma or sepsis.
- Another group are children with known conditions that were thought to be stable. For these children, there may be little or no time available to plan for how death will occur and palliative care may have more to offer the family survivors after the child has died. In one review of circumstances surrounding end-of-life in a PICU, it was found that decisions to forgo life-sustaining treatment required one to two meetings before consensus was reached. For the many children who die in the ICU after a decision to withdraw life-sustaining therapies, it is often possible to guide families as to what to expect and to offer options for different ways that the end of life can happen.
- As the time of withdrawal of life-sustaining therapies approaches consider:
  - The family may appreciate being transferred to a private room.
  - For some families, it is important that the extended family get to say goodbye and to hold the child in their arms before extubation.
  - For other families, it may be important to have very few people present in the room at the time of withdrawal.
  - Some PICUs take pictures of the child and family, make footprints of infants, and/or cut a locket of hair to give to the family to keep as physical memories.
  - Some families are keen for the child to go home or to a hospice on ventilator support with removal of the ventilator occurring once the child is at home or in a hospice.

- Many parents find it both hard and at the same time, comforting to have their child in their arms before and while the tracheal tube is being removed. Some mothers have commented that they were present for the entry of their child into the world and they want to be present when they leave.
- Once the decision has been made to withdraw mechanical ventilatory support, the child and family should be guided through how the process will unfold. It is important to be sure that family as well as ICU staff understand that the child is not having care withdrawn, but is instead having a treatment removed that no longer has more benefits than burdens.
- For children on full ventilator support, it is important to establish a plan for the control of dyspnoea and secretions upon withdrawal of the ventilator.

After the death

- Allow the family to stay with their child in the room until they are ready to leave.
- Prior to bathing/washing the body, ICU staff can remove sutures holding catheters in place and medical devices can be removed.
- Some parents appreciate being offered the opportunity to clean and bathe the body with staff.
- A discussion should take place concerning the possible benefits of an autopsy, which will usually have been considered before death.
- Most institutions have a forum for the team to review morbidities and mortalities that happened in the unit. These reviews are often orientated around medical issues pertaining to pathology and symptom control and lessons learnt for the future. They also offer the opportunity to look at the psychological impact of deaths on the families and the health care professionals. They also allow staff not on duty at the time of the child's death to be brought up to date and understand the full circumstances surrounding the child's death, and to ask questions and consider unresolved issues.
- After a child dies, there are a number of ways to commemorate the child:
  - One way is for staff to write messages for the family in a card that can be sent to them in the following weeks. This also gives staff who were absent at the time of death the opportunity to offer their condolences to the family. Staff may wish to create a 'communication book' for the unit in which those who were present at the time of death can write down what happened as well as their thoughts and feelings about the child.
  - A memorial book may be placed in the unit, chapel, or elsewhere in the hospital and some families may wish to co-design a commemorative page in the book. Offering parents different options on how to commemorate their child who died in the PICU can also help avoid creating a large 'memorial wall of plaques' in the PICU that parents of other temporarily hospitalized children may find uncomfortable.

- The senior physician may arrange to see the family a few weeks after the child's death. This provides an opportunity to review events on the unit and address any unanswered questions about their child's care. Some parents may appreciate telling the 'story' one more time to the doctor who was involved with their child's life at such a vulnerable time, and allows misconceptions to be addressed. If an autopsy was performed, this will need to be reviewed together with an explanation of the significance of its findings. This also allows the physician to review how the family is coping with their bereavement and if additional assistance might be beneficial.
- Many families welcome bereavement follow-up from a suitable health care professional who knew the family in the ICU. Providing this family counselling requires both training and ongoing support for those who participate in the often difficult phone calls and meetings with the bereaved family in the subsequent year or two. Important times to make contact with the family are the child's birthday, anniversary of the death, and during important religious and other holiday periods.

Further reading

1. Goldman A, Hain R, Liben S (eds) (2006). *Oxford textbook of palliative care for children*. Oxford University Press, Oxford.
2. Truog R (2006). Toward interventions to improve end-of-life care in the paediatric intensive care unit. *Crit Care Med* **34**(11Suppl), S373–9.
3. Carter BS, Hubble C, Weise KL (2006). Palliative medicine in neonatal and paediatric intensive care. *Child Adolesc Psychiatr Clin N Am* **15**, 759–77.

Palliative care in the trauma intensive care unit

Introduction

The trauma ICU is one of the most important and challenging places to provide quality palliative care. Life-threatening illness and death are sudden and usually completely unexpected. The typical history is of violent injury, not exacerbation of chronic disease. Patients are often young and previously healthy, yet now at high risk of dying on a rapid trajectory. Families are traumatized in their own way by the suddenness and severity of a personal tragedy. Meanwhile, aggressive resuscitation and other restorative efforts potentially divert attention from distressing symptoms for patients and from the needs of their families. Intensivists who are trauma surgeons also face the extraordinary task of providing palliative care when the patient's death may be perceived—not only by the family, but by the surgeons too—as a medical failure.

Below are some of the key issues involved in providing palliative care in this unique context.

Who needs palliative care in the trauma ICU?

Every patient and family because:

- Palliative care is patient- and family-centred, and focuses on the relief of suffering, communication, and shared decision-making while aggressive resuscitation and critical care is ongoing. As such, it is appropriate for all patients in the trauma ICU.
- Risk of death is high. Despite a clear positive association between age, rising injury severity score, and mortality, the prognosis for individual patients remains uncertain.
- There is also a high disability rate among survivors, particularly those with neurologic injury.
- Acute patient distress from pain and other symptoms is highly prevalent.
- Most families are psychologically traumatized.

Thus, empathetic and effective communication, quality symptom control, and patient/family-centred care should be the standard of care, especially for those patients with high risk of death.

When should palliative care start in the trauma ICU?

Within 24 hours of admission

- Even if prognosis for recovery is excellent, pain and symptom management and family psychosocial support and communication should begin as soon as possible. Palliative care and trauma critical care are not mutually exclusive, but should instead be provided together from the beginning.
- Mortality after injury occurs in a bimodal distribution in the trauma ICU, with the majority of deaths occurring in the first 48 hours after admission to ICU, primarily from brain injury or massive haemorrhage. Attention to family bereavement needs, end-of-life decisions, and organ donation should start early.

- Another group of patients will survive resuscitation, but die two or three weeks later from sepsis and multiple organ failure. In this group, prognosis is more uncertain and goals of restorative and of palliative care must be simultaneously pursued. Waiting for the moment before death is too late for effective palliative care.

What are the components of good palliative care for trauma patients?

- Aggressive management of pain and other symptoms.
- Effective communication with patients and families.
- Bereavement and psychosocial support for families.
- Shared decision-making.
- Continued balancing of benefits and burdens of treatment, with forgoing of life-supporting therapies when burdens outweigh benefits.

What are effective strategies for integrating palliative care into trauma ICU care?

- Processes can be integrated into the usual critical care, both in nursing and medical practice.
- Scheduled palliative care interventions are important (Table 12.1). Evidence suggests that early communication, family meetings, and attention to pain and suffering provide better family satisfaction and decrease conflict around end-of-life decisions as well as the number of days of non-beneficial life support and critical care.

Table 12.1 Palliative care pathway for the critically injured

Within 24 hours	Within 72 hours	Beyond 72 hours
Palliative care assessment: • Likely outcomes/ prognosis. • Pain and symptoms. • Patient preferences/ advance directives.	Family meeting: • Discuss patient condition, prognosis, uncertainty, patient preferences, benefits and burdens of therapy.	• Family support. • Spiritual support.
• Family support and communication.	• Goals of care discussion. • Plan of care to meet goals.	• Update goals of care. • DNR discussion. • Stop therapies that do not meet goals of care.
• Pain and symptom management.	• Pain and symptom management.	• Pain and symptom management.

How should the trauma ICU patient be assessed for palliative care needs?

An interdisciplinary assessment should be performed to guide the implementation of an appropriate palliative care plan. This assessment should consist of several components.

Pain and symptoms
- Pain and anxiety should be assessed using objective scores and criteria. In unconscious patients or those who cannot self-report, a behavioural pain score should be used.
- Anticipate painful procedures (suctioning, blood draws, turning) as well as uncomfortable treatments (ventilator, catheters).
- Assess the patient for other symptoms. Thirst and discomfort are two of the most common non-pain symptoms in trauma patients.

Outcome and prognosis
- Is patient likely to die during this hospitalization? Within other time frames?
- What quality of life and functional outcome are expected?

Values and preferences of the patient
- What are the patient's preferences for life-sustaining therapy?
- Has the patient prepared an advance directive?

Family needs
- Who is the appropriate surrogate decision-maker?
- What kind(s) of support does the family need—emotional, practical?
- Has (have) the involved health care team(s) communicated with the family?

Spiritual and cultural assessment
- Is the patient a member of a church or other congregation that might provide support at this time?
- What observances would be comforting to the patient and family?

What are the best ways to communicate and share decision-making with patients and families in the trauma ICU?
- The majority of critically injured trauma patients lack capacity for medical decision-making. Family members are usually required to be surrogates, but their own capacity for decision-making may be strained by the devastating effects of sudden traumatic injury of the loved one.
- Communication must begin early since families usually need time to accept the patient's condition, particularly if the prognosis is described as poor.
- The family meeting that focuses on goals of care is an important way to ensure communication as well as shared decision-making.

The family meeting
- The family meeting ideally is attended by the physician, nurse, and psychosocial support person (social worker, counsellor, pastor). The physician provides medical information on the patient's condition, likely outcomes, uncertainty, and possible therapies and care plan. The nurse

provides information on bedside care, pain and symptom management as well support for families. Support and spiritual care providers are often essential for facilitating the meeting.

- Prepare both yourself and other participants in the meeting—review prognosis, treatment options, and the family situation ahead of time.
- During the meeting, ask what the family understands of the patient's condition.
- Review the medical information, prognosis, possible therapies, and likely outcome, with and without each therapy. Discuss any uncertainty if it exists.
- Ask what the patient would want if he/she could decide for themselves (do not ask what the family would want). As many trauma patients are young, most families have never had a discussion with the patient regarding end-of-life preferences, nor are there advance directives.
- Discuss goals of care in the context of preferences and outcomes, benefits, and burdens of each treatment.
- Listen! Allow time for questions and emotional reaction.
- Make a recommendation on goals of care and therapy. Do not allow the family to be solely burdened with medical decisions such as DNR, withholding or withdrawing of life support. These should be shared decisions. Time-limited trials of certain treatments may be helpful.
- Arrive at a consensus about the treatment plan and goals of care.
- Arrange follow-up meetings.

What special issues arise in the management of grief and bereavement in the trauma ICU?

- Death or life-threatening injury due to a traumatic event can complicate grief for the survivors. This should be taken into account when communicating bad news and supporting families.
- Sudden death, violence, the random nature of event, preventability, and the survivors' sense of their own vulnerability to harm can all complicate the mourning process.
- Death from trauma, particularly homicide or suicide, increases the risk for post-traumatic stress disorder among survivors, and is linked to the inability of loved ones to say goodbye prior to death.
- Brain injury, spinal cord injury, and traumatic amputation can precipitate grief and mourning in both the patient and the family, even if death does not occur.

What are effective ways to address bereavement in the trauma ICU setting?

- Recognize that the way news of death is communicated and the nature of support for family and survivors in the immediate aftermath can avoid and ameliorate (or worsen, if handled without skill and compassion) complicated grief and can have lifelong effects on bereavement.
- Provide opportunities for family to see the patient and say goodbye before death, if possible.
- Consider allowing the family to be present during resuscitation. Several studies of resuscitation suggest a salutary effect of this practice on bereavement. Family has the opportunity to see, touch their loved one

while alive, and can be reassured that all efforts to save the patient were made. A member of the health care team should be assigned to support the family during this process.

• Deliver news in a private and secure setting.
  • Know the identity of family members and ensure that members of the closest family are present. Avoid delivery of news to large groups of friends/relatives.
  • Assume that the family does not know the patient has died and news will be a shock.
  • Alert the family with a 'warning shot': 'I have bad news.'
  • State clearly that patient has died or is dead. Avoid euphemisms such as 'passed away'.
  • Limit the volume of medical information.
  • Allow time for the information to sink in.
  • Listen, answer questions, and provide emotional support.
  • Reassure the family that they can see the patient.

• After death notification, ensure the family has the opportunity to see and touch the body and say goodbye. Parents may want to hold their dead child and this should be supported. Offer clergy or pastoral care support.

Palliative care and organ donation

• Quality end-of-life care and organ donation are compatible. In fact, bereavement outcomes may be improved for families who consent for organ donation after death from trauma, particularly after the death of a child.

• Patients who progress to brain death after traumatic brain injury are candidates for organ donation. Attention to family support, communication, and bereavement throughout the patient's hospitalization stay may increase consent rates for organ donation, and should be considered a part of the palliative care plan.

• In dying trauma patients who are not brain dead, the end-of-life care plan may include the withdrawal of life support. Donation after cardiac death is theoretically possible in appropriate patients. Consideration for donation after cardiac death should only be made after the family has discussed and agreed to the withdrawal of life support.

Further reading

1. Lilly CM, De Meo DL, Sonna LA, et al. (2000). An intensive communication intervention for the critically ill. Am J Med **109**, 469–75.
2. Mosenthal AC, Murphy PA, Barker LK, Lavery R, Retano A, Livingston DH (2008). Changing the culture of end-of-life care in the trauma intensive care unit. J Trauma **64**, 1587–93.
3. Mosenthal AC, Murphy PA (2006). Interdisciplinary model for palliative care in trauma and surgical intensive care unit: Robert Wood Johnson Foundation demonstration project for improving palliative care in the intensive care unit. Crit Care Med **34**(11Suppl), S390–403.
4. Curtis JR, Patrick DL, Shannon SE, et al. (2001). The family conference as a focus to improve communication about end-of-life care in the intensive care unit: opportunities for improvement. Crit Care Med **29**(2suppl), N26–33.
5. Buckman R (1992). How to break bad news: a guide for health professionals. Johns Hopkins University Press, Baltimore.
6. Jurkovich G, Pierce B, Pananen L., Rivara F (2000). Giving bad news: the family perspective, J Trauma **48**, 865–73.

Non-invasive positive pressure ventilation for acute respiratory failure near the end of life: overview and outcomes

Consider this patient

A 68-year old man with severe oxygen-dependent chronic obstructive pulmonary disease (COPD) presents to the emergency department with an acute exacerbation of his COPD. The clinicians caring for this patient determine that he does not want endotracheal intubation and invasive mechanical ventilation. He understands the potential consequences of this decision. He is willing to try treatment with non-invasive ventilation if he has a reversible cause of his COPD exacerbation, provided there is a reasonable chance that he can return home to his previous baseline health.

Background: non-invasive positive pressure ventilation (NPPV) for patients with acute respiratory failure

- NPPV has become the standard therapy for the treatment of acute respiratory failure in select patient populations and is increasingly being used in the critical and acute care setting.
- This increased utilization has been driven in large part by the desire to avoid complications of invasive mechanical ventilation such as:
  - Ventilator-induced lung injury.
  - Ventilator-associated pneumonia and other nosocomial infections.
  - Patient discomfort.
  - Increased sedation needed with invasive mechanical ventilation.
- The addition of NPPV to standard medical management (oxygen therapy, bronchodilators, antibiotics), compared to standard medical management alone, reduces endotracheal intubation and mortality in patients with acute respiratory failure due to exacerbations of COPD.
- NPPV also improves these outcomes in patients with cardiogenic pulmonary oedema and specific subgroups of patients with hypoxaemic respiratory failure.
- However, most patients in the randomized controlled trials supporting these indications were willing to undergo invasive mechanical ventilation, if necessary.

Use of NPPV for patients where there is a do-not-intubate (DNI) or a do-not-resuscitate (DNR) status

In 2001, an international consensus conference concluded that 'the use of NPPV may be justified in selected patients who are 'not to be intubated', with a reversible cause of acute respiratory failure. NPPV may provide comfort and facilitate physician-patient interaction in the assessment of the reversibility of acute respiratory failure … NPPV can reduce dyspnoea and preserve patient autonomy, given careful and selective application.'[1]

Subsequently, there has been increased interest in the use of NPPV for patients who have declined invasive life support measures such as endotracheal intubation and resuscitation or who have chosen comfort measures only. This increased interest raises several issues:

- The use of NPPV in these patients is certainly not standard of care and remains controversial.
- Some of the controversy surrounding the use of NPPV for such patients with a DNI or DNR status may derive from a lack of clarity about goals of care, from the perspectives of both clinicians and patients.
- When administered to patients who have declined other forms of advanced life support or who are near or at the end of life, NPPV may reverse acute respiratory deterioration, relieve dyspnoea, and increase the chances of survival with a possible return to their pre-admission level of function.
- In other cases, NPPV may be used as a short-term measure primarily for palliation (e.g. to relieve dyspnoea or to allow patients time to get their final affairs in order).
- However, the use of NPPV in this population may be viewed as merely prolonging the dying process while diverting critical care resources away from other patients more likely to survive.

Outcomes of NPPV for patients where there is a DNI or DNR status

The true efficacy of NPPV in these patients with acute respiratory failure remains uncertain. However, NPPV may benefit some patients who have chosen a DNR status. Overall:

- Single and multicentre, observational studies of patients with a DNR status treated with NPPV indicate that hospital survival rates range from 35% to 43%.
- Patients with exacerbations of COPD and cardiogenic pulmonary oedema benefit the most, with up to 70% surviving to hospital discharge.

More specifically, observational studies have examined the potential benefit of NPPV in patients with acute respiratory failure who have DNI orders. For example:

- In a single centre study of 17 patients who had a DNI status, NPPV was initially successful in 59% (10/17) of patients, with a hospital mortality of 47% (9/17).[2]
- In a multicentre, observational study of 114 consecutive DNI patients with acute respiratory failure treated with NPPV, 43% survived to hospital discharge, with approximately 50% of patients with COPD and 70% of patients with cardiogenic pulmonary oedema surviving to hospital discharge.[3]
- A recent, single centre, prospective, observational study of the use of NPPV in 131 consecutive DNI patients with acute respiratory failure found a similar overall hospital mortality of 65%.[4]
  - Patients with advanced cancer had a much poorer prognosis with a hospital mortality of 85% (p=0.002).
  - Of those in the non-oncological subgroups, 63% of patients with COPD and 60% of patients with cardiogenic pulmonary oedema were discharged home.

- Long-term follow-up for 80 consecutive patients presenting with an exacerbation of COPD and treated with NPPV was evaluated in one study.[5]
  - A total of 37 COPD patients who had a DNI order were compared to 43 patients without DNI orders, and the one-year survival was 30% compared to 65%, respectively.
  - Patients in the DNI group were significantly older, had worse dyspnoea and APACHE II scores, and were more limited in their activities of daily living.
  - These results may be useful when discussing the longer-term prognosis of a COPD exacerbation treated with NPPV among individuals electing to forgo endotracheal intubation and invasive mechanical ventilation.

While the aforementioned observational studies suggest a survival advantage for some patients treated with NPPV near the end of life (patients with a DNI or DNR status), goals beyond survival may be as or more important to patients and their families. These include:
- Relief of dyspnoea.
- The ability to communicate.
- Time to cope with life closure and acceptance of death.

The potential use of NPPV on a trial basis, even for those with diseases in terminal stages, is explored further in the next section.

Hospital survival for NPPV for DNI patients[3]

Table 12.2 Outcomes for patients with COPD with acute respiratory failure (ARF) declining intubation[5]

Outcome	DNI (n=37)	Resuscitate (n=43)	p value
Median survival (days)	179	Not reached	<0.001
Median event-free (death or ARF) survival (days)	102	292	<0.001
1-year survival (%)	30	65	<0.001
% time hospitalized in subsequent year (median and IQR)	11 (0–81)	9 (0–75)	NS

n=number of patients; p=probability; IQR=interquartile range; NS=not significant

Table 12.3 Predictors of mortality for DNI patients treated with NPPV[3,4]

Predictor	Odds ratio [95% confidence intervals]
Albumin <2.5g/dL	11.3 [3.7, 34.0]
SAPS II >35	3.0 [1.1, 8.3]
Malignancy	2.0 [0.3, 11.5]
COPD	0.3 [0.1, 0.9]
Wakefulness	0.2 [0.1, 0.6]

Table 12.4 Complications of NPPV in DNI patients[4]

Complication	n per 31 episodes (%)
Facial skin breakdown	20 (65)
Eye irritation	5 (16)
Haemodynamic instability	5 (16)
Gastric distension with vomiting	1 (3)

n=number of patients

References

1. ATS, ERS, ESICM, SRLF (2001). International Consensus Conference. *Am J Respir Crit Care Med* **163**, 283–91.
2. Benhamou D, Girault C, Faure C, Portier F, Muir JF (1992). Nasal mask ventilation in acute respiratory failure: experience in elderly patients. *Chest* **102**, 912–7.
3. Levy M, Tanios MA, Nelson D, *et al.* (2004). Outcomes of patients with 'do-not-intubate' orders treated with non-invasive ventilation. *Crit Care Med* **32**, 2002–7.
4. Schettino G, Altobelli N, Kacmarek RM (2005). Non-invasive positive pressure ventilation reverses acute respiratory failure in select 'do-not-intubate' patients. *Crit Care Med* **33**, 1976–82.
5. Chu CM, Chan VL, Wong IW, Leung WS, Lin AW, Cheung KF (2004). Non-invasive ventilation in patients with acute hypercapnic exacerbation of chronic obstructive pulmonary disease who refused endotracheal intubation. *Crit Care Med* **32**, 372–77.

Use of non-invasive positive pressure ventilation for patients who have declined intubation: controversy and justification

'The use of NPPV for patients who are not to receive invasive ventilation is justifiable as long as the patient understands NPPV is being used as a form of life support, albeit non-invasive, and there is some prospect for reversal of the acute process ... one could argue there is nothing to lose ... lessen dyspnoea, preserve patient autonomy, and permit verbal communication with loved ones ... controversial ... could merely prolong the dying process and lead to inappropriate resource utilization.'[1]

Some have suggested that the use of NPPV for patients who have DNI or DNR orders is inappropriate because NPPV:
• Is still a form of life support delivered by mask.
• May cause discomfort while prolonging the dying process.
• Clinicians may be unclear about the goals of care when NPPV is used for patients who have DNI or DNR orders, and any lack of clarity can lead to:
  • Inadequate articulation of the rationale for NPPV.
  • Ambiguous dialogue between clinicians, patients, and families.
  • Misleading recommendations.

Adverse consequences may be serious, including:
  • Unmet or conflicting expectations.
  • Avoidable adverse outcomes associated with NPPV.
  • Inadvertent prolongation of the dying process.
  • Intensification of patient suffering and family duress.
  • Inappropriate use of medical resources.

Use of NPPV in patients receiving comfort measures only
• While NPPV can reverse non-terminal acute respiratory failure, it may be considered inappropriate by some when patients have elected to limit life support near the end of their lives (e.g. patients who have chosen comfort measures only).
• It is important to highlight that not only do we have inadequate clinical research on the benefit of NPPV in these patients compared to standard therapy without NPPV, but also on the potential harm. For example, patients might find NPPV undesirable because:
  • Any potential benefit (e.g. relief of dyspnoea) is outweighed by discomfort from a tight-fitting face mask.
  • The ability to communicate is limited due to the face mask.
• There are no studies comparing NPPV in this setting to pharmacologic therapies such as morphine. Nonetheless, it is theoretically possible that NPPV could be used in the setting of 'comfort measures only' as an adjunct to opiates and other non-pharmacologic therapies in a way that might minimize some side effects of opiates such as decreased level of consciousness (although is no convincing evidence that NPPV will diminish the burden of symptoms compared to opiates).

- However, for occasional patients, the relief of dyspnoea and the improved level of consciousness might allow for:
  - More effective communication, especially during periods when NPPV is temporarily stopped.
  - Symptom palliation for these patients.
  - An opportunity for families to communicate with patients.
- Patients can and must maintain control over the decision to continue support.
- If discomfort exceeds benefit, patients can choose to discontinue NPPV and any additional comfort should be achieved quickly with pharmacologic therapies.
- Anticipatory dosing of opioids may be needed when withdrawing NPPV to ensure patient comfort as is sometimes necessary during the withdrawal of invasive mechanical ventilation.
- If the patient becomes unable to communicate, the benefits of NPPV in this setting will have likely ceased and therefore, NPPV should be stopped.

Physicians' attitudes to the use of NPPV where there is a DNI or DNR status

- More than half of Canadian physicians (critical care or pulmonary) surveyed feel that NPPV:[2]
  - Adds to the relief of dyspnoea provided by analgesics and anxiolytics for DNR patients.
  - Facilitates verbal communication with family members and clinicians.
- The majority preferred to use NPPV for patients with COPD and cardiogenic pulmonary oedema compared to those with malignancy, regardless of the physician's specialty.
- Physicians reported using NPPV for the short-term relief of dyspnoea due to acute respiratory failure at the end of life with the primary goal of allowing more time for the patients or family members to come to terms with the patient's end of life.
- Most physicians stated that in patients with a DNR status:
  - NPPV can provide an additive effect to analgesics and/or anxiolytics for the relief of dyspnoea.
  - NPPV facilitates verbal communication with families and clinicians due to the avoidance of endotracheal intubation.
- Following the initial successful use of NPPV in patients who are DNI, most physicians will:
  - Continue NPPV as long as the patient is comfortable.
  - Withdraw NPPV, but not restart if the patient deteriorates.
- Many believe that NPPV allows patients time to get their personal affairs in order and come to terms with death.

Decision-making: communication with patients and family members about NPPV

- A shared approach exchanging clinical information and patient preferences may be especially important for decisions about the use of devices unfamiliar to patients and families such as NPPV.
- Provide a clear, understandable description of NPPV, including its potential risks and benefits.

- Outline the goals of care associated with NPPV use that are relevant for the patient.
- Elicit from patients and/or families the patient's values and preferences, to understand, through dialogue, the treatment goals that are most consistent with the patient's values.
- Summarize these points and outline the agreed-upon plan of care, should NPPV succeed or fail in meeting the treatment goals.
- Continually reassess whether NPPV is succeeding or failing to meet the goals of care.

If NPPV is failing, the task of communicating the next step in care is especially important:

- Be clear with families that the patient is likely to be going to die from his/her disease and that NPPV has either failed to improve the patient's physiologic parameters or that those improvements have been achieved at too great a cost of discomfort to the patient.
- When NPPV fails, physicians should:
  • Clearly communicate that NPPV is not working.
  • The goals of care should be changed.
  • Other treatments to achieve palliation of symptoms should be stepped up.

Setting goals with the patient and family members or substitute decision-maker

- Clinicians must be certain about the goals of care for these patients near the end of life.
- Patients and their families must have an adequate discussion with the clinical team and a clear understanding about the role of NPPV and the goals of care.
- NPPV should be applied only after careful discussion of the goals of care, with explicit parameters for success and failure, by experienced personnel and in appropriate health care settings.
- It is important that patients' dyspnoea is well managed so that patients are comfortable on NPPV.
- Patients may also be encouraged to tolerate some discomfort if the NPPV is improving ventilation or oxygenation.
- NPPV is discontinued when:
  • NPPV is no longer needed to support ventilation or oxygenation.
  • NPPV is determined not to be working.
  • NPPV is not being tolerated by the patient.
- In the later two circumstances, the health care team, patient, and family decide together that NPPV is not producing the desired response and that the burdens outweigh the benefits. At this point, the patient's preference for ongoing comfort measures without life-sustaining therapies is called forth.

References
1. Mehta S, Hill N (2001). State of the art non-invasive ventilation. *Am J Respir Crit Care Med* **163**, 540–77.
2. Sinuff T, Cook DJ, Keenan S, *et al.* (2008). Non-invasive ventilation for acute respiratory failure near the end of life. *Crit Care Med* **36**, 789–94.

Chapter 13

Organ and tissue donation

Organ and tissue donation in the ICU *342*
Sam D Shemie

Organ and tissue donation in the ICU

Introduction

There has been an evolution in our understanding that quality palliative care in the ICU should include providing the opportunity to donate organs and/or tissues after death. Transplantation saves and preserves lives and donation is important to many patients and families during the dying process and the grieving stages. Health care providers who regularly manage dying patients, including practitioners of palliative care, should be aware of the criteria and considerations for organ and tissue donation and incorporate these practices. This role in donation is related to managing the dying process, understanding donation criteria, determining death, providing counsel to families, and maintaining the best interests of the dying patient (which may or may not include donation) until they leave the ICU. This is distinct and separate from roles of procurement and transplant professionals, whose involvement may begin with consent discussions but subsequently focuses on arranging surgical procurement and the allocation of organs. This section will assist in the recognition of potential donors within the ICU setting, distinctions between death as determined by neurological and cardiac criteria, and distinctions between organ and tissue donation.

Characteristics of death in critical care

- May be determined by neurological (brain death) or cardiac criteria.
- Most often preceded by the withdrawal or withholding of life-sustaining therapies.
- 5–15% of deaths are brain death, depending on individual ICUs.

Organ and tissue donation after death

- Donation is a voluntary choice in most countries.
- The option of organ and tissue donation should routinely be provided and incorporated into end-of-life practices:
  - In most countries, the general public strongly supports donation and transplantation.
  - Generally influenced by altruism or preceding expressions of the desire to donate.
  - Provides a sense of 'something good' coming out of a tragic situation, helps with the grieving process in follow-up studies, provides meaning.
  - Attitudes vary by social demographics, culture, and religion.
- Consent discussions should be held by knowledgeable staff (ICU or donor coordinators) in a compassionate, but factual and non-coercive fashion.
  - Multiple discussions may be required, given the emotional circumstances.
  - Any preceding wishes of the deceased should be morally and legally respected.
  - Chaplaincy, spiritual advisors, and/or social workers should be included according to family needs.
- Death must be established prior to donation/procurement procedures.

- Solid organs (kidney, liver, lung, heart, pancreas, intestine) and/or tissues (cornea, heart valves, bone, skin) may be donated after death.
  - Organs are vulnerable to ischaemic injury around the time of death and thus must be removed relatively quickly.
  - Tissues are very resistant to ischaemic injury and may be procured hours to days after death.
- There is no predefined age limit or organ dysfunction threshold precluding the eligibility to donate.
- Contraindications to donation in Canada include HIV/AIDS and active malignancy (in the UK, corneal donation from patients with solid tumour malignancy may be acceptable). In the UK, absolute contraindications include patients with spongiform encephalopathies, e.g. Creutzfeld–Jakob disease (CJD).

Patient and family support

- Donation options should be offered in the context of maintaining respect for the beliefs and values of the individuals involved.
- Patient interests are the first and foremost priority:
  - Life, dying, and dignity should be respected.
  - Psychological, emotional, and spiritual well-being should be advanced.
- Support for the patients' families should continue through all phases of dying: before, during, and after any removal of support technologies and regardless of consent to donation.
- There are occasions when families wish to override pre-stated patient wishes for organ donation. While this is a subject of ongoing review in many jurisdictions, an offer to explore these issues further may provide some additional clarity to the decision-making process.

Neurological determination of death (brain death)

- Principle source of transplantable organs.
- Most common aetiologies: cerebrovascular accidents, traumatic brain injury, hypoxic-ischaemic post-cardiac arrest, tumours, hydrocephalus, metabolic conditions (e.g. hepatic failure, diabetic ketoacidosis).
- Most often related to uncontrolled intracranial hypertension leading to downward herniation of the brainstem and stoppage of brain blood flow.
- Better understood as brain arrest or the complete and irreversible loss of all clinical functions of the brain.
- Respiration and oxygenated circulation are maintained through artificial support therapies.
  - Source of confusion to hospital staff and families as the body is warm, tidal movements of lungs and heartbeat are maintained.
- Clinically suspected by GCS ≤5 with fixed and dilated pupils.

Brain death is characterized by the following prerequisites:
  - Absence of clinical brain function with a known, proximate cause that is irreversible.
  - Must have definite clinical and/or neuroimaging evidence of an acute central nervous system (CNS) event that is consistent with the irreversible loss of neurological function.
  - Reversible conditions must be excluded such as barbiturate intoxication, severe hypothermia, locked-in syndromes.

- Deep unresponsive coma:
  - Lack of spontaneous movements and absence of movement originating in the CNS such as cranial nerve function, CNS-mediated motor response to pain in any distribution, seizures, decorticate and decerebrate responses.
  - Spinal reflexes or motor responses confined to a spinal distribution may persist—can be quite dramatic at times and thus disturbing to staff and family— and often requires explanation.
- Absent brainstem reflexes as defined by:
  - Absent gag and cough reflexes and the bilateral absence of: motor responses, excluding spinal reflexes; corneal responses; pupillary responses to light with pupils at mid-size or greater vestibulo-ocular responses.
- Loss of the capacity to breathe, based on apnoea testing in response to $PaCO_2 \geq 60mmHg$ (or 8kPa).
- No confounding conditions:
  - Unresuscitated shock.
  - Significant hypothermia.
  - Severe metabolic disorders capable of causing a potentially reversible coma.
  - Peripheral nerve, muscle dysfunction, or neuromuscular blockade potentially accounting for unresponsiveness.
  - Clinically significant drug intoxications (therapeutic levels and/or therapeutic dosing of anticonvulsants, sedatives, and analgesics do not preclude the diagnosis).
  - Acute post-resuscitation phase after cardiorespiratory arrest.
- Clinical examination may be supplemented by demonstrating the absence of brain blood flow by neuroimaging techniques or the absence of electroencephalogram activity.
  - Repeat determinations may be required by another qualified physician(s) (depending on patient age and regional practices).
- Fluid resuscitation, haemodynamic support, and hormonal therapies will be required to sustain and optimize organ function.

Donation after cardiac death (DCD)
- Also referred to as 'non-heart beating donation'.
- Was the original means by which organ donation occurred (prior to widespread adoption of brain death criteria).

In many jurisdictions, DCD is now being reconsidered on a broader basis as a means by which to honour wishes for organ and tissue donation.
- After cardiac arrest and death, the circulation is arrested prior to organ procurement which results in progressive ischaemic organ injury.
- Organs must be removed urgently after cardiac arrest.
- Distinct from brain death (heart-beating donation).
  - Oxygenated circulation to organs is present prior to surgical procurement—not an urgent circumstance and better graft outcomes.
  - Consent discussions occur after death is established.

Controlled DCD applies to ICU practice. Organ donation may be considered when **death is anticipated** in patients who have:

- A non-recoverable injury/illness.
- Dependence on life-sustaining therapy.
- A consensual decision to withdraw life-sustaining therapy (WLST).
  - Decision agreed to between family and staff.
  - The decision should be supported by WLST guidelines or by supporting medical opinions.
- Anticipation of imminent death following WLST.
- CPR will not be provided.
- Patient conditions may include severe brain injury of diverse aetiology, end-stage neuromuscular failure, high cervical spinal cord injury, and/or end-stage organ failure.
- The option of organ and tissue donation should be **presented** to patients/families **after the consensual decision** to WLST, but **prior to the act** of WLST.
  - Consent discussions are preferably conducted by staff not involved in the decision to WLST.
- Management of the dying process, including procedures for WLST, sedation, analgesia, comfort care, should proceed according to existing ICU practices in the best interests of the dying patient and must not be influenced by the donation potential.
- The ICU/patient care team is responsible for all aspects of management during the interval of care leading to death.
- The organ donation/procurement/transplant team must not be involved in procedures of WLST, management of the dying process, or the determination of death.
- WLST may occur in the ICU or operating room.
  - Psychosocial, spiritual, and bereavement support should be provided for families regardless of the WLST location.
- A maximum time limit of 1–2 hour(s) from the withdrawal of support to death beyond which organs will not be offered or procured:
  - Important to clarify family expectations.
  - Related to family factors, ICU/operating room logistics, and organ viability limits.
- Death after cardiac arrest generally requires five minutes of observation to document the absence of cardiorespiratory function (international variation in observation time from 2–10 minutes).
- Some DCD centres provide low-risk interventions prior to death to maintain donation potential.
  - Heparin, vasodilators, preparation for procurement.
  - Variable international practice.
  - Requires specific and informed consent.
- Even when organ donation is not an option, tissue donation may occur after cardiac arrest regardless of circumstances; no time urgency.

Experience with DCD in Canada has been limited to a few centres and usually in response to family requests for donation in the setting of WLST. Elsewhere in the world, it occurs more frequently and may provide up to 10–20% of transplantable organs.

Further reading

1. Shemie SD (2006). Brain arrest to neurological determination of death to organ utilization: the evolution of hospital-based organ donation strategies in Canada. *Can J Anaesth* **53**, 747–52.
2. Shemie SD, Doig C, Dickens B *et al.*; on behalf of the Paediatric and Neonatal Reference Groups (2006). Severe brain injury to neurological determination of death: Canadian forum recommendations. *CMAJ* **174**, S1–13.
3. Shemie SD, Baker AJ, Knoll G, *et al.* (2006). National recommendation for donation after cardio-circulatory death in Canada: donation after cardiocirculatory death in Canada. *CMAJ* **175**, S1–24.

Research issues

Conducting research at the end of life *348*
Damon Scales, Niall Ferguson

Randomized controlled trials and ethical principles at the end of life: a personal view *352*
Didier Dreyfuss

Conducting research at the end of life

Overview

Medical research involves applying scientific methods and inquiry to obtain new knowledge that will improve the care of patients, including patients who are approaching the end of their lives. Dying patients comprise a broad range of patients, including critically ill patients who are receiving life support, hospice patients receiving palliative care, and patients at home with terminal illnesses. Excluding such dying patients from clinical research is undesirable because it violates the principle of beneficence by denying patients the opportunity to participate in and benefit from research, and it makes it difficult or impossible to advance knowledge about the care of these patients, thus compromising the development of end-of-life care as an evidence-based specialty. Moreover, exclusion of patients near the end of their lives could be construed as a form of discrimination against this population. The ethical principle of justice supports inclusivity in the conduct of research, and provides a moral imperative to conduct research to improve the care of patients who are near the end of their lives.

Nevertheless, there are several factors that can make dying patients particularly vulnerable. They often experience great psychosocial distress, and they are often surrounded by family members who are desperate for any measures that might potentially change their prognosis. Despite palliative care measures, these patients may also be experiencing physical symptoms or discomfort, and their desire to alleviate these symptoms may be great. These factors may cause patients, who are at the end of their lives, to misunderstand the likelihood of benefit or the potential risks of the research. Furthermore, in many situations, dying patients may not be capable to provide first-person consent for such research. These and other considerations have caused some ethicists and researchers to consider dying patients as a particularly vulnerable population, and therefore, special procedures are required to protect their interests. This chapter discusses special considerations for ensuring that the conduct of research involving these patients is ethical and free of coercion.

Ethical principles to guide research at the end of life

Research involving any patients, including dying patients, should adhere to the ethical principles outlined in the Declaration of Helsinki. Important principles that are relevant to the conduct of research at the end of life include the following:

- Protecting patients' dignity: it is the duty of the researcher to protect the life, health, privacy, and dignity of the research subject.
- Scientific validity: medical research involving humans must conform to accepted scientific principles and be based on a thorough knowledge of the scientific literature.
- Expected benefit: the research should be preceded by careful assessment of predictable risks in comparison with foreseeable benefits to the subject or to others. Medical research is only justified if there is a reasonable likelihood that the targeted populations (though not necessarily the participants themselves) might benefit from the results of the research.

- Minimizing harm: researchers must be confident that the risks involved have been adequately assessed and can be satisfactorily managed. The research should be stopped if the risks are found to outweigh the potential benefits or if there is conclusive proof of positive and beneficial results.
- Informed consent: the participants should be adequately informed about their rights to accept or decline to participate in the research, and every precaution should be taken to respect the privacy of the subject (see the section on informed consent below).
- Research ethics board approval: medical research involving humans should always be approved by a specially appointed and independent ethical review committee.

Barriers to conducting research in dying patients

Most studies that have measured preferences of dying patients have confirmed that many still want to participate in research. However, physicians may be reluctant to allow such patients to be approached for research participation. Similarly, research ethics boards may have concerns about research involving patients who are perceived as being vulnerable to coercion or susceptible to overestimating the likelihood that the research might alter their prognosis. To overcome these challenges, special attention should be paid to ensuring that careful and sensitive wording is used on recruitment materials and that appropriate informed consent is sought from prospective participants.

Informed consent

Informed consent is one of the most important requirements for conducting ethical research to ensure each potential subject is adequately informed of the research goals, methods and interventions, the anticipated benefits and potential risks of the study, and perhaps most importantly, the right to abstain from participation in the study or to withdraw consent without fear of reprisal.

The essential components of informed consent are the following:

- Persons giving consent must be competent to make decisions.
- Relevant information must be disclosed.
- Persons giving consent must be able to understand and comprehend the information.
- This consent must be voluntary and free from coercion or false expectations.
- This consent must provide formal authorization to be treated or included in clinical investigations.

Much debate regarding the conduct of research involving dying patients has stemmed from concerns that these patients might agree to participate out of desperation. This has caused many investigators to consider patients near the end of their lives a particularly vulnerable population. Specifically, because of their poor prognosis for survival, many patients (or their families) may be willing to accept unusually large risks or may be prone to overestimating potential benefits.

Patients who lack capacity

A challenge arises when dying patients are incapable of providing informed consent. This situation may arise due to the underlying condition, the severity of illness (e.g. patients are receiving life support for catastrophic conditions), or due to side effects of sedatives, narcotics, or other palliative drugs.

Research involving patients lacking capacity should only be done if the following conditions are met:

- The research is necessary to promote the health of the population represented.
- The research cannot be performed instead on legally competent persons (or excluding incapable patients would introduce important selection bias, compromising the integrity of the study).
- The condition that prevents obtaining informed consent should be a necessary characteristic of the research population (e.g. the study involves patients who are comatose or patients who have delirium).

A common approach to conducting research involving patients lacking decisional capacity is to seek consent from a substitute decision-maker, e.g. a partner/spouse or family member. Obtaining consent from a substitute decision-maker promotes the concept of patient autonomy and self-determination. Family members may be imperfect in providing substituted judgement, but they can still speak accurately for many patients; even when their judgements might disagree, surveys have found that patients would still prefer a family member be involved.

Other frameworks for enrolling incapable patients have been proposed for emergency situations in which the study intervention is time-sensitive.

- Deferred consent: the patient is enrolled, and consent is later sought from either the patient when they become capable or from a substitute decision-maker.
- Waived consent: the need for informed consent is waived after review by a research ethics board.
- Community consent: the need for individual consent is waived after consultation and approval from representatives of the community.

Practical considerations

- Research involving dying patients can encompass a broad range of patients and different types of research, making it important for research ethics boards to provide individualized and contextualized ethical oversight and reviews.
- Is it necessary to involve dying patients in the proposed research? Many research ethics boards will request reassurance that the proposed research cannot be feasibly conducted in other less vulnerable populations.
- Language used in consent forms should be simple and concise, recognizing the physical, emotional, and mental fatigue of dying patients.
- The patient/substitute decision-makers should be given sufficient time to read and consider study materials.
- Fluctuations in mental status may be common in dying patients. The researcher should ensure that the patient is competent and fully

understands the research project at the time that consent is provided; a formal assessment of capacity may be helpful in some studies.
- Patients or their substitute decision-makers must be allowed to withdraw from research at any time.
- Investigations should be limited to those that are absolutely necessary. For example, measuring the long-term toxicity of an intervention is of little relevance to the terminally ill and such assessments should not be conducted in these populations. Similarly, lengthy questionnaires that will be burdensome to dying patients should be avoided.

Summary

Research involving patients near the end of their lives should adhere to accepted ethical principles. In particular, such research must respect patients' dignity, it must be scientifically valid, it should have the potential to benefit the targeted population, and it should minimize any potential for harm. Precautions should be taken to ensure that informed consent is obtained from patients who are capable, free from coercion, and not harbouring false expectations about the likelihood of benefiting from the study intervention. Adhering to these principles will help ensure that dying patients can participate in research that has the potential to advance knowledge and improve future care.

References

1. Beauchamp TL, Childress JF (2001). *Principles of biomedical ethics*, 5th edn. Oxford University Press, New York.
2. Bruera E (1994). Ethical issues in palliative care research. *J Palliat Care* **10**, 7–9.
3. Kendall M, Harris F, Boyd K, *et al.* (2007). Key challenges and ways forward in researching the 'good death': qualitative in-depth interview and focus group study. *BMJ* **334**, 521.
4. Luce JM, Cook DJ, Martin TR, *et al.*; American Thoracic Society (2004). The ethical conduct of clinical research involving critically ill patients in the United States and Canada: principles and recommendations. *Am J Respir Crit Care Med* **170**, 1375–84.
5. World Medical Association Declaration of Helsinki: Ethical principles for medical research involving human subjects. Adopted by the 18th World Medical Association General Assembly, Helsinki, Finland, June 1964.

Randomized controlled trials and ethical principles at the end of life: a personal view

Introduction

Care at the end of life should benefit from the same high-quality clinical research as in other clinical settings. However, it is particularly important at the end of life that the goal of research is kept clearly in mind. In the Belmont report, 'research designates an activity designed to test a hypothesis, permit conclusions to be drawn, and thereby, to develop or contribute to generalizable knowledge (e.g. expressed in theories, principles, and statements of relationships)'. Practice, from which research was separated, was defined as 'interventions that are designed solely to enhance the well-being of an individual patient or client and that have a reasonable expectation of success.' As medical practice becomes increasingly complex, many new interventions may be implemented without prior rigorous testing (for instance, some new surgical procedures) and other simple improvements in the quality of routine care that occur in daily practice may not be amenable to research as defined above. Improving the quality of palliative care, and particularly in the ICU, probably relies more on a continuous process than on any single breakthrough made according to the usual standards of research.

Randomized controlled trials (RCTs) and vulnerable populations: a historical perspective

Ethical principles that govern all kinds of research must be fulfilled with particular scrutiny among patients at high risk of imminent death. RCTs pose specific ethical problems that may be particularly relevant to research in dying patients. To understand this, it is necessary to examine the history and the socio-economic role of RCTs and discuss some ethical issues in general practice before discussing the specific problems of the end of life.

Has the value of the RCT been over-emphasized from the outset (relative to other research methodologies)?

The two famous early RCTs, (1) streptomycin for the treatment of tuberculosis and (2) testing of the polio vaccine which heralded the general conversion of clinical scientists to the concept of randomization, were conducted in conditions where observational studies would have led to similar conclusions. In the streptomycin trial, the methodology of a RCT was preferred simply because the very small amount of streptomycin available made it ethically permissible to administer the drug not to all patients, but on the basis of randomization. In the polio vaccine trials, a RCT was preferred because of political considerations linked to the raging controversy between Salk and Sabin regarding the type of vaccine that should be developed. An observational study conducted at the same time as the RCT yielded similar results. It would be highly unlikely that either RCTs would be accepted by patient associations nowadays.

Academic and non-academic pressures that favour RCTs as a study design

- Large RCTs are vital for the pharmaceutical industry, in particular for obtaining regulatory approval and marketing licenses for drugs.
- Large RCTs conducted by industry are likely to be published in major medical journals that wish to disseminate potential pharmacological breakthroughs.
- RCTs are considered by many methodologists as the gold standard against which other methodologies are thereby judged inferior. As a consequence, the major medical journals are more likely to favour studies using the RCT design. Nevertheless, recent revisions of the grading of evidence have acknowledged that grade IA recommendations (strong recommendation with high-quality evidence) may in fact stem from 'overwhelming evidence from observational studies'.
- Academic pressure favours methodological conformism and risk avoidance in study design.
- Huge financial incentives and academic stakes can pose risks to patients by possibly promoting haste in the conduct of trials.
- Results of RCTs may be accepted without due consideration of whether treatment in the control or placebo arm was an inappropriate comparator (e.g. a drug known to be inferior or given at too low a dose or suboptimal 'standard care'), making the new intervention seem better.

How does all this apply to research conducted at the end of life?

Research may be especially difficult to conduct at the end of life (see Conducting Research at the End of Life, p348). Ethical protection must be particularly strong given the environment in which research is conducted and the fragility of proxies from whom surrogate consent is usually sought.

- There is no doubt that we need sound research to improve care of patients at the end of life.
- As indicated above, RCTs cannot be considered as the only approach in all circumstances.
- Indeed, investigators must strongly consider whether continuous improvement of the quality of care and comparison with historical controls may be not the best way to attain the goals of research, at least in some instances or for example, before and after studies and interrupted time series studies).
- Investigators must carefully weigh advantages and disadvantages of different research methods, including RCTs. As stated by Jerome Cornfield (inventor of both the odds ratio and logistic regression): 'good scientific practice … places emphasis on reasonable scientific judgement and the accumulation of evidence, and not on dogmatic insistence on the unique validity of a certain procedure.'
- RCTs may pose important ethical problems among patients at the end of life:
  - Who benefits from the intervention—the patient or his/her proxies?

- Are proxies at ease with the concept of surrogate consent? They are often highly anxious and may have feelings of guilt, as is frequently encountered during the process of separation from a loved one.
- Should a new intervention (e.g. a new protocol for taking care of patient distress or of anxiety of proxies) be given to all patients in the study or only to half of them in an RCT? What would be the risk/disadvantage of implementation of this new approach in all cases?
- What is the concern with a retrospective comparison (rather than an RCT) if it concludes falsely to the superiority, the inferiority, or the lack of effect of the new approach if this new approach consists of the implementation of more compassionate attitudes?
- Finally, is there a risk concluding that a new approach is superior only because the control group received suboptimal care (as discussed above)?

If RCTs pose ethical problems, what are the solutions?

Research on the care of patients at the end of life may benefit from less rigid methodologies than RCTs. Several issues should be considered:

- The potential emotional trauma that ensues from seeking consent from highly anxious proxies may be ethically more relevant than the purity of the study. If so, it is mandatory to turn to alternative methodologies:
  - Observational studies: it has been shown several times that the results of such studies do not necessarily differ from those of RCTs. The higher occurrence of type 1 or 2 errors in a non-randomized study is not always a reason to perform an RCT.
  - Randomization by clusters comparing two approaches in different units when both approaches can be considered as two modalities of usual clinical care.
  - An alternate possibility, which is also not devoid of ethical problems, may be studies with pre-randomization (Zelen design), in which consent is sought only if the patient is randomized to the new approach. If consent is refused, the patient receives the usual approach.

Conclusion

My purpose in this chapter is not to contend that RCTs are inappropriate or unethical among patients at the end of life, but that the risk-benefit analysis of all different research strategies must be seriously weighed. RCTs should not be performed simply to favour methodological purity, but only in the (probably) rare circumstances when alternative designs would not be suitable.

Further reading

1. Beecher HK (1996). Ethics and clinical research. *N Engl J Med* **274**, 1354–60.
2. Beauchamp TL, Childress JF (2001). *Principles of biomedical ethics*, 5th edn. Oxford University Press, New York.
3. Dreyfuss D (2005). Is it better to consent to an RCT or to care? *Intensive Care Med* **31**, 345–55.
4. Smith R (2005). Medical journals are an extension of the marketing arm of pharmaceutical companies. *PloS Medicine* **2**, e138.
5. Wee B, Hillier R (2008). Interventions for noisy breathing in patients near to death. *Cochrane Database Syst Rev* **23**, CD005177.

Chapter 15

Web-based resources

Web-based resources *356*
Judith E Nelson

Web-based resources

In the age of the internet, many valuable resources about palliative care are available online. These include resources that will be of primary interest to professional caregivers, or to patients and families, or to all. Included here are some of these web-based resources from Australia, North America, and Europe, with an emphasis on sites that have both extensive content and links to other sources of information, including ICU-specific materials.

Australia

- The Respecting Patient Choices programme site has useful links to guides/policy documents (mostly related to advanced care planning and decision-making) and professional organizations within Australia and its various states.
  - http://www.respectingpatientchoices.org.au

Canada

- The Canadian Hospice Palliative Care Association.
  - www.chpca.net/
- Family caregiving for people at the end of life.
  - www.coag.uvic.ca/eolcare/index.htm
- Canadian Researchers at the End of Life Network (CARENET).
  - www.thecarenet.ca/
- End-of-Life Care and Vulnerable Persons New Emerging Team (VP-Net).
  - www.umanitoba.ca/outreach/vpnet/index.htm

Europe

- European Association for Palliative Care (Council of Europe).
  - www.eapcnet.org/
- World Health Organization Regional Office for Europe.
  - www.euro.who.int/healthtopics/HT2ndLvlPage?HTCode=palliative_care
- National End-of-Life Care Programme.
  - www.endoflifecareforadults.nhs.uk/eolc/
- The National Council for Palliative Care
  - www.ncpc.org.uk/
- The Association for Palliative Medicine of Great Britain and Ireland.
  - www.palliative-medicine.org/
- A joint venture between St. Christopher's Hospice and Help the Hospices; this site is an information service for health professionals and members of the public on UK and international hospice and palliative care.
  - www.hospiceinformation.info/
- Association for Children's Palliative Care.
  - www.act.org.uk/

France

- French Society of Palliative Care.
  - www.sfap.org/content/view/126/180/

- Fondation de France (soigner, soulager, accompagner).
  - www.fdf.org/jsp/site/Portal.jsp?page_id=208
- Site francophone de soins palliatifs.
  - www.palliatif.org/content/view/30/29/

USA

- Adult ICU Comfort Care Orders for the Withdrawal of Life Support, UCSF.
  - http://nursing.ucsfmedicalcenter.org/docshares/ComfortCareOrders.pdf
- The following three sites contain comprehensive lists of additional web resources, as well as serving themselves as rich repositories of information.
  - www.chestnet.org/about/links/endOfLife.php
  - www.capc.org/research-and-references-for-palliative-care/add-resources-websites/
  - depts.washington.edu/eolcare/

Other general international resources

- International Association for Hospice and Palliative Care.
  - www.hospicecare.com/
- International Observatory on End-of-Life Care.
  - www.eolc-observatory.net/global/

Additional resources that are particularly relevant to critical care nursing (available through the American Association of Critical Care Nurses)

- AACN Protocols for Practice. Palliative care and end-of-life issues in critical care (Justine Medina, Kathleen Puntillo, eds).
  - my.aacn.org/ecomtpro/timssnet/products/tnt_products.cfm
- Innovative models and approaches for palliative care promoting excellence in intensive care and end-of-life care.
  - www.aacn.org/AACN/PalCare.nsf/vwdoc/RWJ/
- Courses for 2009–2010, including the End-of-Life Nursing Education Consortium, Critical Care programme.
  - www.aacn.nche.edu/ELNEC/

Appendix

Adult ICU Comfort Care Orders for the Withdrawal of Life
  Support *360*

Adult ICU Comfort Care Orders for the Withdrawal of Life Support

UCSF Medical Center

○

**ADULT ICU COMFORT CARE ORDERS
FOR THE WITHDRAWAL OF LIFE SUPPORT**

UNIT NUMBER

PT. NAME

BIRTHDATE

LOCATION   DATE

Date: _____ Time: _____

Allergies: _____

The withdrawal of life support is not withdrawal of care. Nursing and medical care continue for the patient and family but the focus of the care changes. During withdrawal of life support, the ICU approach to care is changed to comfort, as cure is no longer possible and curative treatments are no longer desired. Comfort care focuses on quality of dying and relief of symptoms with attention to emotional, psychosocial and spiritual issues for patients. These limitations of life support do not constitute euthanasia.

1. These orders are only for use in Adult ICU's.

○
2. Conditions of initiating and signing order set:

   a. If Critical Care Medicine ICU and Primary Service are jointly providing care for the patient, Critical Care Medicine will complete the entire order set only after consultation and agreement has been reached between both services.

   b. If the Primary Service is the sole provider of the patient, the Primary Service will complete the entire order set.

3. The prescribing physician will notify both the Critical Care Medicine (ICU) Attending and the Primary Service Attending at the time the orders are written.

○
4. Prescribing physician to insure the following:

   a. Do Not Resuscitate (DNR) order form must be completed.

   b. A note must be written in the chart that documents rationale for withdrawal of life support and discussion between Attending physician, patient and/or family.

5. Prescribing physician to contact Palliative Care Services prior to extubation if patient may be transferred to Comfort Care Suites (CCS) after extubation. Prior to transfer to the CCS, the prescribing physician must complete the Comfort Care Order Form (Adults). See Reference Guide on reverse.

○
6. Contact Spiritual Care Services. See Reference Guide on reverse.

7. End of Life Reference Guide for RN's, RT's and MD's is on the reverse side of the order set.

Start Comfort Care medications:

   " √ " in box activates order

8. ☐ Fentanyl infusion at 100 mcg/hr or _____ mcg/hr (current rate)
   Increase Fentanyl infusion by 50-100 mcg/hr every 30 minutes PRN pain, discomfort &/or respiratory distress.

   AND

   Fentanyl bolus 50-200 mcg IV q 5 to 10 minutes PRN **breakthrough** pain, discomfort &/or respiratory distress.

   ☐ None, due to neurological status

○
Signature_____ M.D.# __ __ __ __ __ Time_____ Date_____ Pager#_____

Checked by_____ R.N. Time _____ Date _____

Adult ICU Comfort Care Orders for the Withdrawal of Life Support Page 1 of 3

Fig. A.1 Adult ICU Comfort Care Orders for the Withdrawal of Life Support, University of California, San Francisco Medical Center. This figure contains the order set, but not the educational pages that accompany the UCSF guidelines. The full document can be found at http://nursing.ucsfmedicalcenter.org/docshares/ComfortCareOrders.pdf. Reproduced with permission.

UC_{SF} Medical Center

UNIT NUMBER	
PT. NAME	
BIRTHDATE	

**ADULT ICU COMFORT CARE ORDERS
FOR THE WITHDRAWAL OF LIFE SUPPORT**

LOCATION	DATE

Comfort Care medications continued:

" √ " in box activates order

9. ☐ Midazolam infusion at 5 mg/hr or _____mg/hr (current rate).
Increase Midazolam infusion by 2 -4 mg every 30 minutes PRN anxiety, discomfort &/or respiratory distress.

AND

Midazolam bolus 5 - 10 mg IV every 10 minutes PRN **breakthrough** anxiety, discomfort &/or respiratory distress.

☐ None, due to neurological status

10. ☐ Glycopyrrolate 0.1 - 0.2 mg IV/SQ every 4 - 6 hours PRN excessive secretions.

11. ☐ Acetaminophen 650 mg PO/PR/NG every 6 hours PRN fever.

12. ☐ Anzemet (Dolasetron) 12.5 - 25 mg IV every 1 - 2 hours PRN nausea or vomiting.
Or Medical Center preferred anti-serotonin drug

13. ☐ Promote comfort by discontinuing all medications except for the following: _____

_____

_____

(To continue any medications, the physician must include name, dosage, route and frequency of each).

Institute Comfort Care:

" √ " in box activates order

14. ☐ Promote comfort by discontinuing all laboratory tests, parenteral and enteral feeds, all blood product infusions, Xray's, EKGs, Hemodialysis and CRRT.

15. ☐ Promote comfort by discontinuing devices not needed, such as the NG, feeding tube, blood pressure cuff, segmental compression devices, and anti-embolism stockings. Disable any AICD device.
Other devices to discontinue include: _____

_____

16. ☐ Promote comfort by discontinuing the following neuromuscular blocking agents (NMBAs):

_____

Refer to Reference Guide on reverse side regarding NMBAs.

17. ☐ Promote comfort by discontinuing routine vital signs. Monitor HR and RR prn for signs of distress.

18. ☐ Promote comfort by decreasing the maintenance IV fluid to TKO.

19. ☐ Additional patient treatments to discontinue include: _____

_____

Signature_____ M.D.# _ _ _ _ _ Time_____ Date_____ Pager#_____

Checked by_____ R.N. Time _____ Date_____

Adult ICU Comfort Care Orders for the Withdrawal of Life Support Page 2 of 3

Fig. A.1 (Continued)

UCSF Medical Center

UNIT NUMBER

PT. NAME

BIRTHDATE

LOCATION   DATE

ADULT ICU COMFORT CARE ORDERS
FOR THE WITHDRAWAL OF LIFE SUPPORT

Ventilator Orders: Terminal Weaning or Immediate Extubation

" √ " in box activates order

20. ☐ Current ventilator settings: Mode: _____ Respiratory Rate _____ CPAP_____
Pressure Support level _____cm H20, FiO2 _____ PEEP _____ cmH20.

21. ☐ a. Ensure adequate sedation for patient prior to and continuously during weaning of ventilation.

    b. Adjust apnea, heater, and other ventilator alarms to minimum setting.

    c. Consider reducing FiO2 to .21 over 5 to 10 minutes.

    d. Reduce PEEP to zero cm H2O over 5 to 10 minutes.

    e. Wean respiratory rate to 4 and/or PS to 5 cm/H2O over 5 to 20 minutes.

    f. When patient is comfortable on respiratory rate of 4 and/or PS of 5 cm/H2O, select one:

    ☐ Place patient on room air cool aerosol T-piece

      OR

    ☐ Extubate patient to room air or nasal cannula.

22. ☐ Additional respiratory orders: _____

_____

Signature_____ M.D.# _ _ _ _ _ _ Time_____ Date_____ Pager#_____

Checked by_____ R.N.   Time _____   Date_____

Adult ICU Comfort Care Orders for the Withdrawal of Life Support Page 3 of 3

Fig. A.1 (Continued)

Index

AACN model of moral
distress 176
abandonment 142
abdominal pain 319
ACLS (Advanced
Cardiac Life Support)
guidelines 230
acute pain interventions 64
acute respiratory distress
syndrome see prognostic
uncertainty
acute respiratory failure 35
admission criteria 28, see
also triage
Advanced Cardiac Life
Support (ACLS)
guidelines 230
advance directives 198
cystic fibrosis 318
good death,
principles 252
legal issues 191–2
and liability 198
trauma intensive care
unit 330
withholding and
withdrawal of
treatment 247
see also planning ahead
afferent arm, rapid response
system 186–7
Africa 112
after death care
Australian
perspective 251
Liverpool Care
Pathway 280
paediatric palliative
care 326
afterlife 147; see also
spiritual care
age see older patients
agitation 68
assessment 69, 72–3
causes/risk factors 71
and delirium 76
interventions 69–70
see also anxiety
AIDS patients 6
air hunger 66, 279
alcohol withdrawal 76
algorithms 20; see also
protocols
alien effect 148
allogenic haematopoietic
stem cell
transplantation 34, 36

ALS see amyotrophic lateral
sclerosis
Alzheimer's disease 190
American Association
of Critical Care
Nurses 176, 357
American Society
for Bioethics and
Humanities 210
amyotrophic lateral
sclerosis (ALS) 312, 316
assisted ventilation 313–14
background
information 312
bronchial congestion 315
decision-making 312
discussing palliation 313
family support 315
intubation 314
medical team distress 315
scenario 190
ventilation 314–15
anorexia 321
anoxia 262; see also
vegetative states
antibiotics 352
antipsychotic medication 76
anxiety 68
assessment 68–9, 71
assessment scale 72–3
cancer patients 38
and capacity 114
causes/risk factors 68, 71
chronic critical
illness 308
definition 68
environmental
management 70
family 6, 66, 84–5, 104
interventions 69–70
medical team 315
see also agitation
Asia, social
perspectives 129
assisted suicide 191, 193,
214, 216
assisted ventilation 313–14
Australia
legal issues 192, 195, 200
mechanism of death
statistics 13
web-based resources 356
Australian perspective,
withholding and
withdrawal of
treatment 246, 250
after death 251

mutual support 251
vs. palliative care 250
autonomy, patient 112
amyotrophic lateral
sclerosis 313
cultural issues 130
social perspectives 129

bad death 142; see also
good death
bad news see breaking bad
news
barriers to high quality
care 42
comfort vs. cure 42
empirical evidence 43
fragmentation of
care 42, 44
fundamental/common
threads 44
international
comparisons 43
overcoming 44
beds, demand for 16
Belgian Act on
euthanasia 214
Belgium 246, 247; see also
euthanasia (Belgium)
beliefs
and CPR 222, 238
cultural see cultural issues
spiritual care 140
benzodiazepines 8
bereavement
addressing 331
follow-up 7, 10, 90
paediatric palliative
care 326
patient/family-centred
care 91
trauma intensive care
unit 328, 331
useful books on 90
best practices 194; see
also withholding and
withdrawal of treatment
biochemical markers 265
biomedical model 130
BiPAP 322
blame, attributing 141, 142;
see also self-blame
body language see non-
verbal communication
BOS see burnout syndrome
brain death 130, 343;
see also coma; organ
donation; vegetative states

breaking bad news 92, 94
  conflict resolution 206
  cultural issues 128
  iatrogenic suffering 100–2
  SOLER model 100
  taking in bad news 95,
    101–2
breakthrough pain 64
bronchitis obliterans with
    organizing pneumonia
    see prognostic
    uncertainty
bruising effect 148
Buddhism 129
Burkholderia cepacia 319
burnout syndrome
    (BOS) 163, 176,
    180, 185
  decreasing risk 182
  definition 180
  emotional factors 181
  epidemiology 180
  family conferences 107
  and hope 149
  iatrogenic suffering 95
  impact on families/
    patients 184
  impact on nurses 182
  impact on physicians 183
  organizational factors 181
  and post-traumatic stress
    disorder 183
  risk factors 181–2
  secondary effects on
    staff 183–4
  solutions to reduce 184
  see also moral distress;
    vicarious trauma

cachexia 2
CAM-ICU (Confusion
    Assessment
    Checklist) 75, 113
Canada
  criteria for intensive care
    selection 28
  legal issues 192, 194
  patient/family-centred
    care 88
  shared decision-
    making 104
  web-based resources 356
Canadian perspective,
    withholding and
    withdrawal of
    treatment 135, 246,
    252, 274
  checklists 252
  common ICU
    principles 253
  extubation indicated 255
  extubation not
    indicated 255

feedback, seeking 255
flexibility/adaptation in
    practices 255
good death,
    principles 252
medication provision 254
order/method of
    withdrawal 254
protocol 274
vasopressor
    dependence 255
cancer patients
  breaking bad
    news 94, 102
  CPR 223
  hope 6
  trust 23
  see also decision-making,
    taking time over
cancer patients,
    ICU admission
    decisions 34, 38
  advances in ICU care 35
  advances in supportive
    care 35
  advances in surgical
    care 34
  advances in treatment 34
  benefit of doubt 37
  functional capacity 36
  haematopoietic stem cell
    transplantation 36
  ICU environment 38
  indications/limitations of
    ICU admission 39
  limits of triage
    decisions 36
  malignancy-related
    characteristics 36
  newly diagnosed
    malignancies 36
  psychological issues 38
capacity 196, 350
  surrogate 114–15
cardiac arrests
  anticipating/avoiding 188
  in-hospital arrests 232
  out-of-hospital
    arrests 232, 262
  prognostic
    assessment 263, 264
  see also cardiopulmonary
    resuscitation
cardiac arrest, life support
    after 262, 266
  age 264
  biochemical markers 265
  electrophysiological
    tests 264
  end-of-life care 265
  Glasgow-Pittsburgh
    cerebral performance
    categories 267

hypothermia 264
imaging 265
prognostic
    assessment 263, 264
waiting period 263
cardiac death, and organ
    donation 344
cardio-defibrillators,
    implantable
    (ICDs) 260–1
cardiopulmonary
    resuscitation (CPR)
  appropriateness/
    usefulness 222
  code status mismatch with
    prognosis 228
  consent to withhold 224
  decision aids see below
  demands for
    treatment 227
  dying patients 223
  important
    considerations 235
  indications for 226
  medical staff
    disagreement 227–8
  overview 222
  patient
    preferences 225, 234
  prognostic
    assessment 222
  steps to take
    when likely to be
    ineffective 225
  steps to take when will be
    ineffective 224
cardiopulmonary
    resuscitation decision
    aid 223, 234, 239
  important
    considerations 240
  personal beliefs,
    patient 238
  personal experiences 238
  questions about
    competence to
    communicate
    preferences 238
  questions about
    effectiveness 237
  questions about side
    effects 238
  questions about nature
    of CPR 236
  questions about need for
    discussion 237
  questions about
    outcomes of medical
    discussion 239
  questions about what
    happens during
    CPR 236
  religious beliefs 238

treatment decision process 240
cardiopulmonary resuscitation outcomes
    overview 230, 233
    age/comorbidity 231
    facts/figures 230
    in-hospital arrests 232
    initial cardiac rhythm 230
    nursing homes 232
    out-of-hospital arrests 232, 262
    paediatric 231
    patient factors 230
    and respiratory arrests (RA) 231
    special circumstances 233
    witnessed/ unwitnessed 232
cards, bereavement 91, 168
care of dying patients, current challenges 22
    communication 26
    consumer expectations 22
    doing everything possible 22
    oversimplification of the issues 22
    protocols 25
    providing short periods of intensive care 25
    trust 23
    uncertainty of prognosis 24
care of dying patients, global overview 12
    conflict reduction 20
    decision-making negotiation process 20
    end-of-life decision-making 19
    historical perspective 19
    ICU environment 15
    language, medical 16
    leadership 16
    measures of success 12
    mechanism of death statistics, Australia 13
    objective assessment of survival probability 13
    religion/ethnicity, respect for 15
    subjective assessment of treatment value 14
    trust, earning 16
case law 192
case studies
    non-invasive positive pressure ventilation 334

paediatric palliative care 322
see also conflict resolution; decision-making; hope; organ donation; prognostic uncertainty; sister's tale; Vietnam veteran's story
ceramic hearts 90
CF see cystic fibrosis
Chaplains 140
checklists
    CAM-ICU 75
    family conference 243
    intensive care delirium screening (ICDSC) 75
    see also protocols
chest wall pain 320
children
    care see paediatric palliative care
    hospital visits 92, 250
Christianity 268
chronic critical illness
    common symptoms 308
    communication 306–7, 310
    definition 306
    delirium 310
    dyspnoea 308–9
    integrative palliative care approach 306
    pain interventions 309
    sources of suffering 308
    symptom control 308
chronic obstructive pulmonary disease (COPD) 6, 334
chronic pain interventions 64
civil law 192
clinical ethics committees see ethics consultants
clinical pathways see protocols
closure 136
cognitive behavioural pain interventions 61
cognitive disability
    Glasgow-Pittsburgh cerebral performance categories 267
    post cardiac-arrest 263
collaborative
    teamwork 160
    communication skills 160
    interpersonal skills 160
    trust 161
    see also teams, palliative care
collectivity/ individuality 129–30

coma 262, 263, 266; see also vegetative states
comfort
    centred strategy 43
    Liverpool Care Pathway 278
    vs. cure dichotomy 42
    see also suffering
common law 192
communication 26, 136
    barriers to high quality care 44
    with caregivers 84
    chronic critical illness 306–7
    collaborative teamwork 160
    conflict resolution 206
    cultural issues 130
    education/training 245
    end-of-life care improvement recommendations 135
    and euthanasia 217
    evidence-based approach 105, 110–11
    families 85, 339
    iatrogenic suffering 95
    legal issues 194
    medical staff disagreement 227
    open 130
    and organizational culture 137
    paediatric palliative care 322–3
    patient preferences decision aid see cardiopulmonary resuscitation preferences
    proactive 107
    protocols 107
    sister's tale 296
    skills of physician 94, 95
    teams, palliative care 157
    trauma intensive care unit 330
    VALUES approach 104–5
    withholding and withdrawal of treatment 242
    see also non-verbal communication
community, valuing 141
comorbidity, CPR outcomes overview 231
conferences, end-of-life care 4; see also family meetings; VALUES approach
conflict reduction/ resolution 20, 84–5

conflict reduction/
    resolution (cont.)
  case study see below
  cultural issues 128, 130
  demands for CPR 227
  legal issues see below
  and moral distress 174
  and organizational
      culture 137–8
  staff 247, 260
  triage 28
  withholding and
      withdrawal of
      treatment 245
conflict resolution case
    study 202
  areas of mutual
      agreement 205
  critical insight 205
  defining the problem 203
  Fisher's principles 203
  identifying interests 204
  interests rather than
      positions 204
  objective criteria 205
  separating people from
      problems 203
  shared understandings 206
  working towards
      agreement 206
conflict resolution, legal
    issues 194, 200–1
  demands that relatives
      should not be kept
      fully informed 200
  inappropriate
      requests 200
  see also legal issues
Confucianism 129
Confusion Assessment
    Checklist (CAM-
    ICU) 75, 113
consent, informed 349
consent to withhold
    form 261
consultants, euthanasia 217;
    see also physicians
consumer expectations 22
continuity of care 136
continuum model
    of life 19
control, retaining 142,
    148, 252
COPD (chronic
    obstructive pulmonary
    disease) 6, 334
CoughAssist devices 315
Court of Protection 115
court orders 194
CPR see cardiopulmonary
    resuscitation
creativity, family
    meetings 99

CREDIBLE criteria, CPR
    preferences 234
criteria for intensive care
    selection see triage
    in ICUs
critical care PFCC advisory
    councils 88
  consideration of others'
      roles 90
  council responsibilities 88
  experiences of a
      council 90
  setting up a council 89
cultural issues 128, 130, 132
  attitudes to death/
      dying 128
  financial/social impact on
      families 151
  scenario 130
  social impact on
      families 153
  social perspectives 129
  trauma intensive care
      unit 330
  withholding and withdrawal
      of treatment 243,
      247, 258
  see also Muslim
      perspectives
cystic fibrosis (CF) 318, 321
  abdominal pain 319
  advance directives 318
  airway clearance
      difficulties 318
  anorexia/fatigue 321
  Burkholderia cepacia 319
  chest wall pain 320
  diabetes 319
  dyspnoea 320
  headache 320
  massive haemoptysis 320
  prognostic indicators 318
  symptom control 320

DCD (donation after
    cardiac death) 344; see
    also organ donation
deactivating cardio-
    defibrillators/pacemaker
    implants 260
death
  denial 4, 84, 137
  determination of 193
  as failure of medicine 19
  hastening 57, 191,
      216, 250
  in ICUs, statistics 18
  legal definition 193
  legal issues 197
  neurological
      determination 343
  paediatric palliative
      care 325

preparation for 8, 135
price of 153
reflective practice 162
rounds see below
statistics 18
taboo 270
see also dying; mortality
death rounds 8
  goals/potential
      benefits 171
  impact of death 168
  in non-ICU settings 170
  preparing physicians for
      coping with death 168
  questions for self-
      reflection 171
  reflections on death/
      dying 170
  structure 171
  support/guidance 168
decision-making 4, 19
  amyotrophic lateral
      sclerosis 312
  and cultural
      issues 128, 130
  deferred 316
  family involvement 6
  legal issues 197
  negotiation process 20
  non-invasive
      positive pressure
      ventilation 339
  paediatric palliative
      care 324
  paternalistic 112, 246, 271
  patient-related factors 28
  questions/topics of
      discussion 98
  schemas/guides for
      professionals 4
  surrogate see surrogate
      decision-making
  taking time over see below
  trauma intensive care
      unit 330
  VALUES approach 104, 109
  see also cancer patients;
      cardiopulmonary
      resuscitation decision
      aid; family meetings;
      questions, patient;
      triage
decision-making, taking time
    over 286
  amyotrophic lateral
      sclerosis 312
  differing policies/
      protocols 287
  going home 287
  lessons learnt 287
  non-verbal
      communication 286
  prognosis, discussing 286

decisions to forgo life
sustaining therapies
(DFLSTs) 246
deep vein thrombosis case
study see prognostic
uncertainty
defibrillators, implantable
(ICDs) 260–1
definitions, legal 191, 193
delirium 2, 74
alcohol withdrawal 76
chronic critical illness 310
definition 74
impact 75
incidence 74
interventions 76
key points 77
measurement tools 75
risk factors 74
denial
of death 4, 84, 137
of illness 312
denigration of
colleagues 245
Denmark 216, 247
depersonalization 180; see
also burnout syndrome
depression 85
and capacity of
surrogate 114
families 6, 10, 84, 104
inappropriate requests
for treatment to be
withdrawn 200
mourning before
death 315
physician 183
demand for beds 16
despair 148
determination of death 193
DFLSTs (decisions to
forgo life sustaining
therapies) 246
diabetes 319
dieticians 242
difficult cases see conflict
resolution
dignity 22, 135,
158, 252, 264
Director Survey, ICU 43
distal intestinal obstruction
syndrome (DIOS) 319
domains of
measurement 47
do-not intubate (DNI)
patients
mortality predictors 337
NPPV 334–7, 339
do-not-resuscitate (DNR)
patients
NPPV 334–5, 339
double effect doctrine 57,
191, 216, 250

dry mouth see thirst/dry
mouth
dying
diagnosis 2
experience 153
humanization 4, 19, 15
needs determination 6
phases of 2
worse things than 297
see also death; mortality
dyspnoea 66
anxiety 68
assessment 66
chronic critical
illness 308–9
cystic fibrosis 320
non-pharmacological
management 66
objective signs 67
pharmacological
management 67
risks/causes 66

ECG strips 92
economic considerations/
demand for beds 16
education/training 9
end-of-life care
improvement 138
patient/family-centred
care 92
team roles in palliative
care 157
withholding and
withdrawal of
treatment 245
see also death rounds
efferent arm,
rapid response
system 186–7
electroencephalograms
(EEGs) 264
emergency cover see
medical emergency
teams
emotional exhaustion 180;
see also burnout
syndrome
empathy 100, 180
end-of-life care
family satisfaction 135
importance attributed
by patients 6
improvement
opportunities 136
improvement
recommendations 135
life support after cardiac
arrest 265
and organizational
culture 137
planning ahead 20; see
also advance directives

quality improvement
initiatives 8
Enlightenment 129
environmental
management 8, 15
cancer patients 38
for families 8
global overview 15
healing environments 90
humanization of dying 4,
19, 15
sleep disturbance 79
VALUES
approach 105
errors, medical 22
ethical principles
practice
environment 137, 158
research 348
symptom relief for
imminent death 57
see also randomized
controlled trials
ethics consultants/
committees 208, 212
background
information 208
composition/members
committees 209
difficulties/concerns 210
legal status 210
role/position in
hospital 209
ETHICUS study 246
ethnicity, respect for 15;
see also cultural issues
EURELD 1 study on
euthanasia 215
Europe
autonomy, patient 112
barriers to high quality
care 43
criteria for intensive care
selection 28
shared decision-making 104
social perspectives 129
web-based resources 356
see also below
European perspectives,
withholding and
withdrawal of
treatment 246
advance directives 247
culturally
perspectives 247
decision-making 246
legal frameworks 246
multidisciplinary care 247
prevalence 246
euthanasia
Belgian perspective see
below
consultants 217

euthanasia (*cont.*)
legal definition 191
legal frameworks 246
legal issues 193
LEIF physicians 217
Muslim perspectives 269
euthanasia
(Belgium) 214, 218
Belgian Act 214
communication 217
and clinical practice 218
definitions 214
and ICUs 217
incidence 215–16
practical steps 217, 219
professional roles 217
public attitudes 218
evidence-based
approaches 105, 110,
111; see also research
extubation indications 255

facing the inevitable 245
failure, death as 19
false hope 244; see also
hope
families of dying patients
conflict reduction 20
ICU environment 15
interventional studies 121
observational studies 119
qualitative studies 123
reflective practice 163
research studies 119
satisfaction with care 135
supporting 315
see also financial/social
impact of illness; needs
of families; patient/
family-centred care;
surrogate decision-
making;
family conference
checklist 243; see also
family meetings
Family Medical Leave
Act (US) 151
family meetings 85
conducting 96, 242
contextual features 99
cultural issues 130
patient preferences 98
quality of life 99
questions/topics of
discussion 98
team roles 157
trauma intensive
care 330
withholding and
withdrawal of
treatment 242
see also VALUES approach
fatigue 321

feedback
patient/personal 10
seeking 255
financial/social impact of
illness 84, 150, 153
facts/figures 150
initial impacts 150
interventions to assist 151
longer-term impacts 151
patients who recover 152
price of death 153
role changes 151
social impact 153
specific/individual
needs 151
uninsured
patients (US) 152
Fisher's principles 203,
206, 254
fluid withdrawal 279
follow-up appointments
bereaved families 7,
10, 90
paediatric palliative
care 326
fragmentation of
care 42, 44
France 112–13, 246, 356
funerals 153, 251, 271
future planning see advance
directives; planning
ahead

Germany 247
Glasgow-Pittsburgh
cerebral performance
categories 267
goal-setting
NPPV 340
paediatric palliative
care 325
good death 135, 137
Canadian perspective 252
and hope 147
staff perspectives 137
grief 91, 142, 183, 290, 331
guided imagery 66
guidelines
Advanced Cardiac Life
Support 230
criteria for intensive care
selection 28
pain interventions 62
symptom relief for
imminent death 57
guilt 295
families 84–5, 142
medical team distress 315
moral distress 164
pulling the plug 244,
253, 295
surrogate decision-
making 114

withholding and
withdrawal of
treatment 244, 246

haematopoietic stem cell
transplantation (HSCT)
34, 36
hair locks 90
handprints 90
headache 320
healing environment 90;
see also environmental
management
healthcare team see
collaborative teamwork;
nurses; physicians; teams
heart attacks see cardiac
arrests;
holistic care 140
honesty 99, 148, 253
amyotrophic lateral
sclerosis 312
collaborative
teamwork 160
and hope 147
withholding and
withdrawal of
treatment 244
hope 146, 282
amyotrophic lateral
sclerosis 313
assumptions 147
cancer patients 6, 38
definition 146
end-of-life spiritual
tasks 143
for good death 147
health care team 149
iatrogenic suffering 95
paediatric palliative
care 323
patient/family-centred
care 91
shrinking
hopelessness 148
unrealistic 227
wife's perspective 300
see also prognostic
uncertainty
humanization of dying 4,
15, 19
hypothermia,
therapeutic 264

iatrogenic suffering 94–5
breaking bad
news 100–2
communication 94–5
contextual features 99
family meetings 96
mechanisms 95
patient preferences 98
quality of life 99

questions/topics of
discussion 98
taking in bad news 95,
101–2
working to prevent 166
see also reflective practice
ICDs (implantable cardio-
defibrillators) 260–1
ICDSC (intensive care
delirium screening
checklist) 75
ICU Director Survey 43
ICU environment see
environmental
management
identification with
patient 95
imagery, guided 66
implantable cardio-
defibrillators
(ICDs) 260–1
important issues for
families/patients 136
independent living 40
independent mental
capacity advocates
(IMCAs) 112, 115
individuality/
collectivity 129–30
information provision
chronic critical illness 306
easy to understand 84
end-of-life care 265
good death,
principles 252
leaflets 85
needs of families 134
organizational culture 138
right to 15
sister's tale 294
informed choice 104
informed consent,
research 349
Institute for Family Centred
Care 88
insurance, medical 152
intensive care delirium
screening checklist
(ICDSC) 75
intensive care units
(ICUs) 4, 16
bereavement follow-up 7
education/training 9
feedback 10
health care team
input 7
listening to family
members 7
needs of dying patients 6
needs of families 6
professional initiatives
to promote social
changes 4

providing a favourable
environment for
families 8
quality improvement
initiatives 8
research 5
interdisciplinary involvement
see collaborative
teamwork; teams
international
comparisons 28, 43; see
also cultural issues and
see individual countries
by name
international web-based
resources 357
internet 18; see also
web-based resources
interpersonal skills 160
interventional studies 121
inukshuk 302–3
Islam 268, 269; see also
Muslim perspectives
istislah 269
Italy 216

jargon, medical 7, 91, 242
Jehovah's Witness
scenario 190
journals written by
families 90
Judaism 268

key attributes, quality
measures 47

language, medical 7, 16
lasting power of attorney
(LPA) 198
LATAREA study 246
laughter, value of 299
leadership 136
chronic critical illness 307
and organizational
culture 137
physician 16
legal issues
advance directives 192
assisted suicide 193
best practices 194
case law 192
civil law 192
common law 192
court orders 194
definitions 191, 193
determination of
death 193
euthanasia 193
framework for
analysis 193
legal questions 192
legislation 191
pain/suffering control 193

professional
consultation 194
scenarios 190
sources of legal
obligations 191
withholding and
withdrawal of
treatment 192, 246
see also conflict
resolution; euthanasia
(Belgium); Mental
Capacity Act (MCA)
legislation 191
LEIF (euthanasia advice)
physicians 217
lessons learnt
decision-making 287
sister's tale 296
sudden tragedies 291
Vietnam veteran's
story 299
see also prognostic
uncertainty
liability, healthcare
professionals 198; see
also legal issues
life, sanctity of 269
life shortening
medication 57, 216, 250
life support withdrawal
see withholding and
withdrawal of treatment
listening to family
members 7, 10, 92,
158, 223
liver failure case study see
sister's tale
Liverpool Care
Pathway 274, 280
background
information 277
after death care 280
differing approaches 276
documentation 279
further care 279
ongoing care 278
patient assessment 277–8
rationale 276
transition to palliative
approach 276
living wills 198; see also
advance directives
loss, coming to terms
with 20; see also
mourning
LPA (lasting power of
attorney) 198
Luxembourg 246

malignancy see cancer
patients
massage therapy 322–3
massive haemoptysis 320

mature minors 191
meaning, finding 84
MCA see Mental Capacity Act
measurement tools, delirium 75
measures of success 12, 36, 136; see also quality evaluation
media influences 22
medical emergency teams (METs) 28, 186–7
medical errors 22
medical insurance 152
medicalization of dying 4
medical jargon 7, 91, 101, 242
medication provision see pharmacological management
memory boxes 90
Mental Capacity Act (MCA) 196
 advance directives/living wills 198
 capacity 196
 deciding best interests 197
 decisions about treatment 197
 lasting power of attorney 198
 liability, healthcare professionals 198
 scope 196
METs see medical emergency teams
mismatches, patient preferences/care 134
monotheistic religions 268
moral distress 38, 95, 164, 174, 177
 AACN model 176
 definition 174
 factors associated 175
 and hope 149
 model 178
 and moral dilemmas 174
 outcomes 176
 recommendations for decreasing 176
 staff perspectives 137
 stages of development 175
moral experts 210; see also ethics consultants/clinical ethics committees
mortality/mortality rates
 cancer patients 34
 older patients 37–8
 paediatric palliative care 322

predictors 337
 see also death; dying
motor neurone disease 312
mourning before death 315; see also bereavement
multidisciplinary care 247; see also collaborative teamwork; teams
music 61, 258, 322–3
Muslim perspectives, withholding and withdrawal of treatment 268
 decision-making 270
 Islam foundational values 268
 Islam major branches 268
 major concerns 269
 monotheistic religions 268
 paternalistic decision-making 271
 physician behaviours 270
 sanctity of life 269

needs, dying patients 6
needs, families 6, 84, 86
 interventions to assist 85
 observational studies 84
 and organizational culture 134
 trauma intensive care unit 330
 see also financial/social impact of illness
Netherlands 214, 216, 246–7
neurological determination of death 343
neuropathic pain interventions 64
New Zealand 195
nociceptive pain 64
no code orders 223–4
non-invasive positive pressure ventilation (NPPV) 338, 314
 amyotrophic lateral sclerosis 314
 background information 334
 case study 334
 complications 337
 as comfort measure 338
 ommunication with families 339
 for DNI/DNR status patients 334
 goal-setting 340
 mortality predictors 337
 outcomes 335–6
 physician attitudes 339
non-pharmacological interventions

delirium 76
 dyspnoea 66
 for imminent death 57
 pain 61
 sleep disturbance 79
 thirst/dry mouth 80
non-verbal communication 160
 and decision-making 286
 family meetings 96
 paediatric palliative care 323
 pain 63–4
not for CPR orders 242
NPPV see non-invasive positive pressure ventilation
nurses
 attitudes 134, 137
 burnout syndrome 182–3
 and euthanasia 217
 moral distress 174
 perspectives 137
 and post-traumatic stress disorder 183
 turnover 137
 web-based resources 357
 withholding and withdrawal of treatment issues 242, 247
nursing homes 232
nutrition withdrawal 269, 279

objective criteria 205
observational studies
 ethical practice environment 137
 families 84, 119
OHCAs (out-of-hospital cardiac arrests) 232, 262
older patients 31, 34
 admission criteria 36
 and CPR outcomes 231
 definition 34
 measures of success 36
 mortality after discharge 38
 mortality in ICU 37
 patient preferences 31
 quality of life 38
 self-sufficiency/independent living 40
open code status 226
open communication 130
open-ended questions 105
opioids 309
oral dryness see thirst/dry mouth
organ donation 90, 92, 302, 342

background 302
after cardiac death 344
characteristics of
    death 342
determination of
    death 343
encouraging 303
patient/family support 343
planning ahead 344
shock, family 302
taking comfort from 303
trauma intensive care
    unit 328, 332
organ failure 2, 28
organ failure-orientation
    strategy 43
organizational culture 134
and burnout
    syndrome 181
definition 136
and end-of-life care 137
end-of-life care
    improvement 135–6,
    138
ethical practice 137
family satisfaction 135
good death 135
important issues 136
manifestations 136
mismatches, patient
    preferences/ care 134
and needs of families 134
and outcomes 137
research agenda 138
staff perspectives 137
withdrawal of
    treatment 135
Osler, Sir William 4
out-of-hospital
    cardiac arrests
    (OHCAs) 232, 262
oxygen therapy 314

pacemaker implants 260
paediatric palliative care
approach of death 325
communication 322–3
CPR 231
after death care 326
decision-making 324
goal-setting 325
hope 323
mortality 322
symptom control 323
pain 60
abdominal 319
AIDS patients 6
assessment 60
chronic critical illness 309
control 193
cystic fibrosis 320
definition 60
family satisfaction 135

guidelines 62
and inappropriate
    requests for
    treatment to be
    withdrawn 200
interventions 61; see
    also pharmacological
    management
management
    recommendations 135
non-verbal
    assessment 63–4
paediatric palliative
    care 323
procedural 61, 65
questions/topics of
    discussion 98
suffering 62–3
trauma intensive
    care 330
types 61, 64
palliative care vs withdrawal
    of treatment 250
paranoid delusions 75
parentalism 104
paternalistic decision-
    making 112, 246, 271
pathways, clinical see
    protocols
patient assessment 277–8
patient-centred care 31
patient comfort-centred
    strategy 43
patient/family-centred care
    (PFCC)
bereavement
    follow-up 90–1
children's visits 92
definition 88
evaluation 92
having a voice 92
high tech/high care 90
hope 91
journals written by
    families 90
recommendations 91
staff education/training 92
see also critical care PFCC
    advisory councils
patient preferences
assessment 186
CPR 225, 234
conflict with families/
    surrogates 113
iatrogenic suffering 98
research 349
trauma intensive care 330
see also cardiopulmonary
    resuscitation
    decision aid
Patient Self-Determination
    Act (US) 113
performance status 36

persistent vegetative
    states 262, 263, 265; see
    also coma
personal reflections 294
see also hope; organ
    donation; reflective
    practice; sister's tale;
    Vietnam veteran's
    story
PFCC see patient/family-
    centred care
pharmacological
    management
anxiety/agitation/
    restlessness 68–9
delirium 76
dyspnoea 67
imminent death 56
open-ended
    prescriptions 8
sleep disturbance 79
thirst/dry mouth 80
withholding and
    withdrawal of
    treatment 254
see also double effect
    doctrine; sedation
physician/s
accessibility 135
attitudes 134
behaviours 270
burnout syndrome 183–4
euthanasia advice 217
feedback, seeking 255
leadership 16
moral distress 174
perspectives 137; see also
    prognostic uncertainty
withholding and
    withdrawal of
    treatment 242, 247
see also education/training
physician-assisted
    suicide 214, 216; see
    also older patients
physiological age 28; see
    also older patients
planning ahead 26, 28,
    31, 113, 246; see also
    advance directives
polio vaccine 352
post-traumatic stress
    disorder 10, 84, 104,
    114, 183; see also sudden
    tragedies
potentially life-shortening
    symptom relief 57, 191,
    216, 250
power of attorney 198
power relations 137
practice/theory
    discrepancies 175–6
prayer 259; see also
    spiritual care

preparation for
  death 8, 135
price of death 153; see also
  financial/social impact
  of illness
primary cardiac arrest 231
primary respiratory
  arrest 231
privacy 143, 252
proactive
  communication 107
procedural pain 61, 65
procedures/routines 136
professional
  consultation 194
  initiatives 4
  relationships see
    collaborative
    teamwork; teams
  roles, euthanasia 217
  schemas/guides 4
prognosis
  assessment 263–4
  discussing 106, 227
  indicators 318
prognostic uncertainty
  (case study) 24, 284
  background 282
  clinical course of
    illness 282
  difficulty of accurate
    prognosis 283
  family background 282
  family devotion 282
  outcome 283
Promoting Excellence in
  End-of-Life Care 4
protocols 25
  communication 107
  decision-making 287
  schemas/guides 4
  trauma intensive care
    unit 329
  withholding and
    withdrawal of
    treatment 274
  see also checklists;
    guidelines; Liverpool
    Care Pathway
Public Health Code of Law
  (France) 112–13
pulling the plug 244,
  253, 260
qualitative studies 123
quality evaluation,
  palliative care
  appropriate measurement
    domains 47
  bundle of process
    measures 47, 49
  how to measure 46
  implementing quality
    measures 48

key attributes of quality
  measures 47
  need for measures 46
  operationalizing 47, 49
  quality measure
    denominators 48
  see also measures of
    success
quality improvement
  initiatives 8
quality of life (QoL) 99
  assessment 14, 29
  older patients 38
  triage in ICUs 29
questions about CPR,
  patient 239
  and competence 238
  effectiveness 237
  nature of 236
  other considerations 238
  outcomes of medical
    discussion 239
  side effects 238
  what happens 236
  why need to discuss 237
questions, legal 192
questions for
  self-reflection 171

randomized controlled
  trials 352, 354
  and end-of-life 353
  getting around
    difficulties 354
  historical perspective 352
  pressures favouring 353
  value 352
  see also research,
    end-of-life care
rapid response system 188
  anticipating/avoiding
    cardiac arrests 188
  assessment of patient
    preferences 186
  components 186–7
  criteria for calling 187
  decision-making/setting
    goals 187
  medical emergency
    teams 188
RASS (Richmond agitation
  sedation scale) 73
RCTs see randomized
  controlled trials
reflective practice 92, 166
  amyotrophic lateral
    sclerosis 316
  burnout syndrome 163
  death/dying 162
  death rounds 168, 170
  family history/
    background 163
  moral distress 164

self-reflection 162
  trauma 165
  vicarious trauma 165
relationships
  doctor-patient 224; see
    also iatrogenic suffering
  healing 142
  professional see
    collaborative
    teamwork; teams
religion 15, 238, 268; see
  also spiritual care
renal dysfunction 309
rescue culture 44
research, end-of-life
  care 5, 19, 351
  agendas 138
  barriers to 349
  and capacity of
    patient 350
  ethical principles 348
  families of dying
    patients 119
  informed consent 349
  observational studies 84
  overview 348
  practical
    considerations 350
  triage in ICUs 29
  see also randomized
    controlled trials
respect for patients 84,
  99, 158
  cultural issues 128, 130
  family satisfaction 135
  Muslim perspectives 271
respect for staff
  members 156
respiratory arrests (RA) 231
respiratory nurses 7
responsibility, for pulling the
  plug 244, 253, 295; see
  also guilt
restlessness 68, 69, 70; see
  also agitation
resuscitation
  references 8, 98
return of spontaneous
  circulation (ROSC) 262
Richmond agitation sedation
  scale (RASS) 73
right to information 15–16;
  see also information
  provision
risk
  agitation 71
  burnout
    syndrome 181, 182
  numeric expression 106
  reduction see rapid
    response
rituals 90, 143; see also
  spiritual care

road traffic accident
  scenario 190
Robert Wood Johnson
  Foundation 4
role changes, families of
  dying patients 151
ROSC (return of
  spontaneous
  circulation) 262
routines 136
RRS *see* rapid response
  system

safety culture 137, 174
sanctity of life 269
SAS (sedation-agitation
  scale) 72
saying goodbye 142,
  250, 252
screening for delirium 75
sedation
  decision-making 287
  life support
    withdrawal 250, 254
  Liverpool Care
    Pathway 279
  massive haemoptysis 320
  total, legal definition 191
sedation-agitation scale
  (SAS) 72
selection for intensive care
  see triage
self-blame, patient 141
self-sufficiency 40
self-worth 140; *see also*
  moral distress
sensitivity 160
septic shock 35
shame, physician 95
shared decision-
  making 104, 109; *see
  also* VALUES approach
sharing the story of
  families 89
shock, family 302–3; *see
  also* sudden tragedies
silence 258–9; *see
  also* environmental
  management
sister's tale 294
  dual roles 297
  information
    provision 294
  lessons learnt 296
  staff continuity/
    changes 294
  stepping down to ward
    care 295
  structural problems 296
  sudden changes of
    direction 295
  worse things than
    dying 297

skidding effect 148
sleep disturbance 78
  adverse effects 78
  assessment 78
  causes/risk factors 78
  chronic critical
    illness 308
  common sleep
    patterns 78
  definition 78
  environmental
    management 79
  interventions 79
social changes,
  promoting 4
social impact on families *see*
  financial/social impact
  of illness
social perspectives 129, 132
SOLER model of expressed
  empathy 100
somatosensory
  evoked potentials
  (SSEPs) 264, 266
South America 112
Spain 247
spiritual care in ICUs
  case studies 141–2
  curative to comfort
    measures
    transition 142
  end-of-life tasks 143
  guidance 141
  honesty 142
  interventions to
    assist 141–2
  issues 99
  meaning and practice
    of 140
  needs 153, 252, 278, 330
  ritual 90, 143
  valuing the patient 141
spirituality 94
SSEPs (somatosensory
  evoked potentials) 264,
  266
staff continuity 176, 294;
  see also nurses;
  physician/s; teams
standards 113
statistics
  deaths in ICUs 18
  risk 106
storytelling 258
streptomycin 352
stress
  family 96, 134
  physician 95, 165
  see also post-traumatic
    stress disorder; sudden
    tragedies
structure-process-outcome
  model 46, 216

Study to Understand
  the Prognosis and
  Preferences for
  Outcomes and Risks
  of Treatment
  (SUPPORT) 150
subjective assessment 14,
  28, 71
success measures *see*
  measures of success;
  quality evaluation
sudden tragedies 290
  follow-up
    appointment 291
  grief, unconsolable 290
  lessons learnt 291
suffering 22, 52, 84
  cancer patients 34
  chronic critical illness 308
  dimensions 62–3
  doing everything
    possible 22
  questions/topics of
    discussion 98
  see also comfort;
    iatrogenic suffering
suicide, assisted 214–220;
  see also double effect;
  euthanasia
SUPPORT Study 150
surrogate decision-
  making 26, 104, 112,
  115, 246
  capacity 114–15
  guilt 142
  implications for
    practice 115
  importance of 112
  lack of surrogate 115
  optimizing 114
  research 350, 353
  role of surrogate 113
  standards 113
  VALUES approach 104–5
Sweden 216
Switzerland 216, 247
symposia, end-of-life care 4
symptom assessment,
  trauma 330
symptom control
  chronic critical illness 308
  common symptoms 52
  cystic fibrosis 320
  family satisfaction 135
  improvement 136
  paediatric care 323
  potentially life-shortening
    57, 191, 216, 250
  see also anxiety; delirium;
    dyspnoea; pain; sleep
    disturbance; symptom
    relief for imminent
    death; thirst/dry mouth

symptom recording/
management 8
symptom relief
for imminent
death 54–5, 58
ethics 57
guidelines 57, 360
non-pharmacological
comfort measures 57
pharmacological
management 56
preparation for
comfortable death 54
symptom control 58
symptoms
chronic critical
illness 308
patients at high risk of
dying 52

taboo of death 270
taking in bad news 95,
101–2
talking about
death 148; see also
communication
Taoism 129
teams, palliative care 156
accountability 158
characteristics 157
complementary
skills 157–8
conflict 247, 260
distress 315
essential elements 156
including patients/
families 158
input 7, 114, 107–8
purpose 156
roles 157
size 157
see also collaborative
teamwork
teddy bear programme 90
theory/practice
discrepancies 175–6
thirst/dry mouth 80, 308
assessment 80
causes/risk factors 80
definition 80
interventions 80
time pressure,
physician 95
time triggers 47
tissue donation 342; see
also organ donation
total sedation, legal
definition 191
tracheostomy 286–7, 298
amyotrophic lateral
sclerosis 314
chronic critical
illness 310

sister's tale 295
training of physicians see
education/training
transcendence 143
transition, curative to
comfort measures 142,
279; see also withdrawal
of treatment
transplantation see organ
donation
trauma see post-traumatic
stress disorder; stress;
vicarious trauma
trauma intensive care
unit 328
addressing
bereavement 331
communication/decision-
making 330
family meetings 330
grief/bereavement
issues 331
needs of families 330
organ donation 332
outcomes/prognosis 330
pain/symptom
assessment 330
palliative care 328–9
patient/family-centred
care 328
patient preferences/
values 330
spiritual needs/cultural
assessment 330
triage in ICUs 28–9
criteria, international
comparisons 28
evaluating 29
older patients 36
organizational
factors 28
patient-related
factors 28
phases 28
quality of life
assessment 29
research, end-of-life
care 29
selection procedure 28
see also cancer patients,
ICU admission
decisions
trust 23, 136
collaborative
teamwork 161
earning 16
improvements 136
team roles 156
withholding and
withdrawal of
treatment 244
truth see honesty
tuberculosis 352

UK (United Kingdom)
advance directives 247
criteria for intensive care
selection 28
independent mental
capacity advocates 112
lack of available
surrogate 115
see also Mental
Capacity Act
UK perspective, withholding
and withdrawal of
treatment 242, 246, 274
conflict with families 245
cultural issues 243
denigration of
colleagues 245
difficulties/pitfalls 243
education/training 245
facing the inevitable 245
false hope 244
family conferences 242–3
guilt 244
honesty 244
protocol 274
trust 244
uncertainty of prognosis 24
unilateral withdrawal
and withholding of
treatment 191–2
US (United States)
criteria for intensive care
selection 28
financial/social impact on
families 151
ICU Director Survey 43
legal questions 192
shared decision-
making 104
standards and their
application 113
uninsured patients 152
web-based resources 357
withholding and
withdrawal of
treatment 246, 274

VAD see ventricular assist
device
values 136
assessment 186
cultural 128
and ethics 137
Islam 268
organizational 136, 138
spiritual care 140
trauma intensive care
unit 330
VALUES approach to
conducting a family
conference 104, 108
communication,
importance 104

communication
    protocols 107
decision-making 104, 109
discussing prognosis 106
evidence-based
    approach 105, 110–11
interdisciplinary
    involvement 107
VALUES history 105
vasopressor
    dependence 255
vegetative states 262, 263,
    265; see also coma
ventilation, ALS 314–15;
    see also tracheostomy
ventricular assist device
    (VAD) 258, 261
consent to withhold
    form 261
device withdrawal
    potential 258
stopping VAD 258
team conflict 260

turning off the
    pump 260
vicarious trauma 95, 165;
    see also burnout
    syndrome
Vietnam veteran's story
background
    information 298
fear, patient 298
key memories
    of ICU 298
lessons learnt 299
stepping down to ward
    care 298
visiting hours 84, 90

web-based
    resources 356–7
Western perspectives see
    cultural issues
withdrawal and
    withholding of
    treatment 84, 111

and euthanasia 218
family satisfaction 135
inappropriate requests
    for 200
incidence 19
legal definition 191
legal issues 192
negotiation
    process 20
organ donation 344
procedures 8
protocols 274
spiritual care in ICUs 142
taking responsibility 16
see also Australian/
    Canadian/ European/
    Muslim/UK
    perspectives; conflict
    resolution, case study
worse things than dying 297

xerostomia see thirst/dry
    mouth